60 HIKES
WITHIN 60 MILES

4th Edition

CLEVELAND

60 HIKES WITHIN 60 MILES: Cleveland

Published by Menasha Ridge Press
Distributed by Publishers Group West
Printed in China
Fourth edition, first printing

Cover and interior design: Jonathan Norberg
Cover and interior photos: Diane Stresing
Cartography: Steve Jones
Editors: Holly Cross and Jenna Barron
Proofreader: Emily Beaumont
Indexer: Rich Carlson

Library of Congress Cataloging-in-Publication Data

Names: Stresing, Diane–author.
Title: 60 hikes within 60 miles Cleveland : including Akron and Canton / Diane Stresing.
Other titles: Sixty hikes within sixty miles Cleveland
Description: Fourth edition. | Birmingham, AL : Menasha Ridge Press, 2024. | Includes index.
Identifiers: LCCN 2024007857 (print) | LCCN 2024007858 (ebook) | ISBN 9781634042468 (pbk)
  ISBN 9781634042475 (ebook)
Subjects: LCSH: Hiking—Ohio—Cleveland Region—Guidebooks. | Cleveland Region (Ohio)—Guidebooks.
Classification: LCC GV199.42.O32 C547 2024 (print) | LCC GV199.42.O32 (ebook)
  DDC 796.520977132—dc23/eng/20240301
LC record available at https://lccn.loc.gov/2024007857
LC ebook record available at https://lccn.loc.gov/2024007858

 MENASHA RIDGE PRESS
An imprint of AdventureKEEN
2204 1st Avenue South, Suite 102
Birmingham, AL 35233
800-678-7006, fax 877-374-9016

Visit menasharidge.com for a complete listing of our books and for ordering information. Contact us at our website, at facebook.com/menasharidge, or at twitter.com/menasharidge with questions or comments. To find out more about who we are and what we're doing, visit blog.menasharidge.com.

SAFETY NOTICE This book is meant only as a guide to select trails in the Cleveland area and does not guarantee hiker safety in any way—you hike at your own risk. Neither Menasha Ridge Press nor Diane Stresing is liable for property loss or damage, personal injury, or death that result in any way from accessing or hiking the trails described in the following pages. Please be aware that hikers have been injured in the Cleveland area. Be especially cautious when walking on or near boulders, steep inclines, and drop-offs, and do not attempt to explore terrain that may be beyond your abilities. To help ensure an uneventful hike, please read carefully the introduction to this book, and perhaps get further safety information and guidance from other sources. Familiarize yourself thoroughly with the areas you intend to visit before venturing out. Ask questions, and prepare for the unforeseen. Familiarize yourself with current weather reports, maps of the area you intend to visit, and any relevant park regulations.

Dedication

This book is for all those who dedicate their time to preserving Ohio's natural beauty so that everyone can enjoy it.

60 HIKES WITHIN 60 MILES

4th Edition

CLEVELAND

Including Akron and Canton

Diane Stresing

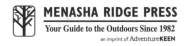

MENASHA RIDGE PRESS
Your Guide to the Outdoors Since 1982
an imprint of AdventureKEEN

60 Hikes Within 60 Miles: Cleveland

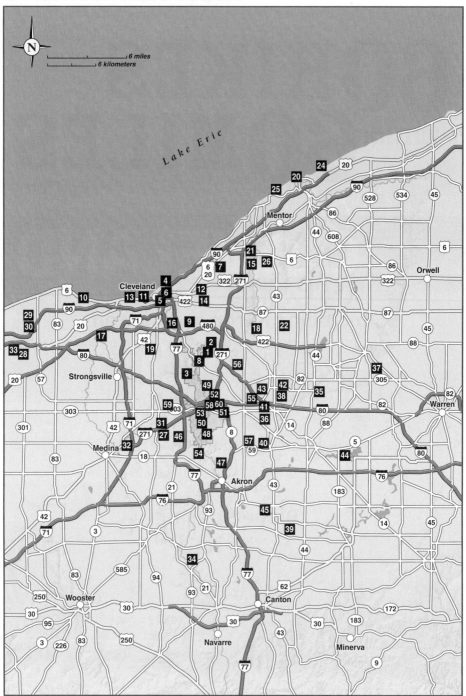

TABLE OF CONTENTS

Worden's Ledges at Hinckley Reservation *(Hike 31, page 148)*

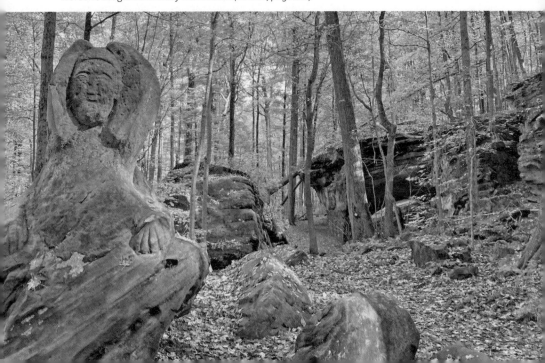

ACKNOWLEDGMENTS

While writing the fourth edition of this book, I again felt extremely fortunate to work with the great team at Menasha Ridge Press, most of whom had worked on the previous editions. Thanks to Holly Cross for wrangling the many files I sent into a manageable text, to Steve Jones for dealing patiently and politely with a nearly endless stream of map and image files, and to Molly Merkle for handling the business stuff in an always friendly manner. Here at home, my family and friends were supportive and encouraging. I appreciate my husband, who, after a long day at work, put up with my complaints when I tried to explain that I'd had a hard day on the trail. I am grateful that same husband and both of my busy, grown-up kids took time to visit a few trails with me, as did some patient friends (Hi Bekah!). I know they share my extreme enthusiasm for all that Cleveland and northeast Ohio have to offer; it is a magical region.

I thank my father for giving me the hiking gene, the inclination to hit the trail for no other reason than to see whatever may be waiting there to be seen. (Thanks, Dad!) I am also grateful for decades of my mother's advice. Because of it, I was careful, wore sunscreen and good shoes, always carried a snack, and drank plenty of water along the way. (Thanks, Mom. See, I was listening.)

Michelle Schultz deserves extra credit for being the best of cheerleaders, telling me that I could meet another book deadline—and that people would actually read it. Janice Sampson is to be commended for slogging through many miles with me, stopping for countless pictures, listening to me snarl at my mapping app the whole time. (Your patience is legendary.) Veronica Jurgena was the editing angel on my shoulder, whispering "you can do it" and sending hundreds of encouraging texts.

I am also indebted to dozens of people in the field, so to speak, who shared with me their time, enthusiasm, and incredible knowledge as I worked on this book. The importance and dedication of people who work in parks and conservation cannot be overstated. I sincerely appreciate their willingness to share everything they know about the properties they manage, the greater ecosystem, and all related local development. I also thoroughly enjoy those brief and casual conversations with people I meet along each trail. Hikers are the best kind of people. Thank you for sharing your view with others you meet along the path. And now, let's hit the trail!

—*Diane Stresing*

FOREWORD

Welcome to Menasha Ridge Press's *60 Hikes Within 60 Miles,* a series designed to provide hikers with the information they need to find and hike the very best trails surrounding metropolitan areas.

Our strategy is simple: First, find a hiker who knows the area and loves to hike. Second, ask that person to spend a year researching the most popular and very best trails around. And third, have that person describe each trail in terms of difficulty, scenery, condition, and other categories of information that are important to hikers. "Pretend you've just completed a hike and met up with other hikers at the trailhead," we tell each author. "Imagine their questions; be clear in your answers."

An experienced hiker and writer, author Diane Stresing has selected 60 of the best hikes in and around the Cleveland metropolitan area. This fourth edition includes new hikes, as well as additional sections and new routes for some of the existing hikes. Diane provides hikers (and walkers) with a great variety of hikes—all within roughly 60 miles of Cleveland—from urban strolls on city sidewalks to aerobic outings in the Cuyahoga Valley.

You'll get more out of this book if you take a moment to read the Introduction, which explains how to read the trail listings. The "Topographic Maps" section will help you understand how useful topos are on a hike and will also tell you where to get them. And though this is a where-to, not a how-to, guide, readers who have not hiked extensively will find the Introduction of particular value.

As much for the opportunity to free the spirit as to free the body, let these hikes elevate you above the urban hurry.

All the best,
The Editors at Menasha Ridge Press

PREFACE

What's the difference between a hike and a walk? I love to ponder this question. Refer to your dictionary and you'll find that *hike* comes right after *hijack,* begging a word-association game. Is a hike just a walk, hijacked by wanderlust? Perhaps.

Merriam-Webster defines *hike* as "a long walk especially for pleasure or exercise," and also "to travel by any means." But walking is a mode of transportation too. Clearly, the difference between a hike and a walk is subject to individual interpretation.

My interpretation, then, is that walking is *primarily* a means of transportation, a point-A-to-point-B kind of thing. Hiking is more a means of *exploration*— even when the ground you're exploring lies between point A and point B. When you define hiking as a means of exploration, you can turn a walk into a hike by altering your perspective. Your perspective will be different than mine, even on the same trail. That's part of the fun of hiking—finding out where the trail takes you.

Land of Plenty (of Variety)

Every hiker has a favorite topography, or three. When I began writing the first edition, I was a hill lover—the steeper and rockier, the better. A view from on high was a bonus, but I was really in it for the climb. I grew to love lake loops, recognizing that they have a serene quality, and forests offer a comfort of their own. And somewhat surprisingly (to me), I've also developed a genuine appreciation—a fascination, really—for wetlands. The sticky goo of a bog and the temporary sheen of a vernal pool create something like a giant petri dish, growing the strangest stuff!

Whatever land type is your favorite, you can probably find it here in northeastern Ohio. Between the muggy bogs and slippery marshes and the edge of Lake Erie, you'll find pretty waterfalls, steep outcrops of shale and the Sharon Conglomerate, boreal forests, and glacial formations, including kames and kettle lakes.

Most of these hikes travel over Ohio's glaciated Western Allegheny Plateau, and a few tread along the Great Lakes eco-region. When you consider an eco-region, you must take into account both land and water systems. The land in the Western Allegheny Plateau is dotted with short, gravelly, dome-shaped hills called kames. These bumps in the landscape were formed by converging glacial lobes. Some of the cool cavelike spots, such as those found at Nelson-Kennedy Ledges State Park and Liberty Park, even support species native to Canada. The Western Allegheny Plateau also boasts some remaining wetlands, most of which are protected as state nature preserves, such as Herrick Fen.

In considering our water systems, the crooked Cuyahoga River gets a great deal of attention, but the Chagrin River, Grand River, and Tinkers Creek watersheds are of equal importance, hosting a significant number of rare and endangered plants and animals.

To learn more about Ohio's eco-regions and the unique species they shelter, spend some time at The Nature Conservancy's website, nature.org, or call the Ohio chapter office at 614-717-2770.

History Underfoot: From Terrible Fish to Trains

About 360 million years before the glaciers made their mark on Ohio's landscape, there was no landscape. All of Ohio was under water. When you visit the Rocky River Reservation, you can see *Dunkleosteus terrelli,* the "terrible fish" that was considerably larger than a shark—and probably ate sharks for breakfast! The nature center at Rocky River is just one of many great places to learn about Ohio's ancient history and more recent events as well.

The first white settlers in northeastern Ohio came here to create the Connecticut Land Company's Western Reserve. Those hardy Easterners built homes, churches, colleges, roads, and railroads when they arrived, and many of these original structures can be seen along the trails described in this book. These settlers also built stations on the "invisible" Underground Railroad. Their legacy remains visible in much of the architecture (and trails) in this area.

The folks who settled here made their mark in other ways too. In addition to inventions and notable "firsts," area artists have also made, and continue to make, an impression on our landscape. Some, like Henry Church Jr. of Chagrin Falls and Noble Stuart of Hinckley, left their signature carvings for us to wonder about. Public art is everywhere in downtown Cleveland and in surrounding towns as well. Many famous Ohioans are buried at Lake View Cemetery and in dozens of smaller, but equally historical, burial sites in the area. In traipsing and researching these trails, I learned more about Ohio's history than I did in all of my school days. What's more, I found these lessons fascinating. I hope you do too. With each edition, I discover new lessons.

Seasons on the Trail

"Winter hiking? Are you crazy?"

All four seasons offer scenic sights on northeastern Ohio trails. Don't let a little number (such as −4°) keep you inside. Properly outfitted, you can be comfortable, have fun, and enjoy something that's hard to find on the trail in the summer months: solitude.

Hike the same trail in each season and you'll discover that it has multiple personalities. What was a serene lake in June is the scene of a raucous party of migrating waterfowl in November. If you think that the woods look dead and drab in the winter, look again. As soon as the leaves fall off the trees, they already have their spring buds. Look closely and you'll see how much tree bud structures differ from each other. And you don't have to look closely in the winter months to spot other features: bird, squirrel, and insect nests are easy to notice on bare limbs. So, too, are the unusual shapes and growth patterns of many branches.

Before spring officially arrives, many wildflowers poke through the snow to reach for the sun. (Skunk cabbage is my favorite!) Get out and see if you can identify them by their leaves, before they bloom.

In the summer, poison ivy, black flies, and mosquitoes may make you think twice before you leave home. Don't let them ruin your fun; the proper repellent will deter them. And here's more good news: Poison ivy is just about the only plant you have to fear in northeast Ohio. Learn to identify its distinctive leaves and habits (it climbs trees as much as it creeps along the ground), and you'll be able to avoid it. Poison oak usually isn't a problem in Ohio, and if you stay away from the mushiest parts of a bog, you're almost certainly safe from poison sumac as well.

People, unfortunately, are far more dangerous to plants than plants are to people. As tempting as it may be, never pick anything along the trail. Even the seemingly innocent action of picking a wildflower on one part of a trail and leaving it on another can upset restoration efforts or hasten the progression of an unwelcome species. Many nonnative species are aggressive (purple loosestrife and garlic mustard, for example), even though they are also pretty. Leave them where they are. In some places, wildlife management experts have decided to control or eradicate the aggressive plants; in others, they remain under observation. In any case, the hiker is bound to follow the trail mantra: "Take only pictures; leave only footprints."

What Do Timberdoodles Do, and Are Nuthatches Really Nutty?

You don't have to be a bird guru to find bird-watching fascinating. The common robin has one of the most beautiful songs of all North American birds. The often-heard catbird can imitate the songs of more than 200 other birds. It can also do impressions of other noises, such as a rusty gate hinge or a crying baby. Once, at Tinkers Creek, I had a rather eerie feeling as I listened to a repeated, panicked call: "Wah! Wah!" If I hadn't been watching the catbird as he called, I would have been certain that I was hearing a human infant! Another time, walking along a city sidewalk, I spotted a backyard-variety blue jay flying very low. He was weighted down by his catch: a fat mole. (Imagine the feast in that nest!)

Birds, both common and rare, offer great entertainment. If you want to learn about them but are overwhelmed by the volumes of bird-watching books, I recommend picking up a chart that identifies a few local varieties for starters. Or visit the children's section of your local bookstore, where you'll find the thinner books an easy starting point. (Several examples are listed in Appendix E. It was from one of these children's books that I learned nuthatches, unlike other birds, can walk both up *and* down tree trunks and branches. Now, I'm always on the lookout for a bird walking the "wrong" way down a tree.) It doesn't take much effort—or much information—to get hooked on birds.

Another great way to learn about our feathered friends is to attend a naturalist-led outing. The rangers and naturalists I've met over the years have all been great sources of information, as well as patient and not the least bit stuffy. Watch your local park listings for events and go, ask questions, and delight in the answers.

Several years ago, I had the good luck to enjoy my first eagle sighting on a group hike hosted by Summit Metro Parks (and more recently, I saw one in a tree in downtown Cleveland). At other park programs, I've learned a tremendous amount from many wonderful naturalists, volunteers, and fellow hikers. So if you are able to attend any similar programs, by all means, go! And don't worry that you'll be surrounded by experienced ornithologists—chances are good that you won't be the only new bird-watcher in the group.

"Bearly" Mentioned Mammals

Are bears back in Ohio? Are coyotes really common in the greater Cleveland area? Probably more so than you think. Do you need to worry? No.

Even if you hike each of these trails several times, it's unlikely that you will see a bear or a coyote. On the other hand, you are quite likely to spot deer, raccoons, and even foxes along these trails. You can also see beavers at work and watch bats zigzagging about in the early evenings.

For more information about bears that occasionally explore our neck of the woods or the coyote population around us, visit the Ohio Department of Natural Resources website (ohiodnr.gov) or that of Cleveland Metroparks

Six script Cleveland signs grace The Land. This one is at Sokolowski's Overlook. *(Hike 5, page 31)*

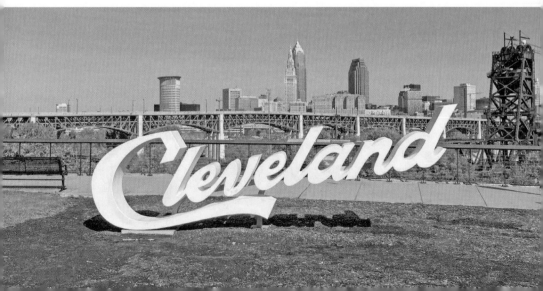

(clevelandmetroparks.com). And try to avoid making snap judgments about either of these "dangerous" animals. After all, if Floridians reside with alligators and crocodiles, we can probably live in harmony with our native species too.

Here a Park System, There a Park System, Everywhere ...

In northeastern Ohio, we enjoy the benefits of many strong park systems and conservation-minded organizations. Most of the hike descriptions in this book include contact information, so you can learn more about the area and the park system that manages it. But if you're really interested in learning about a particular area, the *best* way is to volunteer in it.

Volunteers in parks have increasingly important positions. There's a role for every person and personality. Whether you're inclined to lead a hike, ring up sales in a nature shop, create posters, build a trail, or file paperwork, you'll be greatly appreciated. I have volunteered in city and county park systems and also in the Cuyahoga Valley National Park. Each experience has proven extremely rewarding. Volunteers have the opportunity to learn from a talented pool of workers and other volunteers, and then share their knowledge with others. No matter how much or how little time you may have to offer, a creative volunteer coordinator can help you find your niche. Start by calling your local parks and recreation offices, listed in Appendix D.

Finally, no matter where you hike or visit, take the time to learn where you are and to understand the rules that govern that particular trail. Rules vary. State nature preserves, for example, prohibit pets and anything with wheels, while most state parks welcome pets (on a leash) and even bikes (on some trails). Some city parks do not allow pets; others welcome canine visitors. Rules about drones, geocaching, and, frankly, a lot of things are always evolving. Please remember that the rules of each trail and park system are created for a reason; following them makes outings more pleasant for everyone.

Take a Hike

In assembling a variety of hikes for this book, I walked through parks and creekbeds, on city sidewalks and the shores of Lake Erie. Everywhere I went, I discovered something. In the hike descriptions, I've tried to convey some of the wonder I felt in those discoveries. Now it's your turn. I hope that this book serves as a list of good suggestions, a set of starting points from which you'll discover many pleasures of your own.

60 HIKES BY CATEGORY

REGION Hike Number/Hike Name	Page #	Mileage	Difficulty	Urban	Wheelchair/ Stroller-Friendly	Kid-Friendly	Solitude	Mountain Biking	Running
CUYAHOGA COUNTY									
1 Bedford Reservation: *Bridal Veil Falls & Tinkers Creek Gorge*	16	2.0	E			✓			
2 Bedford Reservation: *Viaduct Park*	20	1.5	M			✓			
3 Brecksville Reservation: *Chippewa Creek Gorge to My Mountain Trail*	23	3.7	E–D		portions		✓		✓
4 Cleveland Lakefront Nature Preserve	27	1.7	E			✓			
5 Cleveland West Side Wanderings	31	2.6	E	✓	✓				
6 Downtown Cleveland Highlights	36	3.5	E	✓	✓				
7 Euclid Creek Reservation	41	5.0	M		portions	✓			
8 Frazee House to Linda Falls on Sagamore Creek Loop	45	4.0	M		portions				
9 Garfield Park Reservation & Mill Creek Falls	50	2.0–5.0	E		✓	✓			✓
10 Lake Erie Nature & Science Center & Huntington Reservation	54	1.9	E		portions	✓			
11 Lakefront Reservation: *Edgewater Park*	58	1.8	E		portions	✓			
12 Lake View Cemetery	62	3.0	E						
13 Lakewood Park Promenade & Solstice Steps	68	1.2	E		portions	✓			
14 The Nature Center at Shaker Lakes	72	1.5	E		portions	✓			
15 North Chagrin Reservation: *Squire's Castle*	77	5.9	M		portions	✓			✓
16 Ohio & Erie Canal Reservation	82	2.8	E		✓	✓			
17 Rocky River Reservation: *Fort Hill Loop Trail*	85	1.2	M–D			✓			
18 South Chagrin Reservation: *Henry Church Jr. Rock*	89	2.0	M			✓			
19 West Creek Reservation	93	2.6	E–M		portions	✓			

DIFFICULTY RATINGS		
E = Easy	M = Moderate	S = Strenuous

60 Hikes by Category (continued)

REGION Hike Number/Hike Name	Page #	Mileage	Difficulty	Urban	Wheelchair/ Stroller-Friendly	Kid-Friendly	Solitude	Mountain Biking	Running
GEAUGA & LAKE COUNTIES									
20 Fairport Harbor Lakefront Park	100	1.0	E	✓	portions	✓			
21 Hach-Otis Sanctuary State Nature Preserve	104	1.2	E				✓		
22 Holbrook Hollows	109	2.2	E		portions	✓			
23 Jordan Creek Park	113	3.0	E–M		portions	✓			
24 Lake Erie Bluffs	117	3.2	E–M		portions	✓			
25 Mentor Lagoons Nature Preserve	121	4.0–5.0	E		portions		✓		
26 Orchard Hills Park	125	2.0	E		portions	✓			
LORAIN & MEDINA COUNTIES									
27 Allardale Park	132	2.3	E–M		portions				✓
28 Cascade Park: *Riverside, Ledges & West Falls Trails*	136	1.0	M			✓			
29 French Creek Reservation: *Nature Center Trail*	140	1.2	E			✓			
30 French Creek Reservation: *Pine Tree Area & Big Woods Trail*	144	1.5	E		✓	✓			✓
31 Hinckley Reservation: *Worden's Ledges*	148	1.0	E			✓			
32 Lake Medina	152	2.5	E			✓			✓
33 Rowland Nature Preserve	156	1.1	E			✓			✓
PORTAGE & STARK COUNTIES									
34 Canal Fulton: *Ohio & Erie Canal Towpath & Olde Muskingum Trails*	162	5.9-10.5	M		portions			✓	✓
35 Headwaters Trail	166	4.5 9.0	E				✓	✓	✓
36 Herrick Fen State Nature Preserve	170	1.6	E				✓		
37 Nelson-Kennedy Ledges State Park	175	2.0	M–D						
38 Paddock River Preserve	179	2.5	M						
39 Quail Hollow Park	183	2.1	E		portions	✓	✓		
40 Riveredge Trail & City of Kent	188	3.0	E	✓		✓			✓
41 Seneca Ponds Park	193	1.0	E			✓			✓
42 Sunny Lake Park	197	2.0	E		portions	✓		✓	✓
43 Tinkers Creek State Nature Preserve	201	2.5	E			✓	✓		

REGION Hike Number/Hike Name	Page #	Mileage	Difficulty	Urban	Wheelchair/ Stroller-Friendly	Kid-Friendly	Solitude	Mountain Biking	Running
44 West Branch State Park: *Michael J. Kirwan Dam*	205	3.0	M		✓		✓	✓	✓
45 Wingfoot Lake State Park	209	1.6	E		mostly	✓		✓	
SUMMIT COUNTY									
46 Bath Nature Preserve	216	3.0	M			✓			✓
47 Cascade Valley Metro Park: *Oxbow Trail & Overlook*	220	1.7	M		✓	✓			
48 Cuyahoga Valley National Park: *Beaver Marsh Boardwalk & Indigo Lake*	225	3.5	E		portions	✓		✓	
49 Cuyahoga Valley National Park: *Brandywine Falls & Gorge Loop*	230	1.7	M	✓		✓			
50 Cuyahoga Valley National Park: *Everett Covered Bridge & Furnace Run*	235	1.9–2.3	M			✓			
51 Cuyahoga Valley National Park: *Haskell Run & Ledges Trails*	239	3.0	M			✓			
52 Cuyahoga Valley National Park: *On the Buckeye Trail from Pine Lane to Boston*	244	3.6–7.0	M				✓		✓
53 Cuyahoga Valley National Park: *Plateau Trail*	248	5.0	M				✓		✓
54 F. A. Seiberling Nature Realm	252	1.9	E	✓	✓	✓			
55 Hudson Springs Park	256	2.0	E			✓		✓	✓
56 Liberty Park: *Twinsburg Ledges*	260	1.6	M		portions	✓			
57 Munroe Falls Metro Park: *Tall- madge Meadows & Lake Areas*	264	5.0	E–M			✓			✓
58 Peninsula History: *Ohio & Erie Canal Towpath & Quarry Trails*	268	3.7	M		portions	✓			
59 Richfield Heritage Preserve	273	3.5	M				✓		
60 Wildlife Woods	277	1.5	M			✓	✓		

DIFFICULTY RATINGS		
E = Easy	M = Moderate	S = Strenuous

60 Hikes by Category (continued)

REGION Hike Number/Hike Name	Page #	Scenic Views	Wildflowers	Wildlife	Waterfalls	Lakes	Steep	Nature Center	Historical Interest
CUYAHOGA COUNTY									
1 Bedford Reservation: *Bridal Veil Falls & Tinkers Creek Gorge*	16		✓		✓		✓		
2 Bedford Reservation: *Viaduct Park*	20	✓			✓		✓		✓
3 Brecksville Reservation: *Chippewa Creek Gorge to My Mountain Trail*	23	✓	✓	✓			✓	✓	
4 Cleveland Lakefront Nature Preserve	27	✓	✓	✓		✓			✓
5 Cleveland West Side Wanderings	31								✓
6 Downtown Cleveland Highlights	36	✓				✓			✓
7 Euclid Creek Reservation	41	✓	✓				✓		
8 Frazee House to Linda Falls on Sagamore Creek Loop	45		✓	✓	✓				✓
9 Garfield Park Reservation & Mill Creek Falls	50		✓		✓				
10 Lake Erie Nature & Science Center & Huntington Reservation	54	✓				✓		✓	
11 Lakefront Reservation: *Edgewater Park*	58	✓		✓		✓			
12 Lake View Cemetery	62	✓	✓			✓			✓
13 Lakewood Park Promenade & Solstice Steps	68	✓				✓			
14 The Nature Center at Shaker Lakes	72		✓	✓		✓		✓	
15 North Chagrin Reservation: *Squire's Castle*	77		✓					✓	✓
16 Ohio & Erie Canal Reservation	82	✓							✓
17 Rocky River Reservation: *Fort Hill Loop Trail*	85	✓	✓	✓			✓	✓	✓
18 South Chagrin Reservation: *Henry Church Jr. Rock*	89	✓	✓		✓		✓	✓	✓
19 West Creek Reservation	93	✓	✓					✓	✓
GEAUGA & LAKE COUNTIES									
20 Fairport Harbor Lakefront Park	100	✓				✓			
21 Hach-Otis Sanctuary State Nature Preserve	104	✓	✓	✓					

REGION Hike Number/Hike Name	Page #	Scenic Views	Wildflowers	Wildlife	Waterfalls	Lakes	Steep	Nature Center	Historical Interest
22 Holbrook Hollows	109		✓	✓					
23 Jordan Creek Park	113	✓	✓		✓			✓	
24 Lake Erie Bluffs	117	✓	✓	✓		✓			
25 Mentor Lagoons Nature Preserve	121	✓	✓	✓		✓			
26 Orchard Hills Park	125	✓	✓	✓					
LORAIN & MEDINA COUNTIES									
27 Allardale Park	132	✓	✓						✓
28 Cascade Park: *Riverside, Ledges & West Falls Trails*	136	✓			✓				
29 French Creek Reservation: *Nature Center Trail*	140	✓		✓				✓	
30 French Creek Reservation: *Pine Tree Area & Big Woods Trail*	144		✓	✓					
31 Hinckley Reservation: *Worden's Ledges*	148	✓	✓						✓
32 Lake Medina	152		✓			✓			
33 Rowland Nature Preserve	156		✓			✓			
PORTAGE & STARK COUNTIES									
34 Canal Fulton: *Ohio & Erie Canal Towpath & Olde Muskingum Trails*	162		✓						✓
35 Headwaters Trail	166		✓	✓					✓
36 Herrick Fen State Nature Preserve	170		✓	✓		✓			✓
37 Nelson-Kennedy Ledges State Park	175	✓	✓	✓	✓		✓		✓
38 Paddock River Preserve	179	✓	✓	✓					
39 Quail Hollow Park	183		✓	✓					✓
40 Riveredge Trail & City of Kent	188		✓						✓
41 Seneca Ponds Park	193		✓			✓			
42 Sunny Lake Park	197			✓		✓			
43 Tinkers Creek State Nature Preserve	201		✓	✓					
44 West Branch State Park: *Michael J. Kirwan Dam*	205		✓	✓		✓			✓
45 Wingfoot Lake State Park	209	✓				✓			✓
SUMMIT COUNTY									
46 Bath Nature Preserve	216	✓	✓	✓					
47 Cascade Valley Metro Park: *Oxbow Trail & Overlook*	220	✓	✓					✓	

60 Hikes by Category *(continued)*

REGION Hike Number/Hike Name	Page #	Scenic Views	Wildflowers	Wildlife	Waterfalls	Lakes	Steep	Nature Center	Historical Interest
SUMMIT COUNTY *(continued)*									
48 Cuyahoga Valley National Park: *Beaver Marsh Boardwalk & Indigo Lake*	225	✓	✓	✓		✓		✓	
49 Cuyahoga Valley National Park: *Brandywine Falls & Gorge Loop*	230	✓	✓		✓		✓		✓
50 Cuyahoga Valley National Park: *Everett Covered Bridge & Furnace Run*	235	✓	✓				✓		✓
51 Cuyahoga Valley National Park: *Haskell Run & Ledges Trails*	239	✓	✓	✓			✓		✓
52 Cuyahoga Valley National Park: *On the Buckeye Trail from Pine Lane to Boston*	244	✓	✓	✓			✓		
53 Cuyahoga Valley National Park: *Plateau Trail*	248		✓	✓		✓			
54 F. A. Seiberling Nature Realm	252		✓	✓				✓	
55 Hudson Springs Park	256		✓			✓			
56 Liberty Park: Twinsburg Ledges	260	✓	✓				✓	✓	
57 Munroe Falls Metro Park: *Tall-madge Meadows & Lake Areas*	264	✓	✓	✓		✓	✓		
58 Peninsula History: *Ohio & Erie Canal Towpath & Quarry Trails*	268	✓					✓		✓
59 Richfield Heritage Preserve	273	✓	✓	✓					
60 Wildlife Woods	277	✓	✓	✓			✓		

INTRODUCTION

Welcome to *60 Hikes Within 60 Miles: Cleveland!* If you're new to hiking or even if you're a seasoned trekker, take a few minutes to read the following introduction. We'll explain how this book is organized and how to get the best use of it.

How to Use This Guidebook

OVERVIEW MAP AND MAP LEGEND

Use the overview map on page iv to assess the general location of each hike's primary trailhead. Each hike's number appears on the overview map and in the table of contents facing the overview. As you flip through the book, a hike's full profile is easy to locate by watching for the hike number at the top of the first page. The book is organized by region, as indicated in the table of contents. A map legend that details the symbols found on trail maps appears on page 2.

REGIONAL MAPS

The book is divided into regions, each prefaced by a regional map. These maps provide more detail than the overview map, bringing you closer to the hikes.

TRAIL MAPS

A detailed map of each hike's route appears with its profile. On each of these maps, symbols indicate the trailhead, the complete route, significant features, facilities, and topographic landmarks such as creeks, overlooks, and peaks.

To produce the highly accurate maps in this book, the author used a handheld GPS unit to gather data while hiking each route, then sent that data to the publisher's expert cartographers. However, your GPS is not really a substitute for sound, sensible navigation that takes into account the conditions you observe while hiking.

Further, despite the high quality of the maps in this guidebook, the publisher and author strongly recommend that you always carry an additional map, such as the ones noted in each entry's listing for "Maps."

ELEVATION PROFILES

For trails with significant elevation changes, the hike description will include this graph. Entries for routes with 100 feet of elevation gain or less will *not* display an elevation profile.

For hike descriptions that include an elevation profile, the diagram represents the rises and falls of the trail as viewed from the side, over the complete distance (in miles) of that trail. On the vertical axis, or height scale, the number of feet indicated between each tick mark lets you visualize the climb. To avoid making flat hikes look

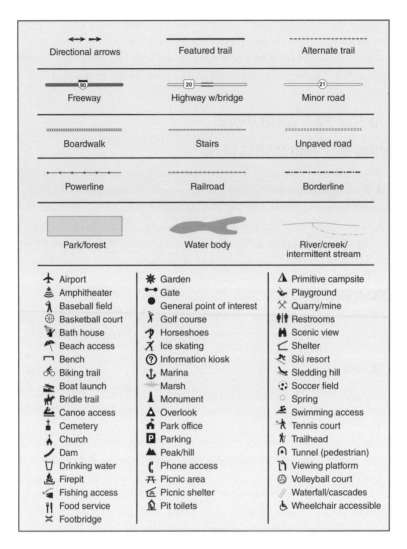

←→ →➤ Directional arrows	——— Featured trail	------------ Alternate trail
Freeway (90)	Highway w/bridge (20)	Minor road (21)
Boardwalk	Stairs	Unpaved road
Powerline	Railroad	Borderline
Park/forest	Water body	River/creek/ intermittent stream

✈ Airport	✳ Garden	⛺ Primitive campsite
♨ Amphitheater	●–● Gate	⚒ Playground
🏃 Baseball field	● General point of interest	✕ Quarry/mine
🏀 Basketball court	⛳ Golf course	🚻 Restrooms
🛁 Bath house	Horseshoes	⚲ Scenic view
🏖 Beach access	Ice skating	⌐ Shelter
⊓ Bench	⑦ Information kiosk	⛷ Ski resort
🚲 Biking trail	⚓ Marina	⛷ Sledding hill
🚣 Boat launch	Marsh	⚽ Soccer field
🐴 Bridle trail	1 Monument	○ Spring
Canoe access	Δ Overlook	🏊 Swimming access
⊺ Cemetery	🏠 Park office	🎾 Tennis court
Church	P Parking	Trailhead
Dam	▲▲ Peak/hill	∩ Tunnel (pedestrian)
Drinking water	℄ Phone access	Viewing platform
Firepit	⊼ Picnic area	Ⓢ Volleyball court
Fishing access	Picnic shelter	// Waterfall/cascades
Food service	Pit toilets	♿ Wheelchair accessible
Footbridge		

steep and steep hikes appear flat, varying height scales provide an accurate image of each hike's climbing challenge. For example, one hike's scale might rise to 600 feet, while another goes to 1,100 feet. Elevation profiles for loop hikes show total distance; those for out-and-back hikes show only one-way distance.

HIKE PROFILES

Each hike contains a brief overview of the trail, a description of the route from start to finish, a key at-a-glance information box, GPS coordinates for the trailhead, directions for driving to the trailhead area, and notes on nearby activities. Each profile also includes a map (see "Trail Maps," page 1) and an elevation profile (if applicable). Combined, the maps and information provide a clear method to assess each trail from the comfort of your favorite reading chair.

IN BRIEF

Think of this section as a snapshot focused on the historical landmarks, beautiful vistas, and other sights you may encounter on the hike.

KEY INFORMATION

The information in this box gives you a quick idea of the specifics of each hike.

DISTANCE & CONFIGURATION The length of the trail from start to finish (total distance traveled) and a description of what the trail might look like from overhead. Trails can be loops, out-and-backs (taking you in and out via the same path), figure eights, balloons (a loop with an out-and-back portion), or a combination of shapes. There may be options to shorten or extend the hikes, but the mileage corresponds to the described hike. Consult the hike description to help decide how to customize the hike for your ability or time constraints.

DIFFICULTY The degree of effort an average hiker should expect on a given route. For simplicity, the trails are rated as easy, moderate, or difficult.

SCENERY A short summary of the attractions offered by the hike and what to expect in terms of plant life, wildlife, natural wonders, and historical features.

EXPOSURE A quick check of how much sun you can expect on your shoulders during the hike.

TRAFFIC Indicates how busy the trail might be on an average day. Trail traffic, of course, varies from day to day and season to season. Weekend days typically see the most visitors. Other trail users that you might encounter are also listed here.

TRAIL SURFACE Indicates whether the trail surface is paved, rocky, gravel, dirt, boardwalk, or a mixture of elements.

HIKING TIME The length of time it takes to hike the trail. A slow but steady hiker will average 2–3 miles per hour, depending on the terrain.

DRIVING DISTANCE Indicates expected distance from an easily identified point—in this case, from the I-77/I-480 exchange.

ACCESS A notation of fees or permits needed to access the trail (if any) and whether the trail has specific hours.

MAPS Resources for maps other than those in this guidebook are listed here.

FACILITIES What to expect in terms of restrooms, water, and other amenities at the trailhead or nearby.

WHEELCHAIR ACCESS Notes on whether the trail is wheelchair compatible.

CONTACT Listed here are phone numbers and websites for checking trail conditions and other information.

LOCATION The address for the trail.

DESCRIPTION

This is the heart of each hike. Here, the author provides a summary of the trail's essence and highlights any special traits the hike offers. The route is clearly outlined, including landmarks, side trips, and possible alternate routes along the way. Ultimately, the hike description will help you choose which hikes are best for you.

NEARBY ACTIVITIES

Look here for information on nearby activities or points of interest. This includes nearby parks, museums, restaurants, or other nearby hikes.

DIRECTIONS

Used in conjunction with the GPS coordinates, the driving directions will help you locate each trailhead. If you're using a mapping app, such as Google Maps, note that its directions may vary depending on current traffic conditions. Before you set out, always confirm that the app is taking you to the correct location, and consult the directions in this book should you lose cell service. Once at the trailhead, park only in designated areas.

TRAILHEAD GPS COORDINATES

In addition to highly specific trail outlines, this book also includes the latitude (north) and longitude (west) coordinates for each trailhead. The latitude–longitude grid system is likely quite familiar to you, but here's a refresher, pertinent to visualizing the coordinates.

Imaginary lines of latitude—called parallels and approximately 69 miles apart from each other—run horizontally around the globe. Each parallel is indicated by degrees from the equator (established to be 0°): up to 90°N at the North Pole and down to 90°S at the South Pole.

Imaginary lines of longitude—called meridians—run perpendicular to lines of latitude and are likewise indicated by degrees. Starting from 0° at the Prime Meridian in Greenwich, England, they continue to the east and west until they meet 180° later at the International Date Line in the Pacific Ocean. At the equator, longitude lincs also are approximately 69 miles apart, but that distance narrows as the meridians converge toward the North and South Poles.

In this book, latitude and longitude are expressed in decimal degrees. For example, the coordinates for Hike 1, Bedford Reservation: Bridal Veil Falls & Tinkers Creek Gorge (page 16), are as follows: N41.37188° W81.54893°. For more on GPS technology, visit usgs.gov.

TOPOGRAPHIC MAPS

The maps in this book have been produced with great care. When used with the hike description in each profile, the maps are sufficient to direct you to the trail and guide you on it. However, you will find superior detail and valuable information in the United States Geological Survey's (USGS) 7.5-minute series topographic maps.

Topo maps are available online in many locations. At mytopo.com, for example, you can view and print topos of the entire Unites States free of charge. Online services, such as trails.com, charge annual fees for additional features such as shaded relief, which makes the topography stand out more. If you expect to print out many topo maps each year, it might be worth paying for shaded-relief topo maps. The downside to USGS topos is that most of them are outdated, having been created 20–30 years ago. But they still provide excellent topographic detail. Of course, Google Earth (earth.google.com) does away with topo maps and their inaccuracies—replacing them with satellite imagery and its inaccuracies. Regardless, what one lacks, the other augments. Google Earth is an excellent tool whether you have difficulty with topos or not.

If you're new to hiking, you might be wondering, "What's a topographic map?" In short, a topo indicates not only linear distance but elevation as well, using contour lines. Contour lines spread across the map like dozens of intricate spiderwebs. Each line represents a particular elevation; at the base of each topo, a contour's interval designation is given. If the contour interval is 20 feet, then the distance between each contour line is 20 feet. Follow five contour lines up on the same map, and the elevation has increased by 100 feet.

In addition to the places listed in Appendixes A and B, you'll find topos at major universities and some public libraries, where you might try photocopying what you need. But if you want your own and can't find them locally, visit national-map.gov or store.usgs.gov.

Weather

Spring, summer, and fall have obvious allure for hikers in northeastern Ohio. On average, August has the clearest days, followed closely by July, September, and October. If there is a best month to hike around here, it might be October. Most of the summer bugs are gone, but some of the late-summer and fall wildflowers remain. Temperatures tend to be quite nice in the afternoons, and the trees are at their colorful best. But there is no reason to stay inside during any month. Consider your destination in terms of the day's weather. A wetland trail may be impassable on a wet spring day, yet stunningly beautiful in December. Black flies bite hard (really hard!) in August; you

AVERAGE DAILY TEMPERATURE BY MONTH						
	JAN	FEB	MAR	APR	MAY	JUN
High	34°F	38°F	47°F	59°F	69°F	79°F
Low	22°F	24°F	30°F	40°F	50°F	60°F
	JUL	AUG	SEP	OCT	NOV	DEC
High	83°F	81°F	74°F	62°F	51°F	38°F
Low	64°F	63°F	56°F	45°F	37°F	26°F

Source: usclimatedata.com

may want to hit an urban trail then. And April–October you'll probably want to wear mosquito repellent when you're on the trail in the early mornings and evenings.

Water

How much is enough? Well, one simple physiological fact should convince you to err on the side of excess when it comes to deciding how much water to pack: A hiker working hard in 90° heat needs approximately 10 quarts of fluid every day. That's 2.5 gallons. A good rule of thumb is to hydrate prior to your hike, carry (and drink) 16 ounces of water for every mile you plan to hike, and hydrate again after the hike. For most people, the pleasures of hiking make carrying water a relatively minor price to pay to remain safe and healthy. So pack more water than you anticipate needing, even for short hikes.

If you are tempted to drink found water, do so with extreme caution. Many ponds and lakes encountered by hikers are fairly stagnant and the water tastes terrible. Drinking such water presents inherent risks for thirsty trekkers. Giardia parasites contaminate many water sources and cause the dreaded intestinal giardiasis that can last for weeks after ingestion. For information, visit the Centers for Disease Control and Prevention's website: cdc.gov/parasites/giardia.

In any case, effective treatment is essential before using any water source found along the trail. Boiling water for 2–3 minutes is always a safe measure for camping, but day hikers can consider iodine tablets, approved chemical mixes, filtration units rated for giardia, and UV filtration. Some of these methods (for example, filtration with an added carbon filter) remove bad tastes typical in stagnant water, while others add their own taste. As a precaution, carry a means of water purification to help in a pinch, if you realize you have underestimated your consumption needs.

Clothing

There is a wide variety of clothing from which to choose. Basically, use common sense and be prepared for anything. If all you have are cotton clothes when a sudden rainstorm comes along, you'll be miserable, especially in cooler weather. It's a good idea to carry along a light wool sweater or some type of synthetic apparel (polypropylene, Capilene, Thermax, and so on) as well as a hat.

Be aware of the weather forecast and its tendency to be wrong. Always carry raingear. Thunderstorms can come on suddenly in the summer. Rainy days really aren't that bad. They cut down on the crowds and can drive bugs away, at least temporarily. With appropriate raingear, a normally crowded trail can be a wonderful place of solitude. Do, however, remain aware of the dangers of lightning strikes.

Footwear is another concern. Though tennis shoes may be appropriate for paved areas, some trails are rocky and rough; tennis shoes may not offer enough support or traction. Waterproofed or not, boots should be your footwear of choice. Sport sandals are more popular than ever, but because much of your foot is exposed, you're vulnerable to hazardous plants and thorns or the occasional piece of glass. And always be sure to pair your footwear with good socks!

Essential Gear

One of the first rules of hiking is to be prepared for anything. The simplest way to be prepared is to carry the "10 Essentials." In addition to carrying the items listed below, you need to know how to use them, especially navigational items. Always consider worst-case scenarios such as getting lost, hiking back in the dark, broken gear (for example, a broken hip strap on your pack or a water filter getting plugged), a twisted ankle, or a brutal thunderstorm. The items listed below don't cost a lot of money, don't take up much room in a pack, and don't weigh much, but they might just save your life.

- ➤ **Extra clothes** (Raingear, warm hat, gloves, and change of socks and shirt)
- ➤ **Extra food** (Trail mix, granola bars, or other high-energy foods)
- ➤ **Flashlight or headlamp with extra bulb and batteries**
- ➤ **Insect repellent** (For some areas and seasons, this is vital.)
- ➤ **Maps and a high-quality compass** (Even if you know the terrain from previous hikes, don't leave home without these tools. And, as previously noted, bring maps in addition to those in this guidebook, and consult your maps prior to the hike. If you are versed in GPS usage, bring that device, too, but don't rely on it as your sole navigational tool, as battery life can dwindle or die, and be sure to compare its guidance with that of your maps.)
- ➤ **Pocketknife** and/or multitool
- ➤ **Sunscreen** (Note the expiration date.)
- ➤ **Water** (As emphasized more than once in this book, bring more than you think you will drink. Depending on your destination, you may want to bring a container and iodine or a filter for purifying water in case you run out.)
- ➤ **Whistle** (This little gadget is more effective than your voice in the event of an emergency.)
- ➤ **Windproof, waterproof matches** and/or a lighter, as well as a fire starter

FIRST AID KIT

In addition to the aforementioned items, those below may appear overwhelming for a day hike. But any paramedic will tell you that the products listed here—in alphabetical order because all are important—are just the basics. The reality of hiking is that you can be out for a week of backpacking and acquire only a mosquito bite. Or you can hike for an hour, slip, and suffer a bleeding abrasion or broken bone.

Fortunately, the listed items collapse into a very small space. You can also purchase convenient, prepackaged kits at your pharmacy or online.

➤ **Adhesive bandages** (Band-Aid or the generic equivalent)

➤ **Antibiotic ointment** (Neosporin or the generic equivalent)

➤ **Antihistamine** (Benadryl or the generic equivalent, for allergic reactions)

➤ **Athletic tape**

➤ **Blister dressing** (such as Moleskin/Spenco 2nd Skin)

➤ **Butterfly-closure bandages**

➤ **Elastic bandages or joint wraps**

➤ **Epinephrine** in a prefilled syringe (typically by prescription only, for people known to have severe allergic reactions to bee stings)

➤ **Gauze** (one roll and a half dozen 4x4-inch pads)

➤ **Hydrogen peroxide or iodine**

➤ **Ibuprofen or acetaminophen**

➤ **Snakebite kit**

Note: Consider your intended terrain and the number of hikers in your party before you exclude any article listed above. A botanical garden stroll may not inspire you to carry a complete kit, but anything beyond that warrants precaution. When hiking alone, always be prepared for a medical need. And if you are a twosome or with a group, one or more people in your party should be equipped with first aid material.

General Safety

The following tips may have the familiar ring of your mother's voice.

➤ **Always let someone know where you will be hiking and how long you expect to be gone.** It's a good idea to give that person a copy of your route, particularly if you are headed into any isolated area. Let them know when you return.

➤ **Always sign in and out of any trail registers.** Don't hesitate to comment on the trail condition if space is provided; that's your opportunity to alert others to any problems you encounter.

➤ **Do not count on a cell phone for your safety.** Reception may be spotty or nonexistent on the trail, even on an urban walk—especially if it's embraced by towering trees.

➤ **Always carry food and water, even for a short hike.** And bring more water than you think you will need. (It cannot be said often enough!)

➤ **Ask questions.** State forest and park employees are there to help. It's a lot easier to solicit advice before a problem occurs, and it will help you avoid a mishap away from civilization, when it's too late to amend an error.

➤ **Stay on designated trails.** Even on the most clearly marked trails, there is usually a point where you have to stop and consider which way to go. If you become disoriented, don't panic. As soon as you think you may be off track, stop, assess your current direction, and then retrace your steps to the point where you went astray. Using a map, a compass, and this book, and keeping in mind what you have passed thus far, reorient yourself, and trust your judgment on which way to proceed. If you become absolutely unsure, return to your vehicle the way you came in. Should you become completely lost and have no idea how to find the trailhead, remaining in place along the trail and waiting for help is most often the best option for adults and always the best option for children.

➤ **Always carry a whistle,** another precaution that cannot be overemphasized. It may be a lifesaver if you do become lost or sustain an injury.

➤ **Be especially careful when crossing streams.** Whether you are fording the stream or crossing on a log, make every step count. If you have any doubt about maintaining your balance on a log, ford the stream instead: use a trekking pole or stout stick for balance, and face upstream as you cross. If a stream seems too deep to ford, turn back. Whatever is on the other side is not worth risking your life to see.

➤ **Be careful at overlooks.** While these areas may provide spectacular views, they are potentially hazardous. Stay back from the edge of outcrops, and make absolutely sure of your footing; a misstep can mean a nasty and possibly fatal fall.

➤ **Standing dead trees and storm-damaged living trees pose a significant hazard to hikers.** These trees may have loose or broken limbs that could fall at any time. While walking beneath trees and when choosing a spot to rest or enjoy your snack, look up!

➤ **Know the symptoms of subnormal body temperature, known as hypothermia.** Shivering and forgetfulness are the two most common indicators of this stealthy killer. Hypothermia can occur at any elevation, even in the summer, especially when the hiker is wearing lightweight cotton clothing that has gotten wet. If symptoms present themselves, get to shelter, hot liquids, and dry clothes as soon as possible.

➤ **Know the symptoms of heat exhaustion (hyperthermia).** Light-headedness and loss of energy are the first two indicators. If you feel these symptoms, find some shade, drink your water, remove as many layers of clothing as practical, and stay put until you cool down. Marching through heat exhaustion leads to heatstroke, which can be fatal. If you should be sweating and you're not, that's the signature warning sign. Your hike is over at that point—heatstroke is a serious condition that can cause seizures, convulsions, and eventually death. If you or a companion reach that point, do whatever can be done to cool the victim down, and seek medical attention immediately.

➤ **Take along your brain.** A cool, calculating mind is the most important asset on the trail. It allows you to think before you act.

9

➤ **In summary:** Plan ahead. Watch your step. Avoid accidents before they happen. Enjoy a rewarding and relaxing hike.

Animal and Plant Hazards

TICKS

Ticks like to hang out in the brush that grows along trails. Their numbers seem to explode in the hot summer months, but you should be tick-aware during all months of the year. Ticks, which are arachnids and not insects, need a host on which to feast in order to reproduce. The ticks that light onto you while hiking will be very small, sometimes so tiny that you won't be able to spot them. The two primary varieties, deer ticks and dog ticks, both need a few hours of actual attachment before they can transmit any disease they may harbor. Ticks may settle in shoes, socks, or hats, and they may take several hours to actually latch on. The best strategy is to visually check every half hour or so while hiking, do a thorough check before you get in the car, and then, when you take a posthike shower, do an even more thorough check of your entire body. Also, throw clothes into the dryer for 10 minutes when you get home, and be sure to check your pet for any hitchhikers. Ticks that haven't attached are easily removed but not easily killed. If you pick off a tick in the woods, just toss it aside. If you find one on your body at home, dispatch it and then send it down the toilet. For ticks that have embedded, removal with tweezers is best.

The blacklegged deer tick is the culprit behind Lyme disease. Experts advocate abundant repellent containing permethrin on footwear and pant legs because the nymphal-stage blacklegged tick often lurks in dead leaves, and ticks rarely climb higher than 18–24 inches off the ground. They can grab on to your shoes and are quite quick to climb up. Get more information from the American Lyme Disease Foundation at aldf.com.

MOSQUITOES

Though it's not a common occurrence, individuals can become infected with the West Nile virus by being bitten by an infected mosquito. Culex mosquitoes, the primary variety that can transmit West Nile virus to humans, thrive in urban rather than in natural areas. They lay their eggs in stagnant water and can breed in standing water that remains for more than five days. Most people infected with West Nile virus have no symptoms of illness, but some may become ill, usually 3–15 days after being bitten.

In the Cleveland area, late spring and summer are the times thought to be the highest risk periods for West Nile virus. At those times of year—and anytime you expect mosquitoes to be buzzing around—you may want to wear protective clothing, such as long sleeves, long pants, and socks. Loose-fitting, light-colored clothing is best. Spray clothing with insect repellent. Remember to follow the instructions on the repellent and to take extra care with children.

SNAKES

Very few of the venomous snakes found in the United States live in the Cleveland area. Although two species of rattlesnakes do reside in Ohio, they are endangered and have not been seen in the Cleveland area for several decades. So, most of your snake encounters will be with the 100-plus nonvenomous species and subspecies. Though you could spend some time studying the snakes in the area, the best rule is to leave all snakes alone and give them a wide berth as you hike past.

BLACK BEARS

It's unlikely that you will meet a bear on any of these trails; however, there are always a few sightings in Ohio, and while most occur in the spring, it pays to be alert to their presence year-round. In most cases, a bear will detect you first and leave. Should you encounter a bear, here is some advice, based on suggestions from the National Park Service:

➤ **Stay calm.**

➤ **Move away,** talking loudly to let the bear discover your presence.

➤ **Back away** while facing the bear.

➤ **Avoid eye contact.**

➤ **Give the bear plenty of room to escape;** bears will rarely attack unless they are threatened or provoked.

➤ **Don't run or make sudden movements;** running will provoke the bear, and you cannot outrun a bear.

➤ **Do not attempt to climb trees to escape bears,** especially black bears. The bear will pull you down by the foot.

➤ **Fight back if you are attacked.** Black bears have been driven away when people have fought back with rocks, sticks, binoculars, and even their bare hands.

➤ **Be grateful that it is not a grizzly bear.**

POISON IVY, OAK, AND SUMAC

Recognizing poison ivy, oak, and sumac and avoiding contact with them is the most effective way to prevent the painful, itchy rashes associated with these plants. Poison ivy ranges from a thick, tree-hugging vine to a shaded ground cover, 3 leaflets to a leaf; poison oak occurs as either a vine or shrub, with 3 leaflets as well; and poison sumac flourishes in swampland, each leaf containing 7–13 leaflets. Urushiol, the oil in the sap of these plants, is responsible for the rash. Usually within 12–14 hours of exposure (but sometimes much later), raised lines and/or blisters will appear, accompanied by a terrible itch. Refrain from scratching because bacteria under fingernails can cause infection, and you will spread the rash to other parts of your body. Wash and dry the rash thoroughly, applying a calamine lotion or other product to help dry the rash. If itching or blistering is severe, seek medical attention. Remember that oil-contaminated garments, pets, or hiking equipment can easily cause an irritating rash on you or someone else, so wash not only any exposed parts of your body but also clothes, gear, and pets.

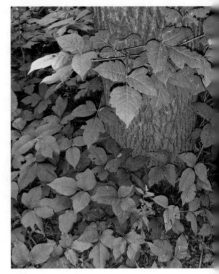

Poison ivy   *Tom Watson*

STINGING NETTLES

Stinging nettles are common in disturbed areas, moist woodlands, and partially shaded trails. The toothed leaves are oval, ribbed, and covered with "hairs." When you brush past stinging nettles, sharp, tiny spines covering the leaves and stems penetrate your skin and release histamine and formic acid. The result is an itchy rash relieved only with hydrocortisone creams and cool compresses.

Hiking with Children

No one is too young for a hike in the woods or through a city park. Be careful, though. Flat, short trails are probably best with an infant. Toddlers who have not quite mastered walking can still tag along, riding on an adult's back in a child carrier. Use common sense to judge a child's capacity to hike a particular trail, and always consider the possibility that the child will tire quickly and need to be carried.

When packing for the hike, remember the needs of the child as well as your own. Make sure children are adequately clothed for the weather, have proper shoes, and are protected from the sun with sunscreen. Kids dehydrate quickly, so make sure you have plenty of fluid for everyone.

Hikes suitable for children are indicated in the table on pages xv–xvii.

Finally, when hiking with children, remember the trip is bound to be a compromise. A child's energy and enthusiasm alternates between bursts of speed and long stops to examine snails, sticks, dirt, and other attractions. Have patience, and know that one day they'll be miles ahead of you.

The Business Hiker

Whether you're in the Cleveland area on business as a resident or visitor, these 60 hikes offer perfect, quick getaways from the busy demands of commerce. Many of the hikes are classified as urban and are easily accessible from downtown areas. Instead of eating inside, pack a lunch and head out to one of the many links in the Emerald Necklace (Cleveland Metroparks) for a relaxing break from the office or convention floor. Consider taking a small group of your business associates on a nearby hike in the Cleveland Lakefront State Parks or along the canal. A well-planned, half-day getaway is the perfect complement to a business stay in northeastern Ohio.

Trail Etiquette

Whether you're on a city, county, state, or national park trail, always remember that great care and resources (from volunteers, nature, and your tax dollars) have gone into creating these trails. Treat the trail, wildlife, and fellow hikers with respect. Here are some helpful reminders.

➤ **Hike on open trails only.** Respect trail and road closures (ask if not sure); avoid possible trespassing on private land; obtain all permits and authorization as required. Also, leave gates as you found them or as marked.

➤ **Leave no trace of your visit other than footprints.** Be sensitive to the dirt beneath you. This means staying on the trail and not creating any new ones. Be sure to pack out what you pack in. (*Note:* Some people believe that there's a special place in heaven for hikers who gather rubbish while on the trail and pack that out too.)

➤ **Never spook animals.** An unannounced approach, a sudden movement, or a loud noise startles most animals. A surprised snake or skunk can be dangerous for you, for others, and to themselves. Give animals ample time and space to adjust to your presence.

➤ **Plan ahead.** Know your equipment, your ability, and the area in which you are hiking—and prepare accordingly. Be self-sufficient at all times; carry necessary supplies for changes in weather or other conditions. A well-executed trip is a satisfaction to you and to others.

➤ **Be courteous to other hikers, or bikers, you meet on the trails.**

➤ **Finally, a little safety advice that goes a long way:** File a "flight plan" with a friend or family member. Let them know which trailhead you're starting from, and when you expect to return—and don't forget to check in with them when you've finished your hike!

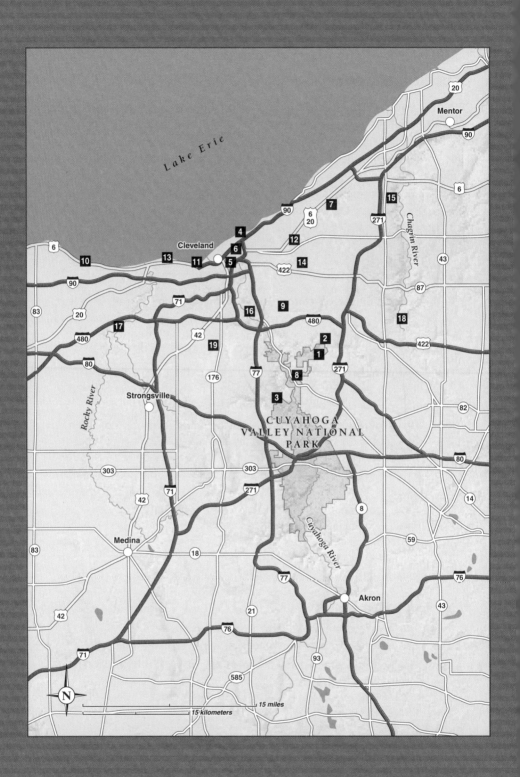

Lake Erie

Mentor

20

90

6

20

7

6
20

271

15

Chagrin River

43

Cleveland

12

6

87

90

4

6

13

11

5

422

14

18

422

6

10

90

20

83

16

9

480

71

42

17

19

2

1

480

8

271

271

176

77

80

82

3

Strongsville

CUYAHOGA
VALLEY NATIONAL
PARK

303

303

271

8

14

80

Medina

42

71

Cuyahoga River

59

18

83

77

43

76

21

Akron

76

42

93

71

585

N

585

15 miles

15 kilometers

CUYAHOGA COUNTY

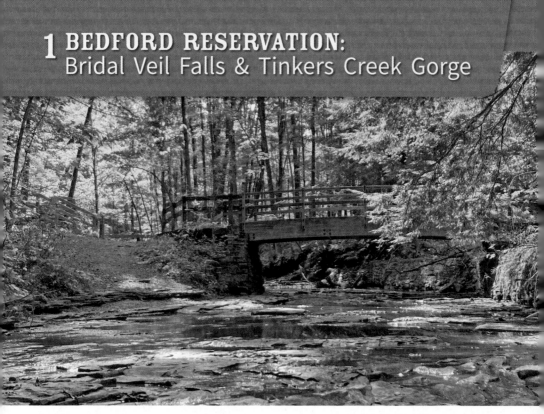

Tinkers Creek Gorge is cool and green and shady.

THIS IS AN easy hike with a big-view payoff: Enjoy cascades and waterfalls on the way to see one of Ohio's grandest canyons, nearly 150 feet deep.

DESCRIPTION

From the parking lot, cross Gorge Parkway and the paved All Purpose Trail to start your hike, following signs for the Buckeye and Bridle Trails. You'll probably hear mountain bikers rolling by—a trail just for them runs east of the hiking trails. Almost immediately, you'll see the long wooden staircase that will take you to the falls viewing area. Along the way, stop and admire the water gently bathing the shale as it trips along to the falls. This is Deerlick Creek.

At the bottom of the steps, the walking and bridle paths meet. Horses cross the shallow water on hoof; the rest of us use the bridge. As you look north from the bridge, notice the layers of Bedford shale that line the side of the hill.

At the bottom of the 85-foot drop, you'll find a small observation deck with benches. Stop here to enjoy the view.

Once you've had a good look, step onto the Bridle Trail, continuing west. You'll roll up and down several gentle hills, under the shade of thick maple, oak, and hemlock trees. The eastern hemlock is common in this area and often simply lumped in

DISTANCE & CONFIGURATION: 2.0-mile out-and-back or loop, hiker's choice

DIFFICULTY: Easy

SCENERY: Waterfall, gorge, lush forest, fall color, wildflowers in spring

EXPOSURE: Completely shaded except for overlook

TRAFFIC: Moderate–heavy

TRAIL SURFACE: Dirt and gravel on north side, paved on south side

HIKING TIME: 45 minutes

DRIVING DISTANCE: 9 miles from I-77/I-480 exchange

ACCESS: Daily, 6 a.m.–11 p.m.; parking lots that close at sunset are clearly posted.

MAPS: USGS *Shaker Heights* and USGS *Northfield;* also at park website

FACILITIES: Pay phone, water, and restrooms at Egbert Road ranger station; portable restrooms at gorge overlook; water and restrooms at Hermit's Hollow Picnic Area; emergency phones along Gorge Parkway

WHEELCHAIR ACCESS: No, but overlook is fully accessible from Gorge Parkway.

CONTACT: Cleveland Metroparks: 216-635-3200, clevelandmetroparks.com/parks/visit/parks /bedford-reservation/bridal-veil-falls-trailhead

LOCATION: Gorge Pkwy., Walton Hills

with the evergreen family. Hemlocks can be distinguished by their tiny opposing leaves, deep green in color, that lie flat along their branches. Look for narrow white stripes on the leaves' undersides.

The well-marked, wide dirt-and-gravel trail you're on performs double duty here: It is both the park district's Bridle Trail and a portion of the Buckeye Trail. A mile west of the falls, you'll rise up to meet the parkway again, soon reaching Tinkers Creek Gorge Overlook. A small parking lot at the overlook is wheelchair- and stroller-accessible; it's a popular spot.

The gorge overlook is awe-inspiring at any time but most picturesque in the fall. While the view is the main attraction, the history is also interesting.

Tinkers Creek, the largest tributary of the Cuyahoga River, begins in Kent, Ohio—about 15 miles southeast. Once it reaches this area, it winds its way nearly 5 miles through Bedford Reservation. In 1965, public officials planned to dam the gorge, intending to create a large inland lake called Lake Shawnee. A five-year study by naturalist William F. Nimberger, however, highlighted the valley's unique blend of plant and animal species. Public opinion, swayed in large part by Nimberger's study, convinced politicians to abandon their plans to build the dam. Today the gorge is a National Natural Landmark.

To return to your car, retrace your steps on the Bridle Trail or cross the parkway to the south and take the All Purpose Trail back to the parking area at Bridal Veil Falls. The difference in the two paths is negligible (about 0.1 mile).

NEARBY ACTIVITIES

Shawnee Hills Golf Course is just south of here; enter from Egbert Road. To arrange a tee time, call 440-232-7184 or go to clevelandmetroparks.com/golf/courses/shawnee -hills-golf-course. If you'd prefer to walk without clubs, head to Viaduct Park (page

Bedford Reservation: Bridal Veil Falls & Tinkers Creek Gorge

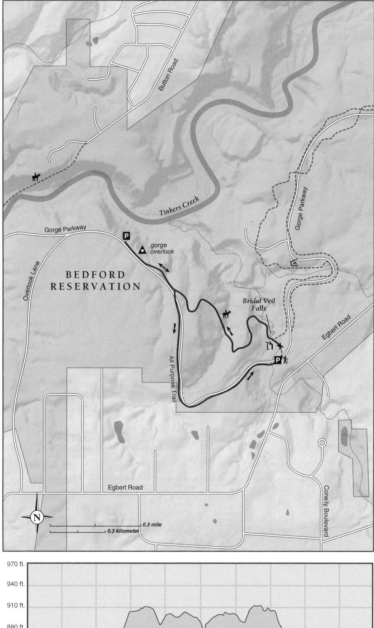

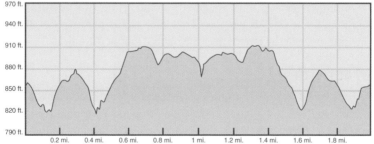

20), in the northeast section of Bedford Reservation, where another chapter of the area's history has been preserved.

• •

TRAILHEAD GPS COORDINATES: N41.37188° W81.54893°

DIRECTIONS From I-480 E, take I-271 S to Exit 23 (Broadway Avenue/Forbes Road). Turn right onto Forbes Road and then make an immediate right onto Broadway. At about 1 mile, turn left onto Bedford Chagrin Parkway/Egbert Road, and then in about 0.5 mile, make a quick right onto Gorge Parkway. Head west about 2 miles to the parking area for Bridal Veil Falls Overlook, on the left.

Bridal Veil Falls offers an always-serene scene.

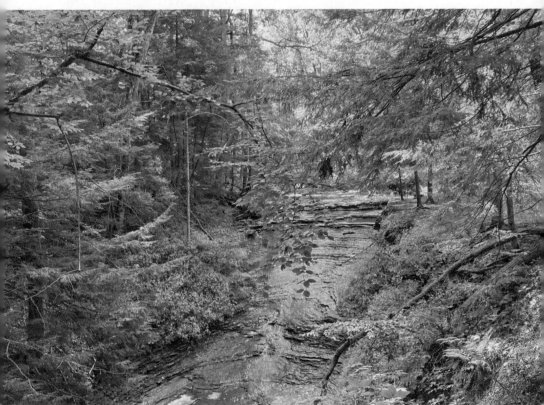

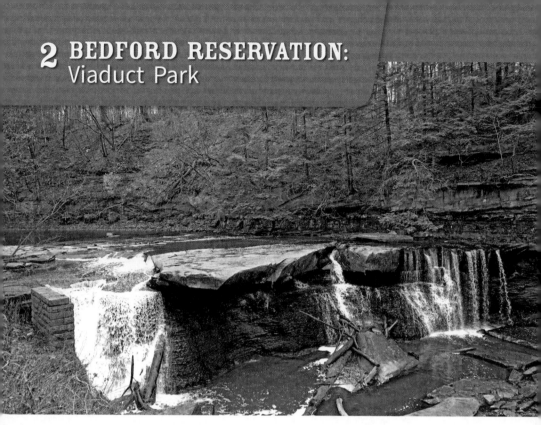

You don't have to hike far to reach the falls.

THIS SHORT TRAIL offers a glimpse into Bedford's industrial past and the Great Falls that provided power in the city's earliest days.

DESCRIPTION

From the parking lot, you can see the viaduct for which this park is named, but much lies beyond that first glimpse from the trailhead.

Follow the wide gravel trail as it takes you gently downhill at first, then a little more steeply toward the creekbed. You'll hear the falls before you see them, and once you catch a glimpse, you may have a hard time being patient and staying on the trail until you can get a better look. We have proof that the Great Falls of Tinkers Creek has been calling to people in this area since at least 1821; it's probably safe to assume that it was an important part of the landscape long before that.

The falls are only 17 feet high but an impressive 50 feet wide. The short trail is popular year-round, as the falls offer great scenery in every season.

The main path remains wide and is fairly level until you reach the creekbed, where it takes you almost to the water's edge via a couple of short staircases, less than 0.5 mile from the trailhead. But even before you reach those stairs, you'll have at least two opportunities to stop and gaze at the falls.

DISTANCE & CONFIGURATION: 1.5-mile balloon

DIFFICULTY: Moderate, with optional walking on creekbed and on rocks

SCENERY: Historic viaduct, waterfalls, rock formations, Tinkers Creek

EXPOSURE: Almost completely shaded

TRAFFIC: Fairly busy

TRAIL SURFACE: Limestone and dirt trails

HIKING TIME: Allow at least an hour

DRIVING DISTANCE: 7 miles from I-77/I-480 exchange

ACCESS: Daily, 6 a.m.–11 p.m.

MAPS: USGS *Shaker;* also posted at trailhead

FACILITIES: Emergency phone, restrooms, and water at trailhead

WHEELCHAIR ACCESS: No

CONTACT: Cleveland Metroparks: 216-635-3200, clevelandmetroparks.com/parks/visit/parks /bedford-reservation/viaduct-park

LOCATION: Willis St., Bedford

One of those opportunities comes with something of a dare. Visitors are invited to walk through the millrace tunnel that was used from 1821 to 1913, when the viaduct was the site of an active sawmill, gristmill, and electric power plant. The tunnel, about 0.25 mile from the trailhead and about 4 feet high, is not nearly as scary inside as it may look from the entrance. Besides, it's only about 10 feet long, so you can make a quick escape if you start to feel panicky.

Most first-time visitors are surprised that such a sweet, natural spot exists in the middle of long-developed Bedford—especially because this Cleveland Metroparks property is effectively surrounded by an industrial park. While there are no picnic shelters or other structures here, save for a few benches on the trail, the park sees a good bit of traffic during the week, as well as on weekends. During warm weather, you'll almost always catch a few folks with their feet in Tinkers Creek, enjoying splashing around on its sandy bottom. The water on the east side of the trail is fairly inviting, but closer to the falls, its power is more evident, and visitors are cautioned to stay on dry land there.

While the path indicated on the trailhead map is a balloon, several well-worn footpaths (and the Metroparks' interpretive signage) allow you to gain a little insight into the area's history and to explore the water's edge.

When you're ready to return, you can loop back uphill to the parking lot, where a concrete deck overlooking the viaduct features a few more interpretive signs that will lend a little more understanding of the falls and their contribution to Bedford's natural and industrial history.

NEARBY ACTIVITIES

It's easy to forget that Viaduct Park is situated inside Bedford Reservation, but it is. That means you're just minutes away from the reservation's other attractions, including hiking trails galore (page 23), as well as Shawnee Hills Golf Course. You can book a tee time by calling 440-232-7184, or see what other attractions can be found in the reservation on the park's website.

Bedford Reservation: Viaduct Park

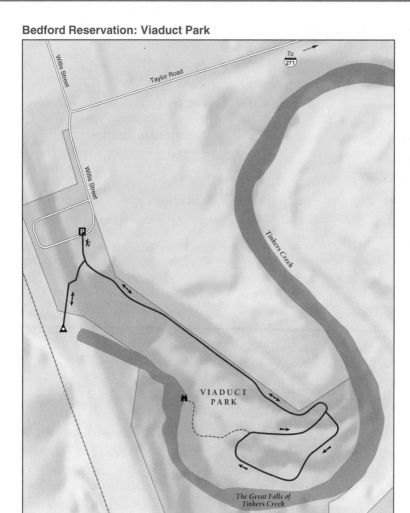

TRAILHEAD GPS COORDINATES: N41.38518° W81.53411°

DIRECTIONS From I-480 E, take I-271 S to Exit 23 (Broadway Avenue/Forbes Road). Turn right onto Forbes Road and then make an immediate right onto Broadway. After 1.3 miles, turn left onto West Taylor Street, and in 0.2 mile, take another left onto Willis Street, where you'll find the park entrance.

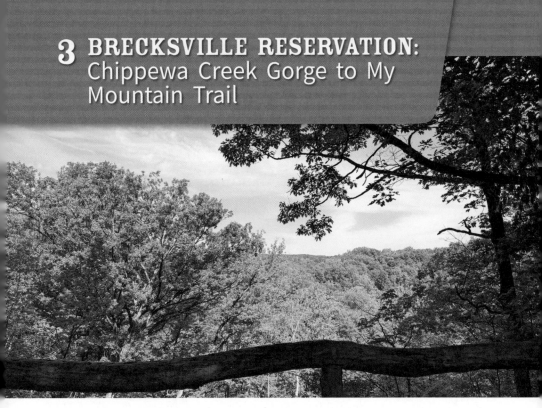

3 BRECKSVILLE RESERVATION: Chippewa Creek Gorge to My Mountain Trail

View from My Mountain Overlook

THIS COMBINATION OF three short trails provides several picture-perfect views, from a scenic stream-and-forest trail to a lovely "mountain" vista, and an opportunity to duck into the nature center for a little education.

DESCRIPTION

Enter the park off Chippewa Road (OH 82) and start from the second parking lot, by the nature center. Follow the signage to NATURE CENTER BUILDING, which is a National Historic Site. If you have time, enter the nature center to learn about the property and local wildlife. Alternatively, you can start from the parking lot for the Harrier Keeler Memorial Picnic Area.

Keeler graduated from Oberlin College in 1870 and then moved to Cleveland, where she was a suffragette and a public-school teacher, eventually becoming the system's superintendent. Keeler was also a prolific nature writer.

From the shelter that bears her name, head east on the All Purpose Trail (APT) toward the Chippewa Creek Gorge Overlook. As you approach OH 82, take a sharp right to follow the short Gorge Loop down a narrow dirt-and-gravel path to get a closer look at Chippewa Creek and the gorge.

The fully shaded trail approaches the overlook via a couple dozen stone stairs. From the overlook, find your way in a clockwise loop around and amid the boulders and ledges that make up the trail as you climb back up to the top, where Gorge

23

DISTANCE & CONFIGURATION: 3.7-mile loop with shorter and longer options

DIFFICULTY: My Mountain Trail segment is moderate–difficult; other trails are easy.

SCENERY: Mature woods, streambed, vernal pools, great views of Chippewa Creek and Gorge

EXPOSURE: Mostly shaded

TRAFFIC: Nature Center and Hemlock Trail are well traveled; My Mountain Scenic Overlook offers solitude.

TRAIL SURFACE: Mostly dirt and natural surfaces, some asphalt

HIKING TIME: 1.5–2 hours

DRIVING DISTANCE: 8 miles from I-77/I-480 exchange

ACCESS: Daily, 6 a.m.–11 p.m., except where otherwise posted

MAPS: USGS *Northfield*; trail map also at nature center and park website

FACILITIES: Restrooms and water at nature center

WHEELCHAIR ACCESS: Nature Center and Harriet Keeler Memorial, yes; other trails, no

CONTACT: Cleveland Metroparks: 440-526-1012, clevelandmetroparks.com/parks/visit/parks /brecksville-reservation/my-mountain-trailhead

LOCATION: Chippewa Creek Dr., Brecksville

Loop intersects Hemlock Trail. Turn left and head east on Hemlock Trail, which hugs the edges of the ravine by Chippewa Creek. It's rooty and rocky in places, and while there is easier footing on the APT (which runs parallel to Hemlock Trail at this point), Hemlock is more shaded and offers better scenery.

As the path levels out you have the option to take a short connector back to the Harriet Keeler Picnic Area and the Andrews Nature Play Area, with climbing structures, swings, and tunnels made of repurposed trees and other natural materials.

For this trek, stay on Hemlock Trail and its carpet of leaves, roots, rocks, and gravel until it ends at the APT, which will eventually lead you to "your" mountain— My Mountain Scenic Overlook, that is.

Follow the APT as it runs along the northern side of Chippewa Creek Drive until you see signs for PLATEAU PICNIC AREA, where you'll cross the parkway to find the trailhead. (If you'd rather skip the pavement of the APT, you can drive from the nature center parking area to the Plateau Picnic Area; let your legs decide.)

From the Plateau Picnic Area, continue heading southeast on the APT until you reach the trailhead sign for My Mountain Trail. It's a short but simple delight for hikers who like hills. Climb up the stairs and keep climbing as the trail becomes narrow and steep. The narrow, uneven path follows the ridge of the hill (it's not really a mountain) until the roadway lies 40 feet below, but you won't be able to see it; the view is splendid. Once you reach the overlook things quiet down, so you can pretend it really is your mountain, if you wish. This oak-hickory forest is thinned at times to encourage wildflower growth, and a few vernal pools dot the land up here, especially in early spring.

Formed like puddles in contained basin depressions, vernal pools have no permanent aboveground outlets. They typically follow the water table—rising with winter and spring runoff, drying in summer, and filling and freezing in fall and winter. Because

Brecksville Reservation: Chippewa Creek Gorge to My Mountain Trail

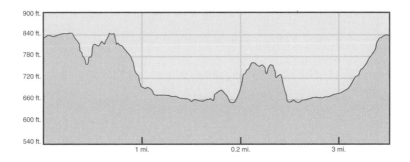

they dry out, they cannot support fish; instead, they are important to other species, such as frogs, salamanders, and fairy shrimp, all of which lay eggs (that fish would eat) in the pools. Depending on the species, the eggs either hatch before the pool dries out or incubate throughout the wet-dry-freeze cycle, hatching the next year.

Continuing along the high point of the trail, you'll make a sharp left and see the blue blazes of the Buckeye Trail (BT). Rather than following the BT, retrace your steps down, taking a sharp right to rejoin the loop, and continue back to the trailhead and the short set of wooden steps leading to the bottom of the picnic area driveway. Cross the parkway to rejoin the APT, then turn left to return to the nature center parking area where you began.

NEARBY ACTIVITIES

Brecksville Reservation offers other hilly trails—Deer Lick Loop, for example, is about 4 miles long. Stop at the nature center, visit the park website, or call 440-526-1012 for more information. You may also want to explore the managed prairie area here, which is dominated by tall grasses and brightened by wildflowers during the growing season. Foxgloves and beardtongue varieties bloom from late spring through midsummer; Shreve's irises bloom in June and July. Tall sunflowers stretch above the grasses from July through early fall, and goldenrods gild the prairie August–October. An observation deck offers lovely views.

History buffs may enjoy the Squire Rich Museum, which was built in 1842 using local black walnut trees. Managed by the Brecksville Historical Association, the museum's entrance is at 9367 Brecksville Road (OH 21). Call 440-526-7165 or visit clevelandmetroparks.com/parks/visit/parks/brecksville-reservation/squire-rich -museum for a schedule of tours and other activities.

• •

TRAILHEAD GPS COORDINATES: N41.31893° W81.61699°

DIRECTIONS Follow I-77 S and take Exit 149A, merging onto OH 82 E/E. Royalton Road. Follow OH 82 1.5 miles, past OH 21 through Brecksville, and turn right onto Chippewa Creek Drive. Parking is available at the Harriet Keeler Memorial/Overlook parking area about 0.4 mile southeast of the park entrance, as well as at the adjacent lot for the nature center.

4 CLEVELAND LAKEFRONT NATURE PRESERVE

Unique city views and natural wonders await at this lakeshore preserve.

PREVIOUSLY A DREDGE impoundment, this peninsula on our Great Lake is now home to—or a popular layover spot for—nearly 300 bird species, and it's a rest stop for thousands of monarch butterflies each fall.

DESCRIPTION

From the parking lot, follow the mulch path along the fenceline and enter through the rotating gate, which helps keep deer and other wildlife out.

Once inside the preserve, you're almost certain to spot a photographer—or a whole photography club. That's not surprising, as the preserve has a unique view of the city skyline and a reputation as one of the area's top bird-watching spots. At least twice a year, however, photographers swarm here for different reasons. Over Labor Day Weekend, they're guaranteed to enjoy a few fly-bys during the Cleveland Airshow, and later in the fall, they're sure to see throngs of monarch butterflies that rest here on their long migration route to Mexico. Don't let a photographer (or 20) dissuade you from taking in this unique preserve; their interests and yours are probably well aligned.

From the gate, turn left and head west as you follow the Perimeter Loop Trail clockwise. You'll soon reach the overlook. With its pergola and decorative wrought iron sculpture, it's a pretty stop. You can see the Cleveland Skyline in the distance

DISTANCE & CONFIGURATION: 1.7-mile loop with inner loops to lengthen or shorten distance

DIFFICULTY: Easy, flat

SCENERY: Cleveland skyline, Lake Erie, monarch habitat

EXPOSURE: Perimeter Loop Trail is mostly exposed; inner trails are mostly shaded.

TRAFFIC: Light–moderate; expect more of a crowd during monarch migration.

TRAIL SURFACE: Dirt and grass

HIKING TIME: 45 minutes

DRIVING DISTANCE: 12 miles from I-77/I-480 exchange

ACCESS: Daily, during daylight hours

MAPS: USGS *Cleveland South;* also at entrance gate

FACILITIES: Restrooms in parking area

WHEELCHAIR ACCESS: No

CONTACT: Port of Cleveland: 216-241-8004, portofcleveland.com/cleveland-lakefront -nature-preserve; ODNR: 216-377-1348, ohiodnr.gov/go-and-do/see-the-sights /lake-erie-birding-trail/cleveland-area-loop /cleveland-lakefront-nature-preserve

LOCATION: 8701 Lakeshore Blvd., Cleveland

and, much closer, the Intercity Yacht Club. Because it's somewhat protected from the winds, the area from East 55th Street Marina all around the Lakefront Preserve sees a fair amount of boating and fishing activity.

As you leave the overlook to follow the Perimeter Loop Trail clockwise, the wide, hard-packed dirt-and-grass trail meanders along the shore about 39 feet above Lake Erie. You might wonder, why so high?

This isn't your typical nature preserve. Whereas most nature preserves are designated for protection from development, this one was rescued and revitalized after suffering the effects of development. In fact, the "land" itself was developed from dumped material—including tens of thousands of cars and industrial waste dumped there and in nearby Gordon Park throughout the 1900s.

In 1975, the U.S. Army Corps of Engineers outlined a plan to utilize the landfill space adjacent to Gordon Park as "Diked Disposal Facility Site Number 14." Thanks to the cooperation of numerous entities, including the Army Corps, the City and Port of Cleveland, the State of Ohio, and countless volunteers, this former confined disposal facility, or CFD, is now a unique, 88-acre Ohio State Nature Preserve. It is also a birding hotspot, and a grand place for a hike or trail run.

At some points on the trail, remnants of the dumping ground and industrial waste can be seen, but in most instances, the metal, concrete, and other material appears almost like modern artworks woven into the environment. And those remnants are clearly being put to good use by the flora and fauna in this somewhat unnatural nature preserve.

Just about 1,000 feet from the overlook, you'll see a sign inviting you to take the aptly named Monarch Trail to the right. If you follow it, you'll head east and meet up with the other interior path, the Northern Harrier Trail. For now, continue clockwise on the Perimeter Loop Trail.

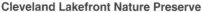

Cleveland Lakefront Nature Preserve

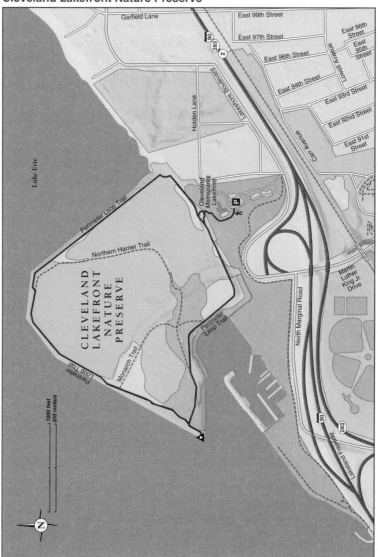

The Perimeter Loop Trail offers the best and broadest views of the lake, along with a weather data collection station and some additional wrought iron creations. As you round out your hike on the Perimeter Loop Trail, you will have a look at the Bratenahl neighborhood before heading up a short flight of stairs to return to the turnstile gate.

After completing the loop trail, you might choose to explore the Monarch and Northern Harrier Trails, either as out-and-backs or by creating a second, shorter loop (connecting with the northern portion of the Perimeter Loop Trail). The interior trails are almost completely shaded, as you're walking through a thick growth of younger woods in the process of "reforesting" a land that didn't exist until recently. If you hike the interior, be aware that it doesn't drain as well as the perimeter trail and typically remains somewhat muddy for several days after a rain.

The Port of Cleveland, Cleveland Metroparks, and Ohio Department of Natural Resources have done a great job here in a relatively short time. By reusing some of the steel and other industrial paraphernalia and letting nature overtake and remake it into "modern art," this nature preserve has developed a distinct city vibe.

For a detailed account of how a dump and dredging site came to be a nature preserve, see Jim Lanese's article, "Cleveland Lakefront Nature Preserve: From Sunken Barges to Nature Preserve," at the Cleveland Historical website at clevelandhistorical .org/items/show/433.

Note for families: While the gate makes it difficult to bring a stroller into the preserve, most of the Perimeter Loop Trail is conducive for an all-terrain stroller. Be aware, however, that any stroller would need to be carried up a short set of stairs on the eastern edge of the loop.

NEARBY ACTIVITIES

Cleveland Lakefront Nature Preserve is just over a mile from Rockefeller Park and Greenhouse. Owned and managed by the City of Cleveland, the greenhouse is worth a visit anytime, and is especially popular for its holiday poinsettia display. Admission to the greenhouse and parking are both free. But if all those lake views have you longing to visit a beach, check out Lakefront Reservation, Wildwood Park, or Edgewater Park (page 58), all of which feature swim beaches.

• •

TRAILHEAD GPS COORDINATES: N41.54163° W81.62907°

DIRECTIONS Take I-77 N to I-90 E and take Exit 177 for Martin Luther King Jr. Drive. Turn left onto Martin Luther King Jr. Drive, which veers right and becomes Lakeshore Boulevard. Turn left onto the access road (East 88th) to the parking lot.

5 CLEVELAND WEST SIDE WANDERINGS

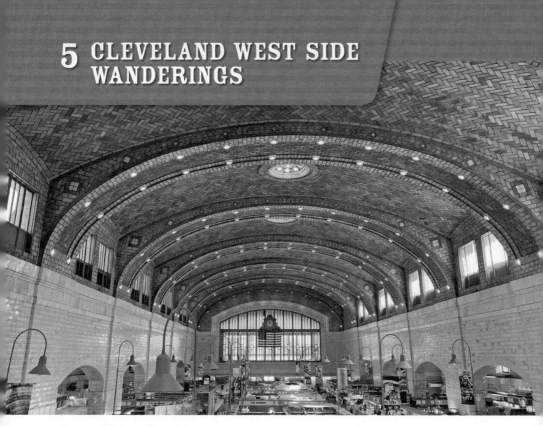

The venerable West Side Market

OHIO CITY, A separate entity from the City of Cleveland from 1836 to 1854, remains a bright and beautiful neighborhood on Cleveland's west side. Take in some of the area's history, public art, iconic architecture, and the splendid smorgasbord that is the West Side Market.

DESCRIPTION

Start at Sokolowski's Overlook, named for the long-loved, family-owned Sokolowski's University Inn Restaurant. While the main attraction now is the view, property adjacent to the overlook is owned by a private developer. At the time of this writing, some residents and Towpath users were feeling anxious about designs being considered for multistory buildings that could alter the view.

But for now, from the overlook you can see the Lorain-Carnegie Bridge and the westernmost of the two Guardians of Transportation statues. Those Guardians, built in Cleveland, have watched over traffic crossing the Cuyahoga since 1932. In the 1970s, when Cuyahoga County Engineer Albert Porter began planning to widen the bridge, he called the Guardians "monstrosities [that] should be torn down." Fortunately, that didn't happen, and in 1976, the bridge was named to the National Register of Historic Places. (Porter left office in 1977, after pleading guilty to 19 counts of theft in office.)

DISTANCE & CONFIGURATION: 2.6-mile loop with optional 2.0-mile out-and-back

DIFFICULTY: Easy

SCENERY: Cleveland skyline, historical bridge and buildings, public art

EXPOSURE: Almost completely exposed

TRAFFIC: Fairly busy

TRAIL SURFACE: City sidewalks and paved Towpath Trail

HIKING TIME: Allow at least an hour, more for shopping at the market

DRIVING DISTANCE: 8 miles from I-77/I-480 exchange

ACCESS: 24/7

MAPS: USGS *Cleveland South*

FACILITIES: Emergency phone and restrooms in Merwin's Wharf parking lot and at West Side Market

WHEELCHAIR ACCESS: Overlook to West Side Market, yes; Columbus Road Bridge, partially

CONTACT: Canalway Partnerships (Towpath overlook): 216-520-1825; West Side Market: 216-664-3387, westsidemarket.org

LOCATION: 1203 University Road, Cleveland

The bridge was closed for widening and revitalization work in the early 1980s, and when it reopened it was renamed the Hope-Memorial Bridge. Bob Hope attended the dedication, in part because the new name was a nod to his father, William Henry Hope. The elder Hope was a stonemason who worked on the construction of the Guardians in the 1930s.

Quite often you will see a barge on the river; sometimes foxes and coyotes are also spotted here. Like many areas along the Towpath in this still-industrial city, people and wildlife are finding a strange balance here.

From the overlook, head west on Abbey Avenue to the Tremont script Cleveland sign. One of six such signs in the city, the shiny script signs grew out of a Destination Cleveland promotional campaign launched in 2014.

From the sign, continue west on Abbey Avenue to West 24th Street and turn right. Before heading into the West Side Market, stop to enjoy the Ohio City mural with the prominent suggestion in bright pink: EXPLORE. The mural was created by students in a Center for Arts-Inspired Learning program.

Now, follow the mural's invitation and explore the West Side Market. Use the crosswalk to cross Lorain Avenue to the market's main entrance. During warmer weather, you'll find multiple vendors in outdoor stalls before you even get inside the landmark building.

Construction began on the market in 1908, and when it opened in 1912, it replaced the Pearl Street Market, which was located across the street. At that time, it was one of three public markets in Cleveland; today, the West Side Market is the only one that remains.

The classic clock in the 137-foot-tall tower was designed and manufactured by the Seth Thomas Clock Company. The clock tower and the market's 44-foot-high Guastavino tile vaulted ceiling (see photo on page 31) may vie for the title of most-photographed architecture in Cleveland. Originally, there were 109 stands inside

Cleveland West Side Wanderings

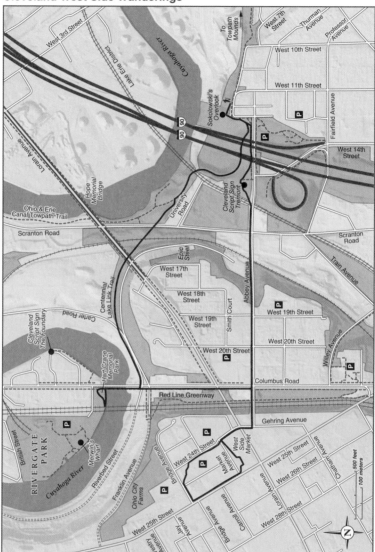

selling meats, dairy products, groceries, and ethnic specialty foods. Produce was sold from curb stands until the outdoor produce aisles were erected a few years later.

Once you've had your fill of the market, exit and cross West 24th Street again, turning left onto Abbey Avenue, then at the next block turn left again onto Columbus Road. Follow it north and downhill to reach two more iconic Cleveland structures: the Cuyahoga Viaduct and the Columbus Road Bridge.

A bridge has been here since the mid-1830s. West Siders apparently weren't too happy about it and tried to take it down in 1836. Three bridges and more than 175 years later, it's pretty certain that this bridge is here to stay. In fact, the current bridge underwent a major renovation in 2014. Walk across this piece of history to explore some newer development on the east side. Continue on Columbus and cross the river to learn about Hart Crane in a small park dedicated to the poet, a native of Garrettsville. You'll also find Merwin's Wharf, the riverside restaurant owned and operated by the Cleveland Metroparks, along with a small skatepark and a kayak launch where paddlers can access the Cuyahoga. It's worth noting that individual boaters are likely to encounter large freighters—and occasional sculling team practice—on this stretch of the river.

Retrace your steps across the river and cross Columbus Road, heading south, to where a sign welcomes you onto the Centennial Lake Link Trail. This trail connects the Cleveland Lakefront Bikeway to the Ohio & Erie Canal Towpath Trail, and it is one of many projects that are successful thanks to the cooperation of multiple government and private organizations. (Thanks, Cleveland!)

The Columbus Street Bridge is raised for the *Nautica Queen*.

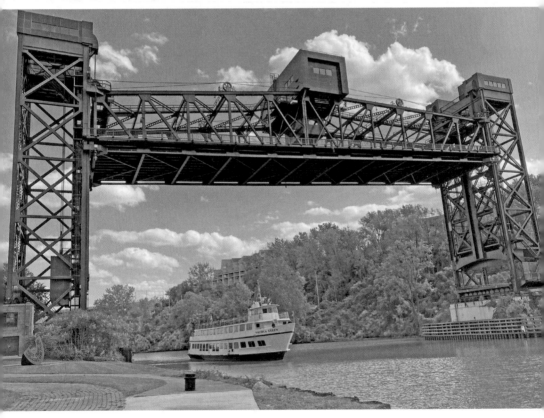

True to form, what goes down must go up, and uphill you'll go, soon joining the Ohio & Erie Canal Towpath, and then, returning to your starting point at Sokolowski's Overlook, possibly with a few treasures from the West Side Market and a new appreciation of the city and its history.

Feel like adding a couple more miles to your total today? Keep walking south on the Towpath. Soon after leaving Sokolowski's Overlook behind, you'll encounter some interesting history from Camp Cleveland, which was the largest of the city's six Civil War training camps. The display includes a replica Civil War–era canon, a structure approximating a barracks, and signage filling in some of the history. More than 15,000 troops trained at the then 35-acre training camp.

Continuing south on the Towpath, you'll soon come to the Roundhouse Overlook, highlighting Cleveland's rail history and fittingly overlooking what remains of Cleveland's roundhouse, where the Midwest Railway Preservation Society works to promote northeast Ohio's railroad history. The volunteer group has periodic open houses and tours. For more information, see midwestrailway.org.

About a mile south of your starting point at Sokolowski's, you'll walk under I-490 and turn right, heading up a short but steep grade. There you'll see the Towpath Mounds, an artistic installation created to mimic some of the resources that built this city: gravel, iron ore, and sand. If you turn around there and return to your starting point, you'll have added about 2.2 miles to your tour of the west side, and hopefully also added a bit to your store of Cleveland knowledge and appreciation.

NEARBY ACTIVITIES

If you haven't been walking in Cleveland for a few years, you might be surprised at just how many hiking and biking trails link the city now. The Towpath and connector trails run for miles in either direction. If time and energy permit, you can head south to enjoy some more history, turning around at the Towpath Mounds or continuing south through the Cuyahoga Valley. Or continue north on the Towpath to the lake. Perhaps most logical now that you've seen the West Side, however, is to visit some downtown Cleveland landmarks (page 36).

• •

TRAILHEAD GPS COORDINATES: N41.48506° W81.69028°

DIRECTIONS Take I-77 N to Exit 161B for I-490 W. Following signs for I-490/I-71/I-90 W, merge onto I-490 W and take Exit 1B for W. 7th Street. Turn right onto W. 7th, then left onto Literary Road, and right again onto Professor Avenue. Continue straight onto Fairfield Avenue, turn right onto W. 11th Street, and then left onto Abbey Avenue. Parking is available at 1351 Abbey Avenue, and also at 1429 Abbey Avenue.

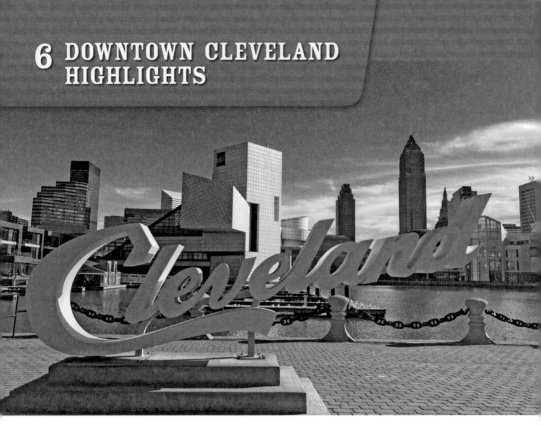

It's OK to act like a tourist here, even if Cleveland is your home!

THIS HIKE IS uniquely Cleveland—and it starts at a historical landmark turned shopping mall. Whether you have out-of-town guests who want to see the north coast, or you haven't been downtown for a while, this mini-tour will put you in a Cleveland state of mind, with stops at stately Public Square, the anything-but-square Rock & Roll Hall of Fame and Museum, the Steamship *William G. Mather,* USS *COD,* and the home fields of the Browns and the Guardians.

DESCRIPTION

From Tower City's lower lot, go inside Tower City Center, up the escalator, and wander north through the shopping center's bright interior. When the Van Sweringen brothers planned the 52-story tower in the 1920s, they worked to sway both public opinion and political decisions to have it constructed to their desired specifications. Built to be the main tower in the Cleveland Union (railroad) Terminal, it was the tallest building outside of New York City from its opening in 1930 until 1967. Today, the tower cum mall-and-office space has far outlived the railroad line for which it was planned (though the Rapid Transit station is still active), yet the building remains a signature flourish on Cleveland's skyline. For the past decade or so, like so many malls, it has struggled to keep tenants and to attract shoppers. What Tower City has

DISTANCE & CONFIGURATION: 3.5-mile loop

DIFFICULTY: Easy

SCENERY: Landmark buildings (both old and new), our Great Lake, public art

EXPOSURE: Mostly exposed

TRAFFIC: Heavy

TRAIL SURFACE: Asphalt

HIKING TIME: 1.5+ hours

DRIVING DISTANCE: 9 miles from I-77/I-480 exchange

ACCESS: 24/7; most shops and all roads and parkways open daily

MAPS: USGS *Cleveland North* and *Cleveland South;* street maps posted at Regional Transit Authority stops and map at Towpath Trailhead

FACILITIES: Public restrooms and water at Tower City Center

WHEELCHAIR ACCESS: Overlook to West Side Market, yes; Columbus Road Bridge, partially

CONTACT: Terminal Tower/Tower City guest services: 216-306-0633; Erie Street Cemetery: 216-348-7217; see "Nearby Activities" on page 40 for additional contact information.

LOCATION: W. Sixth St., Cleveland

that most malls don't is the City of Cleveland—a city that will likely find a new way to use the fabulous building. (Stay tuned.)

Exit Tower City Center onto Euclid Avenue, emerging on Public Square. The Cuyahoga County Soldiers' and Sailors' Monument, built in 1894, sits to your right, on the eastern side of Ontario Street. The monument to the almost 10,000 Cleveland-area soldiers who served in the Civil War is as impressive inside as it is from the outside. Go in to learn from the displays and knowledgeable docents.

Continue north across Public Square to the Old Stone Church. Established on the corner of Ontario Street and Rockwell Avenue in 1834, the church has been rebuilt a couple of times since. The building you see today dates to 1855. If your timing is good (don't interrupt a wedding!), you may be able to go in to appreciate the church's ornate interior. From the church, follow Ontario north, across St. Clair Avenue, continuing to Lakeside Avenue and the Cuyahoga County Courthouse. As you approach, crane your neck to take in six stately sculptures atop the building's facade. Various artists created the marble figures in 1911; each honors an individual for their contributions to English law. Simon de Montfort (1208–1265), for example, sculpted by Herbert Adams, created a parliament with two houses, which became the precursor to the House of Commons. Below, bronze busts of Alexander Hamilton and Thomas Jefferson, both by Karl Bitters, grace opposite sides of the main entrance steps.

With a nod to Hamilton and Jefferson, turn left in front of the courthouse and follow Lakeside Avenue southwest about a block; then turn right onto West Third Street. From the top of the hill, you'll catch a glimpse of Lake Erie. Follow West Third downhill, passing the Port of Cleveland on your left, and wind around the 31-acre site of the Cleveland Browns Stadium. This may be a good place to get some landscaping ideas: The field is heated to extend the growing season of the grass, and the rest of the area features hardy, attractive, low-maintenance plants.

Downtown Cleveland Highlights

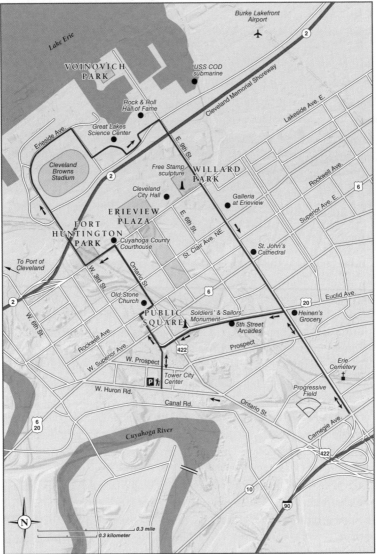

Follow West Third east as it bends right, heading south onto Erieside Avenue; the 171-foot-tall stadium now stands to your right. Several impressive sculptures dot this part of the walk. Turn left onto North Marginal Road, walking east past the Great Lakes Science Center and the Rock & Roll Hall of Fame and Museum. Walk down to Voinivich Park, behind the Science Center, to marvel at the 618-foot-long *William G. Mather* steamship, a piece of history in striking visual contrast to the futuristic Rock & Roll Hall of Fame and Museum, designed by architect I. M. Pei. One of the six script

Cleveland signs is neatly positioned with the skyline as its backdrop. It's a great photo op! You'll also notice signs advertising the *Goodtime III*. When in Cleveland, visiting the *Mather, Goodtime,* and nearby USS *COD* submarine offers a comprehensive education in the city's unbreakable connection to the Great Lakes. Tours on any of the three are enjoyable, but the best choice for hikers is a walk-and-crawl-through tour of the USS *COD*. (See "Nearby Activities" on page 40.)

Continue your walk by turning right, going south on East Ninth Street. You'll cross over busy OH 2, also known as the Shoreway, and begin to head uphill.

Soon you'll see the always-good-for-a-conversation-starter Free Stamp sculpture at Willard Park, on the north side of Lakeside Avenue. And just south of Lakeside, you'll find the Galleria. The beautiful mall, modeled to honor Cleveland's history of interior arcades, has struggled to maintain occupants, but the food court inside the Galleria remains popular with downtown workers and visitors.

Ahead and on your left, at the corner of East Ninth and Superior Avenue, is the Cathedral of Saint John the Evangelist. Originally constructed from 1848 to 1852, the current church is part of a complete rebuilding that took place from 1946 to 1948.

From the church, continue south about 0.2 mile to the eastern corner of East Ninth and Euclid Avenue to find downtown Cleveland's only grocery store. In 2015, Heinen's opened inside the Cleveland Trust Building after restoring many of the historic features, including the oft-photographed rotunda, where shoppers can sit and enjoy wine, ice cream, and other forms of sustenance. Back outside on East Ninth, continue south across Prospect Avenue to reach Bolivar Road. Progressive Field (known for years as Jacobs Field), home of the Cleveland Guardians, is on your right. Take a few minutes here, between Bolivar and Eagle Avenue, to see some of the interesting sculptures designed for the new ballpark in 1994. Once you've peered inside the gates of Progressive Field, return to East Ninth and turn right, heading south again.

On the eastern side of East Ninth (on your left) is Erie Street Cemetery. Created in 1826, when Erie Street was constructed, it was the city's first official cemetery. Many bodies buried at church cemeteries were relocated here when the cemetery opened. And here lies Chief Thunderwater, who advocated on behalf of humane treatment of Indigenous peoples and traditional culture. He participated in *Buffalo Bill's Wild West* show, later ran several businesses, and was a visible public figure until his death in 1950. He's also the most likely inspiration for naming the city's baseball team the Indians (now the Guardians). Today, Thunderwater shares the grounds with his hero, Joc-O-Sot, a chief who fought in the Black Hawk War, as well as myriad early settlers and other folks notable in the city's history.

Of course, now the team is named for the Guardians of Transportation. And if you leave the cemetery and continue south on East Ninth to Carnegie Avenue, you'll face the oft-photographed entrance to Hope Memorial Bridge, which opened in 1932 as the Lorain-Carnegie Bridge. Impressive stone carvings on each entrance represent the progression of transportation. The figures hold various icons: a covered wagon, stagecoach, car, and several trucks. Water transportation isn't represented by the figures, but the bridge itself reminds us—it was built 93 feet above water level to allow for shipping clearance. While fans may need a few seasons to get used to the new name, historically it's a good fit.

Reverse your steps and head north again on East Ninth (or meander through the *Sports Stacks,* taking Huron or Prospect west to East Fourth Street) to reach yet another gorgeous mall: the 5th Street Arcades. More than a century old, the arcades are more fully occupied and see more foot traffic than the Galleria and Tower City, perhaps due to location and because the arcades focus on attracting small, locally owned retail businesses. Go in and marvel at the architecture; you might leave with a handcrafted dog collar or artisan cupcake. The north side of the street is largely occupied by a Hyatt Hotel; its golden stairway makes it a populr wedding spot.

From the 5th Street Arcades, head west on Euclid Avenue to return to Public Square and back to your starting point at Tower City.

NEARBY ACTIVITIES

It's OK to act like a tourist here, even if Cleveland is your hometown. The Soldiers' and Sailors' Monument is open daily, 10 a.m.–5:30 p.m. See soldiersandsailors.com for more information. The USS *COD* is open April–November, but a tour of the World War II submarine is only for the agile. Visitors enter and exit through original hatches and climb ladders inside. For information, call 216-566-8770 or visit usscod .org. Less constraining is the Steamship *William G. Mather,* the 1925 flagship of the Cleveland-Cliffs Iron Company. The floating maritime museum is operated by the Great Lakes Science Center; call 216-694-2000 or visit greatscience.com for information. The *Goodtime III* offers fabulous views of Cleveland's industrial flats and the area's many different bridges. So (ahem) for a *Goodtime,* call 216-861-5110 or visit goodtimeiii.com. For a different view of the skyline, visit Edgewater Park, part of the expanding Lakefront Reservation (page 58).

This walk abuts Cleveland's celebrated theater district and historic Gateway neighborhood. Tours of Cleveland LLC offers walking tours of the city year-round, including Playhouse Square and more. See toursofcleveland.com for more information.

• •

TRAILHEAD GPS COORDINATES: N41.49685° W81.69391°

DIRECTIONS From I-77 N, take Exit 163 (E. Ninth Street). From E. Ninth Street, merge onto E. 14th Street; in 0.2 mile turn right onto US 422/Orange Avenue and follow signs to PUBLIC SQUARE/STADIUM. In 0.7 mile turn left onto W. Huron Road. In 0.3 mile turn right onto W. Sixth Street to park at the Tower City Center parking garage.

7 EUCLID CREEK RESERVATION

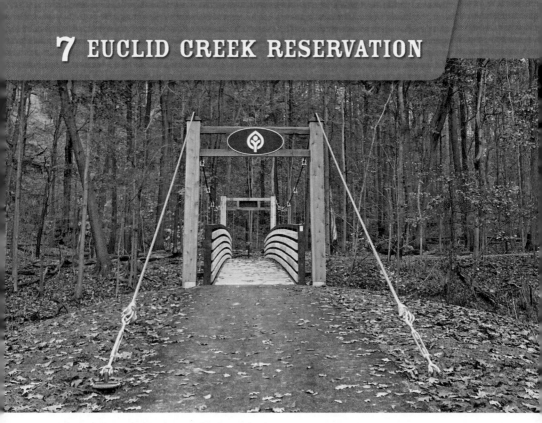

Follow the suspension bridge to reach the overlook.

EUCLID CREEK RESERVATION features hilly, forested trails, multiple picnic areas and basketball courts, and nearly 5 miles of paved All Purpose Trail. The Eastern Ledge Trail takes visitors to a new observation deck 130 feet above the namesake creek, but that's not all this park offers.

DESCRIPTION

Visitors can park at any of the lots along Euclid Creek Parkway to pick up the paved All Purpose Trail (APT) and not be disappointed. Scenery on the shady trail includes stunning sandstone cliffs rising above pretty Euclid Creek. But it's definitely worth the effort to follow the newest path here, Eastern Ledge Trail, to enjoy the view from above.

For this hike, start at Welsh Woods Picnic Area. The Eastern Ledge Trail beckons you to cross the creek on a short wooden suspension bridge, and the trail starts off relatively flat. It's wheelchair accessible to the point where you can see a couple of small but robust waterfalls to your right.

From there, you'll start to climb. The trail is short—just a little over a mile out and back—and smart trail design spreads out the elevation gain, but as you approach the overlook, you will feel the climb. The trail heads north up a short staircase, then soon takes a sharp left to reach the overlook.

DISTANCE & CONFIGURATION: 1.0-mile out-and-back to overlook plus 4.0-mile loop

DIFFICULTY: Moderate with steep sections on both trails

SCENERY: Panoramic overlook, small waterfall, thick woods, sandstone cliffs, excellent spring wildflower display

EXPOSURE: Mostly shaded

TRAFFIC: Moderate–heavy

TRAIL SURFACE: Natural surfaces, mulch, rocks, dirt

HIKING TIME: Allow 2 hours to explore the trails and linger at the overlook.

DRIVING DISTANCE: 19 miles from I-77/I-480 exchange

ACCESS: Daily, 6 a.m.–11 p.m., except where otherwise posted

MAPS: USGS *East Cleveland;* also at park website

FACILITIES: Restrooms at picnic areas

WHEELCHAIR ACCESS: The overlook and nature trails are not, but 4+ miles of the All Purpose Trail is paved and accessible.

CONTACT: Cleveland Metroparks: 440-473-3370, clevelandmetroparks.com/parks/visit/parks/euclid-creek-reservation

LOCATION: Highland Road, Euclid

The trail was designed to drain well, but its natural surface may be somewhat slippery when wet. It's popular with locals and visitors alike, so be courteous and share the (sometimes narrow) path.

When you reach the top, 130 feet above the parkway, don't be surprised if the view takes your breath away. If Euclid Creek is pretty from the trailhead, it'll knock your socks off from here. When you're ready, retrace your steps back down, pausing to appreciate the waterfalls again.

If you're up for more miles, from the Welsh Woods parking area, you can cross the parkway and pick up Squirrel Run Trail, turning right and heading north. Alternatively, when the trails are a little wet, follow the paved APT north a bit—taking in a great view of the observation deck from below—and pick up Squirrel Run at a connection point about half a mile from the Eastern Ledge Trailhead.

Take Squirrel Run north and you'll notice signs indicating you're heading toward Glenridge Loop Trail (marked with a leaf symbol). While you're almost never out of sight—or earshot—of the parkway and busy basketball courts, your scenes are almost entirely wooded, and the trail is mostly shaded thanks to mature maple trees and a few pines along the way. You may also notice that relatively rare Rock Chestnuts grow here as well.

When the trail starts to rise a bit, you're nearing the connection with Glenridge, but it's easy to miss. While it's usually well signed, unfortunately some folks take those signs as souvenirs (please don't). To help hikers navigate, the park system installs "confidence markers" 10–12 feet up on tree trunks, so when in doubt, look up. The intersection of the Squirrel Run and Glenridge Loop Trails looks like a steep root staircase. It's also usually covered in thick leaf litter, making it a little harder to spot.

Follow the "staircase" up to the top of the ridgeline, and for your climb this time, you're rewarded with a view of a residential neighborhood on the corner of Glenridge Road and Grand Boulevard. Never fear, you're still on the trail. Stay on the

Euclid Creek Reservation

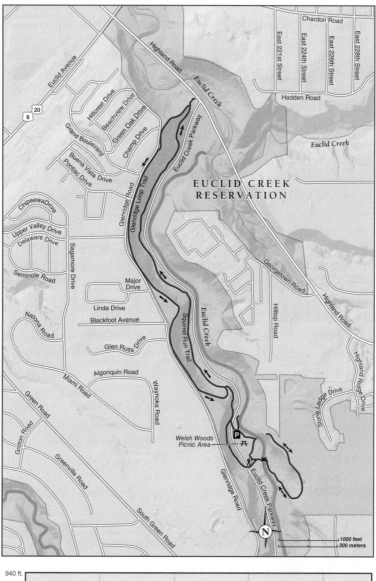

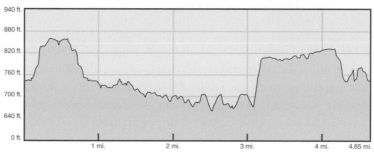

grassy path, where you can see the ravine below and to your left as you continue south. Eventually, within a few blocks' distance—just past Blackfoot Avenue—the trail ducks back into the woods, and you'll descend back into the park to rejoin Squirrel Run Trail. You're likely to see some deer in this quiet area of the park.

Is this the most tranquil and serene hike in Cleveland? No, but this park packs a lot of nice trails into a very natural spot in the middle of an otherwise urban area—something area residents clearly appreciate, based on the number of visitors Euclid Creek Reservation sees.

A small footbridge just north and west of Welsh Woods Picnic Area marks the end of your loop of around 4 miles, plus the 1-mile out-and-back to the overlook, for a total of 5 miles.

Want a little more before you leave? The Upper Highland Trail is a short loop on the west side of the parkway that follows close to Euclid Creek and offers good views of many of the park's spring wildflowers, including jack-in-the-pulpit, red and white trillium, squirrel corn, and bloodroot. (Watch the Metroparks' calendar for naturalist-led wildflower hikes in the spring.)

NEARBY ACTIVITIES

History buffs will want to learn about the ghost town of Bluestone, where Euclid bluestone was quarried in the mid-1800s. The quarry spawned a town of about 400 people, which had its own post office, saloon, and church. While this sandstone was quarried in Euclid, it runs through other parts of the county, including at the northern end of Garfield Park Reservation, where it forms the top of Cataract Falls (page 50).

The reservation is situated among the 'burbs of Euclid, South Euclid, and Richmond Heights, so there are restaurants aplenty nearby. If you're craving more hiking and history, head north about 3 miles to reach Euclid Beach Park. While it's now "just" a swim beach with some short nature trails, it is named for the former amusement park. Euclid Beach is also home to another one of those six script Cleveland signs that dot the city.

• •

TRAILHEAD GPS COORDINATES: N41.54924° W81.52955°

DIRECTIONS From I-77/I-480, follow I-77 N to Exit 163 for I-90 E. Follow I-90 E to Exit 182A and exit onto E. 185th Street. Turn left onto E. 185th and continue on Nottingham Road, then stay straight to continue onto Dille Road, then Highland Road, where you'll turn right into the park. Park at the Welsh Woods Picnic Area to access the trailhead.

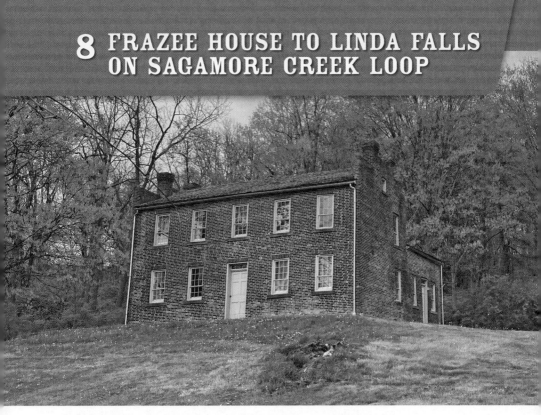

Mehitable and Stephen Frazee made the bricks they used to build their home.

THE TRAIL CROSSES Sagamore Creek—and the county line—several times on its way to Linda Falls and back. Even if the 20-foot waterfall is only a trickle, the trail offers pretty ravine views and a sense of hide-and-seek as it darts into the woods, then reappears on more trafficked routes.

DESCRIPTION

Linda Falls is a beautiful—but hardly dependable—waterfall. (The falls view is best after some steady rains.) However, you can count on the trail here to deliver a fun hike, with several creek crossings as you dart back and forth between Cuyahoga and Summit Counties.

Before detailing the hike, here's the scoop for waterfall seekers: The 30-foot waterfall, which is sometimes called Alexander Falls, is fed by two different tributaries of Sagamore Creek. After the two combine and tumble over the shale ridge atop the ravine, the water eventually makes its way to Tinkers Creek. In spite of the twin sources, the waterfall is at its best only after some fairly steady rain. Then, it's really quite a sight. If you are here for the waterfall—and don't care about shortening your hike—see the "You Have Options" section below for a faster way to reach the falls.

To take the long way to the falls, start your hike from the trailhead on the southwest side of the Frazee House parking lot.

DISTANCE & CONFIGURATION: 4.0-mile loop

DIFFICULTY: Moderate

SCENERY: Creek crossings, ravine, waterfall

EXPOSURE: Mostly shaded

TRAFFIC: Light

TRAIL SURFACE: Primitive trail and paved surfaces, several creek crossings

HIKING TIME: 2 hours

DRIVING DISTANCE: 4 miles from I-77/I-480 exchange

ACCESS: Daily, 6 a.m.–11 p.m. Nature center: Daily, 9:30 a.m.–5 p.m.; closed January 1, Easter, Thanksgiving, and December 25.

MAPS: USGS *Cleveland South;* also at national park visitor centers

FACILITIES: Restrooms at trailhead (no water)

WHEELCHAIR ACCESS: Towpath yes; other trails, no

CONTACT: 216-524-2497, nps.gov/cuva /planyourvisit/the-frazee-house.htm

LOCATION: Canal Road, Valley View

Pause to appreciate the landmark brick home, managed by the National Park Service. In 1812, Mehitable and Stephen Frazee purchased the plot from Moses Cleaveland's land company and built a log cabin there. Between 1812 and 1827, the Frazees worked hard, expanding the farm and selling produce to locals and travelers. Stephen Frazee also sued the state of Ohio for damage to his property brought about by the canal-building process—for which he was awarded $130. The Frazees surely used that sum (and proceeds from the farm) to help finance the stately Federalist-style house that still stands today. However, other than window glass and door hardware, the Frazees didn't pay architects or buy building materials from back East. The couple used bricks made in their own oven and lumber from trees on their property to build the family home, where they lived for 35 years.

Today, if you look carefully, you may be able to see initials and other marks in some of the exposed bricks. Now that you know a bit about the Frazees, find the trailhead (close to Sagamore Road) and head east to traipse through some of their former farmland.

The trail is mostly shaded on the north side of the small stream, and throughout the spring and summer you'll notice a scattering of wildflowers, including mayapples and phlox. This lower portion of the trail is often a little wet.

You'll head east from the trailhead to reach the falls, but not in a straight line. The trail meanders, at first within sight of the creek. You'll probably hear light traffic on Canal Road, but that fades away as you begin to veer north, before making your way back to the creek and crossing it—on this stretch, you're always within sight of the creek.

Shortly after the first creek crossing, you'll see a marker indicating that you're in Cuyahoga Valley National Park. After this crossing, the base of the falls is to your right, just south of the trail. As you continue heading east, you'll soon cross the creek again. It's a little wider here, but only a few inches deep, and you should be able to find rocks to cross on.

Frazee House to Linda Falls on Sagamore Creek Loop

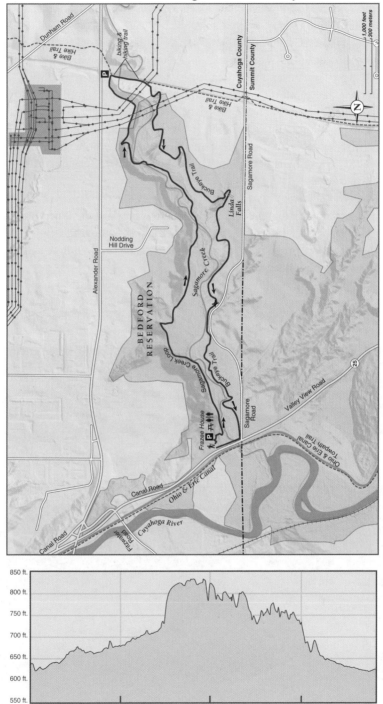

47

After your second crossing, you'll see a diminutive stairstep falls. As the trail climbs on the ravine's edge here, you'll approach private property—heed the signs and stay on the trail. Emerging from the ravine, you'll find yourself walking on a grassy path under power lines. Continue east until you reach the Alexander Road Bike & Hike Trailhead, then turn right onto the paved trail to continue your clockwise hike.

After walking south on the paved Summit County Bike & Hike Trail for about 0.25 mile, you'll see signs to leave the paved trail and turn right. As you head down a short incline to join the Buckeye Trail, you are just 0.8 mile from Linda Falls. Here, high above the creek, you'll see a few small tributaries as you wind along the top of the ravine. The footing is good, but it's uneven in many places due to heavy roots along this portion.

Even if the falls aren't especially impressive on the day you visit, the ravine is lovely, heavily lined with hemlocks and deciduous hardwoods. If the falls are flowing, you'll probably hear them before you see them. As the trail winds around the top of the falls, you'll probably want to take pictures. Be cautious here and know that the leaf litter can be slippery!

There's more than one way to reach Linda Falls.

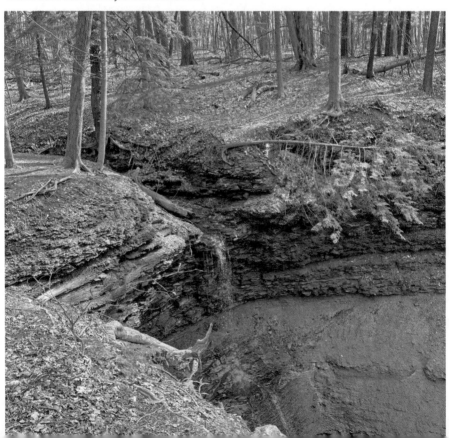

From the falls, continue your clockwise loop by following the Buckeye Trail's blue blazes as the meandering path makes a slow descent. This section is not heavily traveled, so you might wonder if you've lost the trail. Just when you think that, you'll spot a sign that tells you you're doing fine. (Some of those signs will display National Park Service emblems—and at least one or two bear Summit County trail markers. How many different signs did you spot?)

After you cross a footbridge, you'll be trekking parallel to—and just a few yards from—Sagamore Road. Near the corner of Sagamore and Canal Roads, the trail turns right and follows Canal a short distance back to the trailhead.

YOU HAVE OPTIONS

To reach the waterfall in short order, park at the Summit County Bike & Hike Trailhead off Alexander Road, just west of Dunham Road. Take the paved trail south under power lines and watch for a small sign pointing to Linda Falls via the Buckeye Trail. Turn right onto the Buckeye Trail, which meanders left before heading down a slight incline, eventually flattening out and giving you a look at the falls (and the ravine). If you take that route, you'll reach the falls in less than a mile (and skip the creek crossings too). You can turn around at the falls and return to your car for a roughly 1.5-mile out-and-back, or complete the loop from that point.

NEARBY ACTIVITIES

The Ohio & Erie Canal Towpath runs through this park and will take you north all the way to Cleveland's flats, so if you want more miles, you can get them here. Love mountain biking? You may like the trails in Bedford Reservation, just northeast of here. Brecksville Reservation (page 23) is about a 15-minute drive to your west from here.

• •

TRAILHEAD GPS COORDINATES: N41.35237° W81.59257°

DIRECTIONS From I-77/I-480, take Rockside Road west to Canal Road and turn right. Pass Alexander Road and turn left into the Frazee House parking lot on the east side of the canal and roadway.

9 GARFIELD PARK RESERVATION & MILL CREEK FALLS

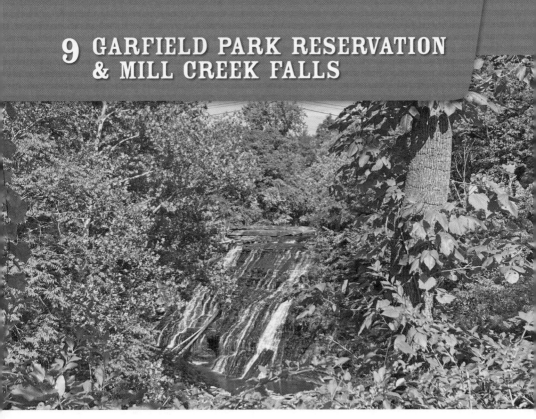

Mill Creek Falls

GARFIELD PARK RESERVATION is rich in both history and features. The paved All Purpose Trail (APT) encircling the park offers two heart-pounding hills for joggers and in-line skaters. Look closely on the nature trails in the middle of the park's 223 acres and you may catch glimpses of the park's former life in remnants of the original stonework and bridges dating back more than a century. At the newly restored boat pond, a new chapter in the park's history is beginning.

DESCRIPTION

Garfield Park was created when the city of Cleveland purchased three farms from the Carter, Dunham, and Rittberger families in 1895. Opened in 1896 under the name Newburgh Park, the property featured tennis, swimming, and boating facilities for many years. It became a part of the Cleveland Metroparks system in 1986. Start your stroll at the historical Trolley Turn Trailhead, immediately south of Garfield Park Boulevard.

The name pays homage to the park's early days, when Cleveland residents could take a trolley to the park that city officials called "an ideal place in the country to get away from it all."

Follow the paved APT counterclockwise as it takes you uphill before looping around and taking you to the east, where you'll see a forest of maples, beeches, and elms on your left. Heading downhill along the southern end of the loop and curving

DISTANCE & CONFIGURATION: 2-mile loop, with option to take interior nature trails and 3-mile out-and-back (or drive) to Mill Creek Falls (also known as Cataract Falls)

DIFFICULTY: Easy, with two steep sections

SCENERY: Natural and historical stonework, waterfall, ravines

EXPOSURE: Mostly shaded

TRAFFIC: Moderate–heavy

TRAIL SURFACE: APT, paved; nature trails, grass and dirt

HIKING TIME: Allow 2 hours to explore the trails, pond, and waterfall at the northern end of the park.

DRIVING DISTANCE: 7 miles from I-77/I-480 exchange

ACCESS: Daily, 6 a.m.–11 p.m., except where otherwise posted

MAPS: USGS *Shaker Heights;* also on park website

FACILITIES: Emergency phones throughout park; water and restrooms at picnic areas

WHEELCHAIR ACCESS: Yes, though steep sections on trail to falls overlook may be difficult

CONTACT: Cleveland Metroparks: 216-206-1000, clevelandmetroparks.com/parks /visit/parks/garfield-park-reservation

LOCATION: Broadway Ave., Garfield Heights

left again, you'll notice the lines of Bedford shale in the ravine walls above Wolf Creek. At this point, Wolf Creek begins to tumble over a series of stone ledges, eventually descending nearly 50 feet. (On the northern side of the park about a mile away, Wolf Creek empties into Mill Creek and eventually into Lake Erie. We'll get to that waterfall soon enough.)

On the eastern side of the park, the APT is actually the old park roadway. As such, it gives wide berth to strollers, bikers, joggers, and skaters. Happily, hikers can find a narrow and slightly higher footpath just inside the loop of the APT that affords better views of the ravine and creek so far below.

Just north of Red Oak Picnic Area, you'll see a stone staircase leading to Iron Springs Trail, one of several entry points along the APT where you can duck off the paved trail and head for the old boating pond, where beautiful stonework remains from the park's early days.

The pond and the stonework were part of a master park plan, developed in the 1890s by landscape architect Ernest Bowditch, who was inspired by Frederick Law Olmsted. The Iron Springs Loop is an unpaved nature trail that intersects with several others nestled inside the larger loop of the APT. While these footpaths can be somewhat damp, especially during the spring, they're worth getting a bit muddy if you want to get a firsthand look at the Olmsted-inspired designs.

Even from the paved APT, you'll be able to appreciate nature's stonework. Once you've finished this loop, but before you return to Trolley Turn, you can follow the APT as it veers north past a baseball field, cuts through a residential block, and continues for almost 1.5 miles before reaching Mill Creek Falls Overlook. It's a steep and hilly stretch of trail, with a big reward: the nearly 50-foot-tall waterfall, also known as Cataract Falls, is the tallest waterfall in Cuyahoga County. A sign at the top of the falls explains that one of the layers of rock that forms the base of the falls is Euclid bluestone, which was quarried north of here, in what is now Euclid Creek Reservation (page 41).

Garfield Park Reservation & Mill Creek Falls

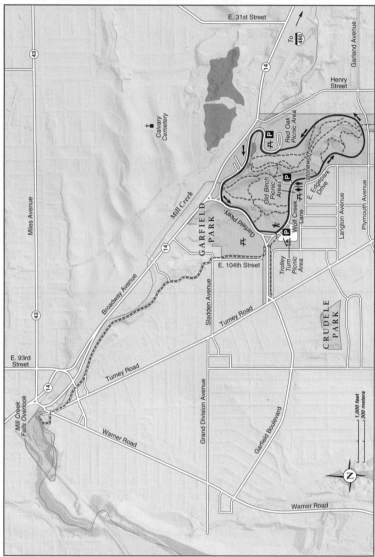

When the city was known as Cleaveland, in the late 1700s and early 1800s, the water powered a mill, and the industry it spawned fueled the area's continued growth. By the falls overlook, you'll find interpretive signage and several decorative ironworks that pay homage to the history of the humans and machines that built this city.

The spur to the falls is an out-and-back, and while it's a good path to give your legs some exercise, the scenery isn't exciting until you get to the falls. So my advice, if you want to see the park and the falls, is to drive to the falls overlook and save the walking for the rest of the reservation. Sometime after 2024, you'll be able to explore a lot more miles around here, on foot or by bike, as several connector trails are planned. One will connect the existing Morgana Run Trail to the Mill Creek Falls area of Garfield Park Reservation and north and west into Slavic Village.

However you decide to explore Garfield Park Reservation, you're bound to learn something about the city and its history, flora, and fauna.

NEARBY ACTIVITIES

Be sure to visit the park website for information about the new boathouse, boat rentals, and education programs, as well as history and wildflower walks at this storied park. For more information about Mill Creek Falls and the surrounding area, contact Slavic Village Historical Society at slavicvillagehistory.org. For more hiking—and history—head to CanalWay Center, just about 3.5 miles west of the falls parking area (page 81).

• •

TRAILHEAD GPS COORDINATES: N41.42996° W81.60997°

DIRECTIONS From I-77/I-480, follow I-480 E and take Exit 23 (OH 14/Broadway Avenue). Turn right and go north on Broadway for about a mile, turning left onto Garfield Park Boulevard just north of the Henry Street intersection. To reach the trailhead, follow Garfield Park Boulevard west and veer left onto Wolf Creek Lane to the Trolley Turn picnic area, approximately 1 mile west of the Broadway Avenue park entrance.

Wrought iron figures grace the walkway at Mill Creek Falls.

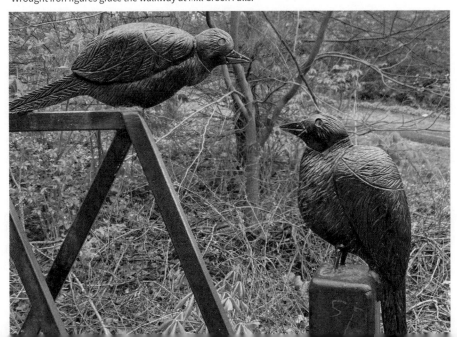

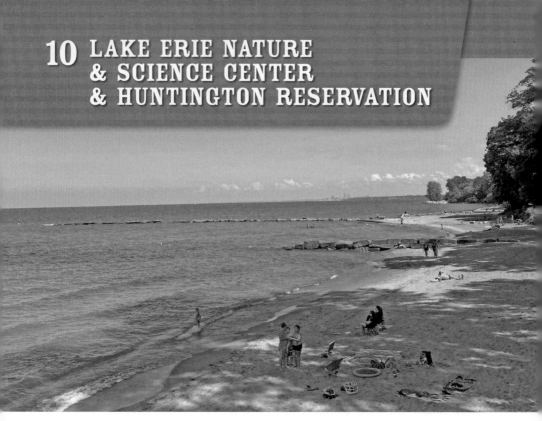

10 LAKE ERIE NATURE & SCIENCE CENTER & HUNTINGTON RESERVATION

The beach is a big draw on clear days; the nearby nature center is a worthy indoor attraction.

CRAWL THROUGH A hollow log, visit the stars, and hit the beach—all in the span of about a mile.

DESCRIPTION

Huntington is one of the oldest Cleveland Metroparks reservations. It gets its name from English immigrant John Huntington, who purchased the land in 1880. He built a distinctive tower used to pump water from Lake Erie to irrigate his grape fields. The water tower still stands; today, it is a concession stand (open seasonally) offering ice cream, sandwiches and other fare, much appreciated by picnickers and beachgoers. A plaque on the side of the concession stand relates the park's history and illustrates some of the improvements made by Cleveland Metroparks after purchasing the land in 1927.

Rather than starting at the lakeshore for this trek, you'll begin on a different property to the south: Lake Erie Nature & Science Center. Brimming with life, from amphibians and insects to birds and mammals, LENSC is a fabulous indoor/outdoor destination for all ages. Start inside, where nimble visitors can crawl through a 15-foot-long hollow tree that lies just inside the center's front door—it's a 200-year-old hickory, but a well-varnished one, so it's likely to last a long time.

DISTANCE & CONFIGURATION: 1.9-mile balloon

DIFFICULTY: Easy

SCENERY: A little creek, a Great Lake, science on display at the nature center

EXPOSURE: Mostly exposed

TRAFFIC: Path lightly traveled; beach very busy during summer

TRAIL SURFACE: Asphalt, dirt, and sand trails

HIKING TIME: 50 minutes, plus playtime at the beach and Lake Erie Nature & Science Center

DRIVING DISTANCE: 20 miles from I-77/I-480 exchange

ACCESS: Daily, 6 a.m.–11 p.m., except where otherwise posted; Lake Erie Nature & Science

Center: Daily, 10 a.m.–5 p.m. No pets allowed on beach.

MAPS: USGS *North Olmsted;* also at Lake Erie Nature & Science Center and park website

FACILITIES: Restrooms and water inside Lake Erie Nature & Science Center, on both sides of Lake Road, and at the beach

WHEELCHAIR ACCESS: Lake Erie Nature & Science Center, yes; trails, no

CONTACT: Cleveland Metroparks: 440-331-8111, clevelandmetroparks.com/parks/visit/parks /huntington-reservation; Lake Erie Nature & Science Center: 440-871-2900, lensc.org; swimming conditions: 216-635-3383

LOCATION: Wolf Road, Bay Village

The center also houses the Walter R. Schuele Planetarium, which offers regular presentations on weekends. Outside, the center's lovely "backyard" is great for bird-watching and relaxing. It's also where the center houses some of the birds of prey being rehabilitated by the center's employees and volunteers.

Once you've soaked up the sights inside and around the nature center, cross the street to the east and turn left, heading north on the All Purpose Trail to the lake. You'll follow the paved trail past the Wolf Picnic Area (at about 0.1 mile), down a slight incline, and across a small bridge over Porter Creek. You'll share the way with light car traffic, so stay on the trail as you make your way back up the hill.

Just over the bridge, there's a lovely view of Porter Creek as it heads east before making its final turn to drop into Lake Erie. You'll lose sight of the creek as you climb up a small hill that serves as a sledding hill when conditions are right. There, on your left (western side of the trail), you'll see the BAYarts building for visual and performing arts. (See the website under "Nearby Activities" for exhibitions and class info.)

You can see the lake from here, but don't cross busy Lake Road to get there. Instead, turn right and follow signs to the pedestrian tunnel underpass. (Restrooms and emergency phones are located near the tunnel's entrance.)

Emerging on the north side of the park, you'll find a shady playground area, a large picnic shelter, and the distinctive tower. Next to the tower (which houses a seasonal concession shop), you'll spot a steep set of stairs—about 50 of them—that lead down to the shore.

Before heading to the beach, stretch your legs on the mostly shaded, paved trail that heads west about 0.25 mile. Situated above the shore, it offers nice, breezy views

55

Lake Erie Nature & Science Center & Huntington Reservation

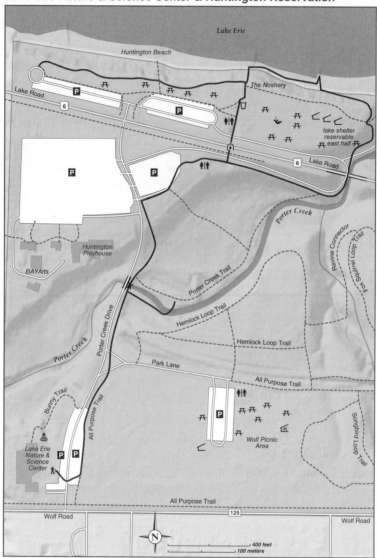

of Lake Erie. Turn around at the park's edge, retrace your steps to the concession stand and staircase, and head down those stairs to walk on the beach.

During the too-short summer season, Huntington Beach is often crowded. But on an early-spring or late-fall day, you may find solitude along the breakwater. On such days, the gulls are the only ones playing in the waves. And if you dare to breach the shore during one of Cleveland's extended cold snaps, you might think that you could walk across the lake to Canada. (Note to adventurous types: Don't try it.)

Walk on the sand following the shore east about 0.2 mile, where you'll find another set of stairs that lead up to the picnic shelter. If you continue walking east on the beach, however, you'll soon find a path that curves to the right and stays low. This narrow path along Porter Creek takes you south through the underpass—not the tunnel—under Lake Road.

Follow the dirt path along the side of the road as it curves west, toward the sledding hill and back to the All Purpose Trail. From here, turn left to retrace your steps back to the LENSC parking area.

Want to add a couple more miles to your outing? Cahoon Park, just east of the beach entrance on US 6 (Lake Road), has a 0.5-mile exercise trail and lovely gardens. And, on the south side of Lake Road, three interconnecting loop trails just east of Porter Creek wind through the wooded ravine, offering about 2 miles of nature trails to explore.

NEARBY ACTIVITIES

Huntington Beach has lifeguards on duty during the main swimming season, and fishing is permitted year-round.

Catch a star-studded show at the Walter R. Schuele Planetarium at Lake Erie Nature & Science Center; call 440-871-2900 or visit lensc.org for a schedule or for information about other programs at the center.

Huntington Playhouse (28601 Lake Road), a part of BAYarts, offers visual and performing arts and art classes throughout the year. For more information, call 440-871-6543 or visit bayarts.net.

• •

TRAILHEAD GPS COORDINATES: N41.48598° W81.93755°

DIRECTIONS Take I-480 W to Exit 7 (Clague Road to Westlake/Fairview Park). Turn right onto Clague Road. In 4.1 miles, turn left onto Wolf Road. In 2.9 miles, you'll see the entrance to Lake Erie Nature & Science Center, at the intersection with Porter Creek Drive.

This tunnel leads to Huntington Beach.

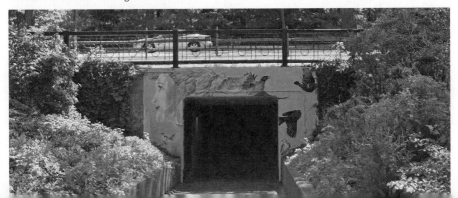

11 LAKEFRONT RESERVATION:
Edgewater Park

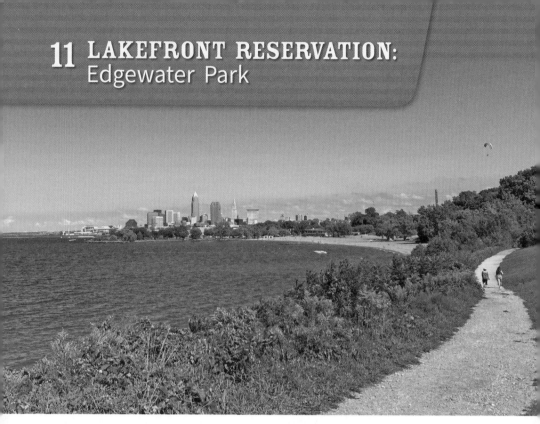

Edgewater boasts skyline views, a popular beach, and what is possibly Cleveland's coolest playground.

ICONIC EDGEWATER PARK is thriving under the management of Cleveland Metroparks. Locals and city visitors alike come to hike along the Lake Erie shore, fish from the pier, and enjoy the 900-foot-long public swimming beach here. The beach still provides one of the best places to watch Cleveland's annual Independence Day fireworks display.

DESCRIPTION

Edgewater Park, known for its swimming beach, is a popular site year-round with dog walkers, trail runners, and families, so why not hikers?

Start at the western edge of the park, at the upper parking area, noted—appropriately—as a scenic overlook on some maps. It's impossible to miss the shiny script Cleveland sign on the eastern edge of the parking lot. From there, turn around to appreciate the oversize statue of German composer Richard Wagner. The statue was a gift to the city from some of Cleveland's many German immigrants. From the base to the top of his hat, Wagner stands 18 feet tall, and he's been looking out over the lake and the skyline since 1911. If only he could talk. . . .

From the upper parking area, make your way to the lower parking area on the grassy path, and then take the short staircase leading to Perkins Beach, where there's

DISTANCE & CONFIGURATION: 1.8-mile figure eight with shorter and longer options

DIFFICULTY: Easy, with one hill and some optional slogging through sand

SCENERY: Lake Erie beach, Cleveland skyline, historical markers, and bird-watching opportunities

EXPOSURE: Mostly exposed

TRAFFIC: Moderately heavy

TRAIL SURFACE: Paved, beach, and dirt trails

HIKING TIME: 1+ hour

DRIVING DISTANCE: 14 miles from I-77/I-480 exchange

ACCESS: Daily, 6 a.m.–11 p.m.

MAPS: USGS *Cleveland South;* also at park website

FACILITIES: Restrooms and water at beach house, concessions and changing area open seasonally

WHEELCHAIR ACCESS: Partially; the paved trail is accessible.

CONTACT: Cleveland Metroparks: 216-635-3200, clevelandmetroparks.com/parks/visit/parks /lakefront-reservation/edgewater-park

LOCATION: West Blvd., Cleveland

rarely a crowd but always a lovely lake view. After enjoying the relative quiet amid driftwood, rocks, and shells, head to the northeast corner of the parking lot and pick up the gravel path that goes down to the dog park. This is the shadiest portion of the trail and park; remember, you're on your way to the beach!

As you continue east on the paved path, several unmarked paths on your left lead down to a sandy dirt trail about 25 feet closer to the lake, and as many feet below you. Stay on the main gravel path heading toward the dog park. On the wide crushed limestone and gravel path you will have a good view of the lake between the trees. Soon, you have a choice between taking the path down to the dog beach and the rest of the beach area or taking the stairs up to West upper level parking. Note that the dog beach is a designated area for dogs, but it is not fenced, so if anyone in your party is uncomfortable around dogs, take the stairs and continue your loop on the paved All Purpose Trail. Otherwise, continue following the signs to the dog beach, where humans are also welcome.

As you continue east, you have your choice of using the sand that's hard packed by the shore or the looser stuff farther from the water—either way, you are heading toward the beach house and concession area. Once you reach the beach house, you'll be able to see the fishing pier, which is usually crowded with anglers and photographers. If you want another panorama of the city from the lake, venture over about 0.1 mile northeast of the beach and concession area.

To follow the hike described here, when you reach the beach house, veer to the right where the paved All Purpose Trail splits and continue east on the paved trail to the main parking area. The grassy fields here host numerous sports team practices, intramurals, and informal games throughout the year, as well as running events. Other times, the grass is dotted with picnic blankets, kids, and dogs playing catch.

Follow the paved trail as it continues east and loops back heading west, past the beach pavilion, and then up a short but steep hill to Upper Edgewater Shelter. The

Lakefront Reservation: Edgewater Park

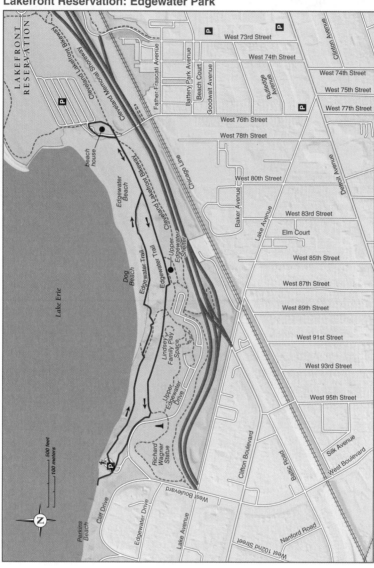

paved trail levels out by a large, Spanish-style reservable pavilion (contact Cleveland Metroparks for information). Here, in the shadier, upper portion of Edgewater, you'll find a fountain honoring Conrad Mizer, who hosted free public concerts at Edgewater and helped support the Cleveland Symphony Orchestra. Continuing west on the path, you'll reach the Lindsey Family Play Space, truly one of the coolest playgrounds in northeast Ohio.

Just past the play area, you'll find yourself back at the Cleveland sign where you began. Wave to Mr. Wagner, assuring him that you'll be back, because how could you not return to a place like this?

NEARBY ACTIVITIES

Downtown Cleveland beckons! (See page 36.) But it may be hard to leave Edgewater—during the summer season, kayaks and stand-up paddle boards can be rented on the beach. Also, during the warmer months, you're likely to find live music and food trucks at the edge of the beach. The park also hosts a variety of naturalist programs year-round. Visit the park website for a calendar of events. Whiskey Island and Wendy Park, situated between Edgewater and downtown Cleveland, are rapidly becoming destinations in their own right. Cleveland Lakefront Bikeway also zips by Edgewater on its 17-mile-long span. The bikeway connects to several other trails. Learn more about that at planning.clevelandohio.gov/bike/lakefront.html.

• •

TRAILHEAD GPS COORDINATES: N41.48856° W81.75085°

DIRECTIONS Take I-77 N to Exit 163 (I-90 E). Follow signs to Erie, PA, and merge onto I-90 E. Take Exit 174B to merge onto OH 2 W, toward Lakewood, which becomes US 20 W/US 6 W. In 4.8 miles, take the West Boulevard exit, and turn right, then left into the Lakefront Reservation: Edgewater Park lot.

There's more to Edgewater than the beach!

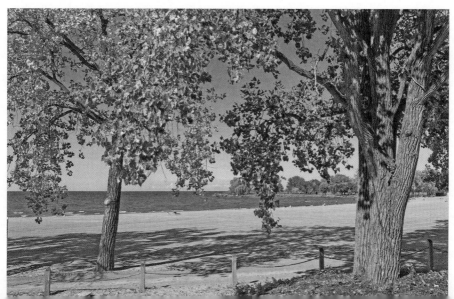

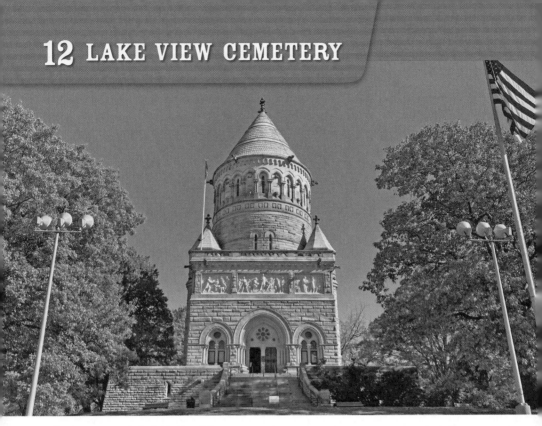

Lake View Cemetery's Garfield Memorial

A CEMETERY IS an unlikely tourist attraction, but Lake View's history and incredible beauty draw thousands each year. Lake View was designed after the garden cemeteries of Victorian England and France. Adding to its European appeal, it lies next to Little Italy, one of Cleveland's tastiest neighborhoods.

DESCRIPTION

Is it appropriate to hike through a cemetery? Lake View Cemetery encourages visitors—tourists, even—and throughout the year offers tours highlighting its unique architecture, geology, history, and horticulture. If you choose to stroll through sans guide, call or stop in at the office for the day's burial schedule, so you won't walk near a burial or where a family is mourning. So how important is the timing of your exploration here? That depends on your interests.

You can walk around the cemetery grounds any time of the year, but it's ideal to plan a visit when the Garfield Monument and the equally impressive Wade Chapel are both open. (Admission to both buildings is free; donations are accepted to be used for building maintenance.) It's also worth noting that the blooms on Daffodil Hill bring throngs of visitors each spring, so if you don't like crowds, plan to come another time.

DISTANCE & CONFIGURATION: 3-mile out-and-back with shorter and longer options

DIFFICULTY: Easy

SCENERY: Splendid architecture, views of downtown and Lake Erie

EXPOSURE: Half exposed

TRAFFIC: Moderate

TRAIL SURFACE: Dirt, grass, stone steps, and paved walkways

HIKING TIME: 1–3 hours, depending on interest and stamina

DRIVING DISTANCE: 13 miles from I-77/I-480 exchange

ACCESS: Cemetery: November–March: Daily, 7:30 a.m.–5:30 p.m. April–October: Daily, 7:30 a.m.–7:30 p.m. Do not walk in areas where there will be a burial, and be respectful of families who are burying or mourning a loved one.

MAPS: USGS *East Cleveland;* also at Euclid Avenue cemetery office

FACILITIES: Restrooms in the cemetery office, Community Mausoleum, and the Garfield Monument

WHEELCHAIR ACCESS: No

CONTACT: Call for burial schedule before visiting; 216-421-2665, lakeviewcemetery.com

LOCATION: Euclid Ave., Cleveland

Regardless of when you visit, there's plenty to see in this stunning "outdoor museum." Included in this description—but not in the total mileage—are some optional out-and-backs to a few notable gravesites.

Established in 1869, the cemetery is a Cleveland landmark. President James A. Garfield and industrialist John D. Rockefeller are both buried here, along with numerous other famous folks with Cleveland ties. A tour booklet available in the cemetery administration office identifies the gravesites of members of The Early Settlers Association of the Western Reserve Hall of Fame who are buried at Lake View. This description highlights only a few of the notable figures buried here and offers a basic introduction to some of Lake View's treasures. When you visit, you will discover many more.

Begin at the James A. Garfield Monument, where you'll enjoy views of Cleveland and the lake. The exterior of the monument is made of Berea sandstone. Constructed between 1885 and 1890, the building features five 7-foot-tall terra-cotta sculpted panels varying in length from 12 to 20 feet. The panels depict important stages of Garfield's life, including teaching, his service during the Civil War, and taking the presidential oath. The bas-relief panels feature the likenesses of more than 100 life-size people. Walk around outside to appreciate the artistry; then, if you can, go inside.

The monument is open April through mid-November. Inside you'll find stained glass windows and windowlike panels, representing the 13 original colonies, Ohio, and war and peace. Also inside, in Memorial Hall, a sculpture of the former president stands watch in the middle of the monument; his and his wife's crypts are on the lower level.

From the Garfield Monument, head southeast on Garfield Road toward the Mayfield Gate. Turn left onto Quarry Road. Along the way, you'll pass beautiful threadleaf Japanese maples on your left and the Mayfield Gate and mausoleum on your right. Stop in for a unique and lovely commemoration of the lives of other less-famous, but quite impressive, Clevelanders.

Lake View Cemetery

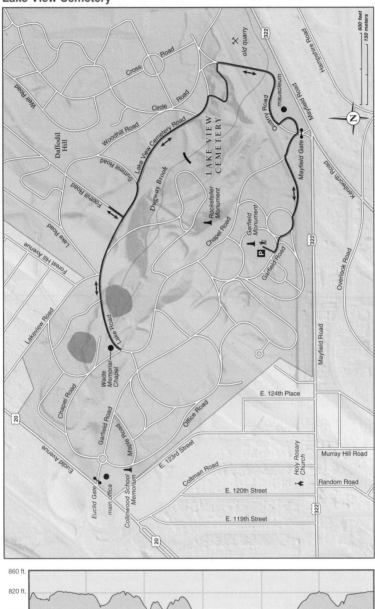

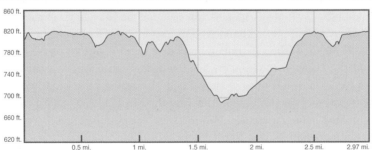

If you opt to explore section 10, to the north, you'll find the obelisk marker for John D. Rockefeller's gravesite. John D. Rockefeller, founder of Standard Oil Company, is laid to rest here along with other notable Clevelanders, including Dr. Harvey Williams Cushing, who pioneered brain surgery techniques, and John Hay, President Abraham Lincoln's personal secretary during the Civil War and Secretary of State to President William McKinley.

After crossing little Dugway Brook, you'll notice an old dirt road, closed to the public. It was once used for traffic coming and going from the quarry. In operation from the 1870s through the mid-1930s, the quarry never wasted its contents. Dust from the quarry was used as the foundation for many of the headstones placed here; rocks from this quarry were incorporated in many of the cemetery's buildings and also form the massive cemetery wall that stretches west from the Mayfield Gate to East 123rd Street.

Continuing, you'll soon reach a traffic island splitting the road. Follow the road left and walk toward section 30, where the Van Sweringen brothers are buried. The Van Sweringens built Cleveland's Rapid transit system and Terminal Tower. You can cross Circle Road to visit their gravesite (no. 117), or continue bearing left to pick up Lake View Cemetery Road, passing section 35 on your right and the ravine on your left. Look left from the edge of the grass, where the Lake View Flood Control Reservoir stands 60 feet high and 500 feet across. It can impound 80 million gallons of water. When it was built in 1978, it was the largest concrete-poured dam east of the Mississippi River. That it only has to hold back mild-mannered Dugway Brook seems odd, but suffice it to say that the waters here are well under control.

Proceed northwest along Lake View Cemetery Road, meandering uphill toward Woodhill and Summit Roads to get a better view of the cemetery's layout and, to the north, a glimpse of Daffodil Hill. Also off Woodhill, you'll find the grave marker for Cleveland Indians' (now Guardians) shortstop Ray Chapman, who died after being hit by a baseball during a game with the New York Yankees. Chapman is one of several famous MLB figures buried here.

Between Summit and Foothill Roads, in section 3, you'll find the monument of Jeptha Wade. Wade was a cofounder of Western Union Telegraph Company and first president of the Lake View Cemetery Association. Just east of his monument is Daffodil Hill. Each spring, more than 100,000 daffodil blooms burst with color.

Return to Lake View Cemetery Road and head northwest until the road intersects Lakeview Road. Turn left to pass between two scenic ponds. Just northeast of the first pond, on the south side of Lake Road, is a memorial to Eliot Ness. After helping bring down Al Capone in Chicago, Ness served as Cleveland's safety director from 1935 to 1942. He modernized the police department, developed an emergency medical patrol, and improved Cleveland's traffic fatality record from second worst in the nation to receiving the National Safety Council's Safest City Award. When Ness died in 1957, he was cremated, and his ashes remained with his family for 40 years. In

1997, he was honored with a memorial service and this memorial stone. The grassy area by the lakes is graced with several pieces of sculpture, creating a good spot to sit, sip some water, and enjoy your surroundings.

When you're ready to continue on Lake Road, turn right at the intersection to follow Chapel Road as it goes north. On your right is Jeptha Wade Memorial Chapel. Stop to admire the windows, designed by Louis Comfort Tiffany. When the chapel is open, go in to appreciate the interior, and to find a docent who can answer questions about the building's design and construction. Also nearby, in section 5-C, are the remains of Carl Burton Stokes, the first African American mayor of a major US city.

For a short excursion, you can head north on Chapel Road, crossing Garfield Road, and then follow Maple Road past the cemetery office. If you stay on Maple as it bears left and circles around section 26, in section 25 you'll find the Collinwood school fire memorial.

When an elementary school in Collinwood caught fire in 1908, 172 students, 2 teachers, and a rescuer died inside. The tragedy caused numerous school inspections nationwide and spurred new, stricter building codes. The lessons of 1908, sadly, are still relevant today. (*Note:* This excursion is optional and is not part of the hike as described or mapped.)

Returning on Lake Road, you'll see Alan Freed's jukebox headstone, which is fitting, as Freed is credited with coining the phrase "Rock and Roll" and was posthumously inducted as a charter member of the Rock & Roll Hall of Fame in 1986. As you continue back along Lake View Cemetery Road, you should also spot the famous Haserot angel. The Haserot family made their fortune in canned food; the iconic sculpture, erected in 1924, holds an inverted torch symbolizing a life extinguished. Heading back on Quarry Road toward the Garfield Monument and the Mayfield Gate, you'll appreciate the intricate gardening work and incredible planning for which Lake View is known. In the late 1800s, many Italian stonecutters and gardeners migrated to Cleveland and helped construct the cemetery.

The neighborhood immediately east of the cemetery, Little Italy, reflects more of the immigrants' heritage, and it's a wonderful place to stop for a hearty meal or delicious pastry.

NEARBY ACTIVITIES

Lake View offers an almost-constant schedule of tours and special events; check the website or call the office for details. For more information about happenings in Cleveland's Little Italy neighborhood, visit littleitalycle.com. Looking for an indoor/outdoor activity nearby? You're just about 3 miles from The Nature Center at Shaker Lakes (page 72), and you're even closer to Cleveland's many museums on Wade Oval (named, of course, for Jeptha Wade) in University Circle. Whichever direction you go from here, you're likely to go with a new appreciation of Cleveland history.

• •

TRAILHEAD GPS COORDINATES: N41.50991° W81.59158°

DIRECTIONS From I-77 N, take Exit 163 (I-90 E). Follow I-90 E to Exit 173B (Chester Avenue). Turn right onto Chester, going about 3 miles before turning left onto Euclid Avenue. In 1 mile, the Lake View Cemetery entrance is on the right, at 12316 Euclid Avenue. Continue southeast on Garfield Road about 0.5 mile to reach parking for the Garfield Monument.

The Haserot Angel at Lake View Cemetery

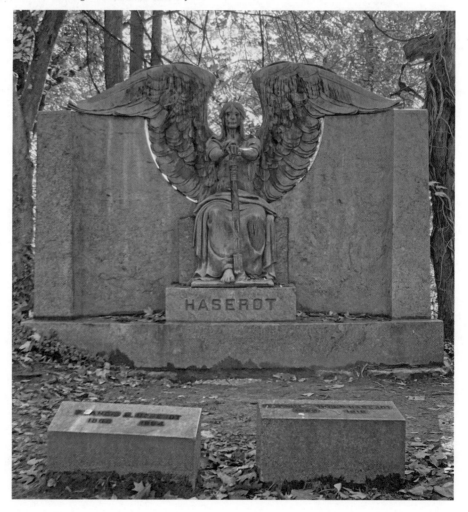

13 LAKEWOOD PARK PROMENADE & SOLSTICE STEPS

It's hard to beat the view from Lakewood's Solstice Steps.

PROMENADE HERE, THEN perch on the Solstice Steps to really bask in the lake view. City parks don't get much better than this.

DESCRIPTION

From the road, Lakewood Park doesn't look like a hiking destination. The first sights you'll see are basketball courts, a city pool, a stage for outdoor concerts, and a few citified wildflower plantings. Keep an open mind; park your car where you can and plan to stay a while—there's a lot to see.

From the large playground to sand volleyball courts, the park is dotted with benches, and from each one, you have an expansive view of the lake. If you're just here for a sunset or to enjoy a brown-bag lunch with a view, you can take one of the paved paths from the parking lot to the Solstice Steps. Most of those paths are shaded by mature pin oaks and other deciduous trees, and in just a few hundred feet, you'll reach the massive concrete steps.

For this hike, however, we start at the southeastern end of the parking lot and follow the brick walkway to the small stage on the park's east side, which was a gift from the Rotary Club of Lakewood and Rocky River. The area around the stage is adorned with native wildflower plantings; at the end of the summer, monarchs can be seen here preparing for their migration.

DISTANCE & CONFIGURATION: 1.2-mile loop with options for more miles

DIFFICULTY: Easy

SCENERY: Lake Erie and Cleveland skyline views, Solstice Steps, gardens

EXPOSURE: Mostly exposed

TRAFFIC: Often busy

TRAIL SURFACE: Sidewalks, bricks, and asphalt

DRIVING DISTANCE: 14 miles from I-77/I-480 exchange

HIKING TIME: 1 hour, plus time to linger at the lake or playground

ACCESS: Daily, 6 a.m.–11 p.m.

MAPS: USGS *Lakewood, OH*

FACILITIES: Restrooms and water

WHEELCHAIR ACCESS: Sidewalks along top of trail, yes; Solstice Steps and lookout point, no

CONTACT: 216-529-5697, lakewoodoh.gov/accordions/lakewood-park

LOCATION: Lake Ave., Lakewood

Continue east a bit, following the paved path as it curls left and north toward the lake, ducking in and out of the shade, and nodding to other visitors. It's a busy park most any day, throughout the year. Just past the sand volleyball court, the path veers slightly to the right, leading to a gazebo and down to the lakeside path—more formally know as the Lakefront Promenade.

Promenade is a noun and a verb. To promenade is to take a "leisurely public walk, ride, or drive so as to meet or be seen by others." A promenade is a "public walk, typically one along a waterfront at a resort." Lakewood Park offers a beautiful example of both forms of the word. The Solstice Steps on the park's northwest corner are a delightful bonus, providing the perfect place to bask in the rays bouncing off Lake Erie or take in a sunset.

Follow the bricked path down to the lookout point. Facing east, the Cleveland skyline looks small, especially compared to the expanse of the lake. When you've had a good look, turn and follow the Promenade west as leisurely or aerobically as you like.

The brick path offers a very civilized way to enjoy the lake—no chance of sand between your toes here—with an almost constant, usually gentle, breeze. You'll promenade less than 0.25 mile before you'll walk across a beautiful brick compass and, looking up, spot the Solstice Steps. From this vantage point, they tower above the path (and you).

The Promenade leads uphill, turning slightly to the left again (south, here); at the top, you'll see the park's baseball field, picnic shelter, and large playground. Follow the path as it takes a sharp turn left, toward the top of the Solstice Steps.

A few benches dot the top of Solstice Steps, and you can take a staircase with a railing down to the bottom. Enjoy the view from here, however, for as long as you like. On a warm sunny day, you'll almost certainly be in the company of other walkers, sunbathers, yogis, and lunch-breakers.

After exploring paths at Lakewood Park, there's still a bit more to take in, including a historical footnote and lovely children's peace monument. A historical marker at the Woman's Club Pavilion notes that Lakewood women were able to vote in

Lakewood Park Promenade & Solstice Steps

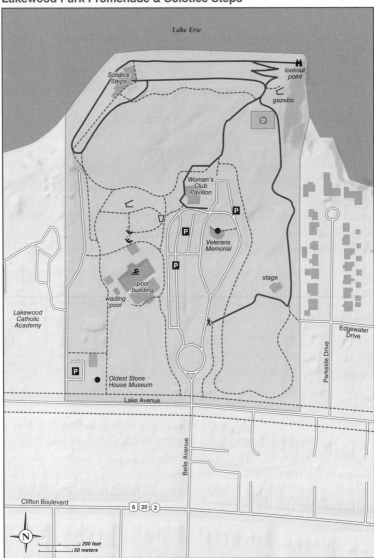

local elections in 1917, 3 years before women got the vote (nationwide) in 1920. The Lakewood League of Women Voters was chartered in 1922 and is still active today.

Now that you've visited the park, consider this: The stunning Solstice Steps sit on what was once a garbage dump and construction landfill during most of the 1900s. With that perspective, you might be interested in learning more about Lakewood's history—and again, this park has you covered: The Oldest Stone House Museum sits on the southwestern edge of the property. Built in 1834 and moved to this location in 1952, the structure has housed a barbershop, doctor's office, shoe repair shop, and upholstery business. Tours are offered seasonally and by appointment.

Like that house, Lakewood Park continues to evolve. The gazebo and Promenade were dedicated in 2006, the steps in 2015, and, in 2024, the city was finalizing plans for a pier and "cobble beach" to offer additional lakefront access. You can visit the city's website for the latest park management plans. To learn more about the Oldest Stone House, visit lakewoodhistory.org.

NEARBY ACTIVITIES

If you want to feel the sand between your toes, don't despair—the beach is close by. Edgewater Park lies just about 4 miles to the east, and Huntington Beach is about 7 miles due west. Cyclists who want to keep moving from here can take Edgewater Drive east to connect to the Cleveland Lakefront Bikeway, or head south to Rocky River Reservation's miles of paved All Purpose Trail.

• •

TRAILHEAD GPS COORDINATES: N41.49413° W81.79658°

DIRECTIONS Take I-480 W to Exit 17A to I-176 N and then I-90 W. Take Exit 165B to Bunts Road, following Clifton Boulevard before turning right onto Belle Avenue, which leads you into the parking lot.

The children's peace monument at Lakewood Park

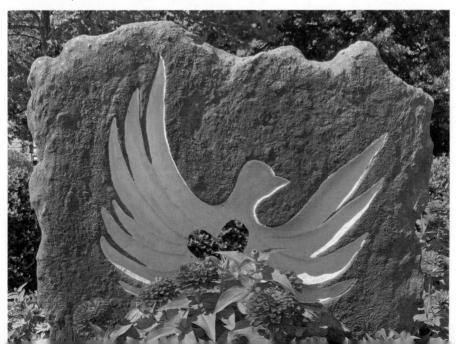

14 THE NATURE CENTER AT SHAKER LAKES

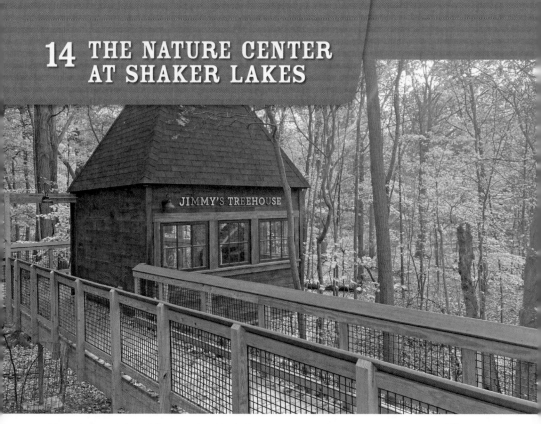

This treehouse would look funny on the side of a freeway.

NESTLED IN THE densely populated Shaker and Cleveland Heights neighborhoods, this preserved wilderness was nearly wiped out in the 1960s by a proposed freeway. Now dirt trails and boardwalks lead visitors past the nature center, a floodplain forest and marsh, a wildflower garden, and an enchanting treehouse.

DESCRIPTION

In the late 1800s, Cleveland city dwellers escaped to the relative countryside of the city's east-side Heights area. In the 1960s, it seemed like a good place to construct a freeway connecting the city and the eastern suburbs. That is, it seemed like a good idea to people who did not live in the Heights area. Residents were so opposed, in fact, that they hustled to establish a nature center and effectively prevented the freeway's placement. Good thing too—a few years later, the National Park Service named the center a National Environmental Education Landmark and a National Environmental Study Area. In short, coming here will probably make you smarter—and you'll have a good time too.

Start exploring on the short All People's Trail. Enter the accessible path from the southwest corner of the parking lot. From here, you'll make a clockwise loop back to the nature center. You'll also get an interesting perspective on the park—from

DISTANCE & CONFIGURATION: 1.5-mile loop; option for shorter or longer loops

DIFFICULTY: Easy

SCENERY: Birds; wetland, marsh, and lake views; wildflower and rain gardens

EXPOSURE: Mixed sun and shade

TRAFFIC: Can be crowded on weekends

TRAIL SURFACE: Wooden boardwalk, dirt, hard-packed gravel, and some asphalt

DRIVING DISTANCE: 13 miles from I-77/I-480 exchange

HIKING TIME: 1 hour, plus time for inside sightseeing and education

ACCESS: Trails: sunrise–sunset; nature center: Monday–Saturday, 10 a.m.–5 p.m. and Sunday, 1–5 p.m. Foot traffic only—no bikes, skates, or pets permitted, though a bike trail does intersect the hiking trail.

MAPS: USGS *Shaker Heights;* also at nature center

FACILITIES: Restrooms and water

WHEELCHAIR ACCESS: Nature center and All People's Trail, yes; Stearns Woodland Trail, no

CONTACT: 216-321-5935, shakerlakes.org

LOCATION: S. Park Blvd., Cleveland

several spots on the All People's Trail, you're surrounded by natural beauty and, at the same time, you can hear the cars go by on North Woodland Road. That is the defining characteristic of this property: its preserved wildness is firmly entrenched in the densely populated, long-developed cities of Shaker and Cleveland Heights.

In 1796, Moses Cleaveland surveyed the land that would become Shaker Heights. In 1822, a Shaker colony was established in three locations, roughly on the intersections of what are today Lee Road and Shaker Boulevard, Fontenay Road north of South Woodland, and North Park Boulevard near Doan Brook. Known as the North Union Shaker Community, they dammed Doan Brook to run their mills, creating Horseshoe Lake first and then Lower Shaker Lake in 1852. In 1889, the colony leased the lands (including the lakes) to Shaker Heights Land Co., which in 1895 donated 279 acres (including both lakes and the Doan Brook Valley) to the City of Cleveland, with the stipulation that the lands be used "for park purposes only."

If you know your Cleveland history, you know that Rockefeller Park was being developed at that time, and the Van Sweringens were formulating a plan for a neighborhood utopia. Although that utopia was threatened by plans to build a freeway through it, the development we see today is largely what the Van Sweringens had in mind, with the notable exception of the lakes. Between 2018 and 2021, both were drained, studied, refilled, and drained again. Here's a bit of trivia for you: until 2019, Lower Shaker Lake was the oldest man-made lake in Ohio.

As of this writing, both lakes are dry and it appears a plan from Northeast Ohio Regional Sewer District, agreed to by the City of Shaker Heights, will see Doan Brook run more-or-less free through here again, as it did for millennia before the Shakers dammed it.

Why does this matter to the casual hiker or nature center visitor? Glad you asked.

The Nature Center at Shaker Lakes

While city trails to Lower Shaker Lake and Horseshoe Lake are presently open (running by the now-dry lakes), they will likely be reimagined as work is being done on Doan Brook. How the project may affect Rockefeller Park as far north as Wade Oval was being discussed as this book was being published. Resources at the end of this section may be illuminating, and a walking tour of Rockefeller Park and Greenhouse and Wade Oval is highly recommended.

So back to the parking lot: head west on the All People's Trail and then north as the boardwalk bears right to the marsh landing and overlook. Follow the boardwalk to the left as it crosses over Doan Brook and you wander through the floodplain forest. Soon you'll have an option to take an offshoot to your left that connects with the neighborhoods and a path to Lower Shaker Lake. For this hike, stay on the All People's Trail as it crosses over Doan Brook again and approaches the front of the nature center. Before you reach the end of the trail, however, you'll be tempted to explore the impressive wood gazebo, with inviting shaded benches. (Go ahead, the nature center will wait.)

After stepping off the All People's Trail, go in and see all that the nature center has to offer—it's a lot, and the knowledgeable folks inside can answer your questions about the current state of Doan Brook. As one of just five brooks in Cleveland that are direct tributaries of Lake Erie, it plays a significant role in drainage, and therefore flood control, on the entire east side of Cleveland.

Exit the nature center and pick up the Stearns Trail from the south end of the parking lot near the entrance to the All People's Trail, following signs to the Nature Play Area—enjoy the play area as long as you like before returning to your hike.

Follow Stearns as it runs alongside and over the south branch of Doan Brook. The trail is a mix of boardwalk and natural surfaces, with a few short staircases, so this portion of the visit isn't wheelchair- or stroller-friendly.

In this actively managed natural area, you will see plants that are being protected from wildlife and people as you walk along Stearns Trail. Although the birds and bugs buzzing have some competition from the neighborhood traffic, it is a serene spot. Most of the flowers here are natives, but a few invasive plants are sometimes identified, and their impact is explained to educate visitors.

Continue on the Stearns Trail in a counterclockwise loop that leads through more marsh and forest land, passing by (or stopping to enjoy) a meditation terrace before reaching the woodland garden, to your right, and an extremely cool treehouse, on your left.

Visitors can explore Jimmy's Treehouse unless it is in use for a park program or a private event. (Ask for rental information at the nature center.)

Your hike can end here at the treehouse or nature center, a short distance from the parking lot. If you wish, you can extend your hike on the sidewalks surrounding the nature center, in the neighborhoods that were planned to be—and many would agree still are—an ideal community.

NEARBY ACTIVITIES

There are plenty of paved paths near here. Consider visiting another urban park, Rockefeller Park and Greenhouse, which lies just a few miles north of here along Martin Luther King Drive. Or take a (self-guided) walking tour of the very pedestrian-friendly community of Cleveland Heights. You are also close to Lake View Cemetery (page 62).

• •

TRAILHEAD GPS COORDINATES: N41.48531° W81.57443°

DIRECTIONS Coming from Cleveland? Take the Rapid. From the Shaker Heights Green Line, take the South Park stop; walk north along South Park Boulevard about 0.3 mile. The nature center is on the left, at the bottom of the hill, at 2600 South Park Boulevard. By car, from the I-77/I-480 exchange, follow I-480 E to I-271 N and take Exit 29 (OH 87/US 422/Chagrin Boulevard), heading west for 0.5 mile on OH 87/US 422/Chagrin Boulevard. Turn right onto Richmond Road and go 1 mile north to Shaker Boulevard and turn left. In 3.9 miles, turn right onto South Park Boulevard. After going down a small hill, the road forks. Veer left; a sign and the driveway to the nature center will be on your left.

The All People's Trail at The Nature Center at Shaker Lakes is completely accessible.

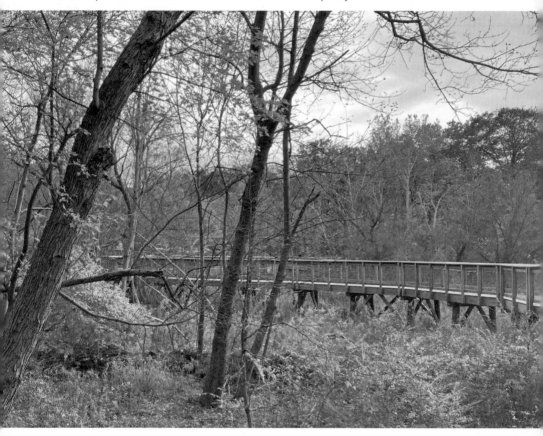

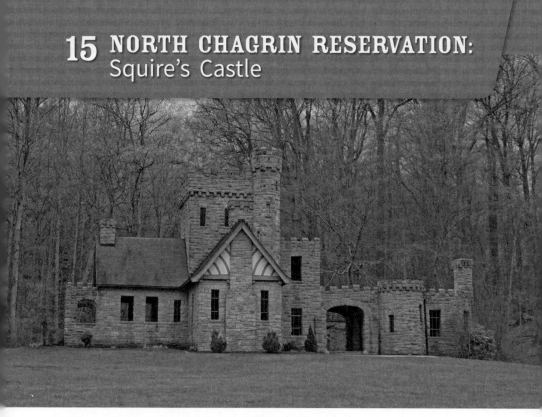

The former caretaker's cottage, better known as Squire's Castle

NORTH CHAGRIN RESERVATION has something for everyone. The nature center's exhibits are fun for all ages. A variety of trails throughout the reservation lead visitors by a gentle waterfall, through fragrant ravines, and to a castle romantically set on a gently sloping hill.

DESCRIPTION

Start at the nature center, stepping onto the paved Sanctuary Marsh Loop Trail, which runs between Sunset Pond and Sanctuary Marsh. Sanctuary Marsh Loop Trail's wide boardwalk is ideal for strollers and wheelchairs. Crisscrossing over the marsh, then looping back to the nature center to join the All Purpose Trail, is a good option offering 4+ miles of accessible paths.

For this trek, head north from the Sanctuary Marsh Loop Trail to connect with Buttermilk Falls Trail. The falls overlook, on the western side of Buttermilk Falls Parkway, is about 0.5 mile from the nature center. (If you'd like to shorten your hike, consider taking the 1.6-mile Hickory Fox Loop for some forest ravine views, then drive to the castle.) The pretty falls tumble over Cleveland shale, which has fractured in such a way that it makes the falls appear to be tumbling down a staircase.

Leave the waterfalls and head east (right), crossing the parkway, where you'll find a trailhead sign pointing to the Hickory Fox Loop (marked by a squirrel symbol),

DISTANCE & CONFIGURATION: 5.9-mile loop

DIFFICULTY: Moderate

SCENERY: Waterfall, deep ravine overlooks, deciduous forest, summer wildflowers, historical country estate

EXPOSURE: Mostly shaded

TRAFFIC: Moderate–heavy

TRAIL SURFACE: Mostly natural surfaces

HIKING TIME: 2.5–3 hours

DRIVING DISTANCE: 24 miles from I-77/I-480 exchange

ACCESS: Daily, 6 a.m.–11 p.m. See website for nature center hours.

MAPS: USGS *Mayfield Heights*; also at nature center and park website

FACILITIES: Restrooms inside nature center; grills, water, and restrooms at picnic areas

WHEELCHAIR ACCESS: Sanctuary Marsh Loop and All Purpose Trails, yes; other trails, no

CONTACT: 440-473-3370, clevelandmetroparks .com/parks/visit/parks/north-chagrin-reservation

LOCATION: SOM Center Road, Willoughby Hills

the Hemlock Trail (marked by a bird symbol), and the Bridle Trail. Many runners train on the Bridle Trail here, which is wider and more level—though just as hilly—as the Hemlock Trail. The Hemlock Trail offers better views of the ravine, though, and sometimes during the year, better wildflower displays. (Note that while a sturdy pair of sneakers will do on the Bridle Trail, you may prefer trail runners or boots on the Hemlock and Castle Valley Trails, as both have rocky, narrow places. Regardless of the trail you take to the castle landmark, you'll probably need to share the path.)

From the trail intersection, follow Hemlock as it wiggles its way north. The trail is appropriately named; plenty of the evergreens grow here, hugging the ravine's edge. Glance between them and you'll see a steep, deep valley—so Castle Valley Trail is a good name too. A few moderate hills and a lot more twisting turns will eventually find you at the intersection of Scenic Loop Trail, which shares the path with Hemlock until Hemlock ends and Scenic Loop veers sharply to the right. Don't follow it; instead, pick up Squire's Lane Trail and continue east. In less than a mile, the trail makes a sharp turn to the right, and you'll reach the storied structure: Squire's Castle. It's not really a castle, but it sure looks like one.

Feargus B. Squire, vice president of the Standard Oil Company, was so taken with the rolling landscape that he purchased 525 acres of land here, planning to build a vast estate. In the 1890s, he, his wife, and his daughter summered in the gatehouse, which we now know as the castle. As it happened, Mr. Squire never built his estate, and the Cleveland Metroparks purchased the land in 1925. To thwart vandals, the park filled in the basement and gutted the inside of the castle. They could not, however, stop reports of Mrs. Squire's ghost. Apparently, one of the reasons plans for the estate were never realized is because Mrs. Squire just didn't like the country. Though folks from the Metroparks explain repeatedly that no one has died in the castle, local legends abound, most of which feature Mrs. Squire taking a nasty fall in the building and dying of her injuries. (Most local records have recorded her death as occurring in 1929, 5 years after the park owned the property.) Still, some say Rebecca Squire can be seen carrying a red lantern through the cottage or wailing along Chagrin River Road on

North Chagrin Reservation: Squire's Castle

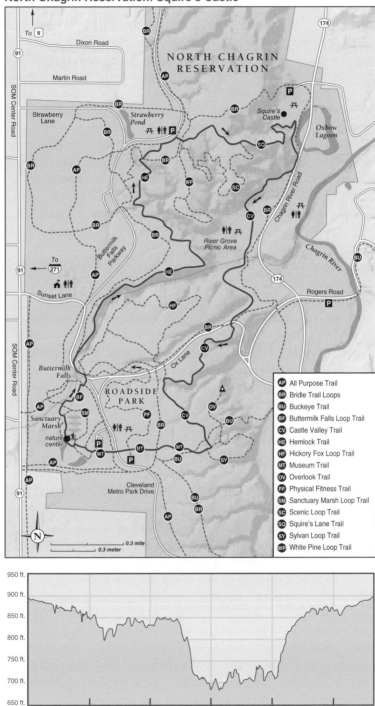

NORTH CHAGRIN RESERVATION

To 6

Dixon Road

91

Martin Road

SOM Center Road

Strawberry Lane

Strawberry Pond

Squire's Castle

Oxbow Lagoon

Chagrin River Road

Buttermilk Falls Parkway

River Grove Picnic Area

Chagrin River

To 271

91

Sunset Lane

174

Rogers Road

Buttermilk Falls

Sanctuary Marsh

nature center

ROADSIDE PARK

Ox Lane

SOM Center Road

91

Cleveland Metro Park Drive

N

0.3 mile
0.3 meter

AP	All Purpose Trail
BR	Bridle Trail Loops
BU	Buckeye Trail
BF	Buttermilk Falls Loop Trail
CV	Castle Valley Trail
HE	Hemlock Trail
HF	Hickory Fox Loop Trail
MT	Museum Trail
OV	Overlook Trail
PF	Physical Fitness Trail
SM	Sanctuary Marsh Loop Trail
SC	Scenic Loop Trail
SO	Squire's Lane Trail
SY	Sylvan Loop Trail
WP	White Pine Loop Trail

950 ft.
900 ft.
850 ft.
800 ft.
750 ft.
700 ft.
650 ft.

1 mi.   2 mi.   3 mi.   4 mi.   5 mi. 5.69 mi.

cool, dark nights. What you believe is up to you, of course, but one way to avoid such supernatural encounters is to visit the castle on a sunny day.

Whenever you visit, you'll surely have company, as the castle and surrounding picnic area are quite popular with the area's living population, especially photographers. While it's hard to imagine the structure now as a warm and cozy cottage, it was that. The westernmost room was reportedly Mr. Squire's library, with books shelved floor to ceiling. It takes more effort to imagine the upstairs and basement, but in its current state, with beams and bricks exposed, it may be more interesting to gawk at now.

After your tour of the "castle," pick up Castle Valley Trail as it runs from the south side of the structure. The path can be muddy through this stretch of woods, and it's slow to dry out after heavy rains. Since you walked mostly uphill to reach this point, you're in for a gentle downhill trek as you leave the castle behind. The trail is well marked, which is good, because it intersects with the Buckeye and Bridle Trails—so mind the signs.

Castle Valley Trail ends at the Museum Trail. Turn right and head west about 0.8 mile. When you reach the All Purpose Trail, you'll see the main parking lot for the nature center.

When's the best time to come? This park offers amazing fall colors, thanks to a mighty mix of deciduous trees and evergreens. The ravine is deep, fragrant, and peaceful, with a nice display of wildflowers, especially in the spring. In my experience, Hemlock Trail is lightly traveled compared to the other trails here. It also has a certain charm—and you're likely to enjoy some solitude—anytime you visit.

NEARBY ACTIVITIES

Why leave? North Chagrin Reservation and the nature center offer programming for all ages and interests, year-round. You can check the schedule at the park website or call 440-473-3370 for information.

If you're looking for more hikes with great views, you're in luck. From North Chagrin Reservation, you're about a 15-minute drive from Orchard Hills Park (page 125), just over the border in Geauga County, and about the same distance from Hach-Otis Sanctuary State Nature Preserve, in Lake County (page 104).

• •

TRAILHEAD GPS COORDINATES: N41.56173° W81.43583°

DIRECTIONS Take I-271 N to Exit 36 (Wilson Mills Road). Head east on Wilson Mills Road about 0.5 mile and turn left (north) onto OH 91/SOM Center Road. Go north about 2 miles and turn right onto Sunset Lane into the park. In 0.3 mile, turn right onto Buttermilk Falls Parkway, and follow the signs 0.5 mile south to the nature center.

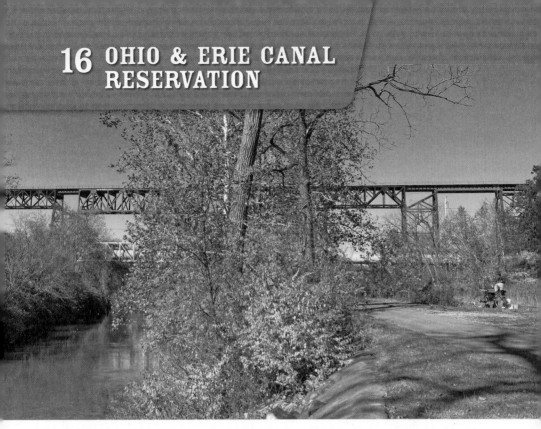

In this tranquil spot below the train trestles, you'll find an inviting visitor center, pollinator garden, and miles of trails.

ONE OF THE most urban outposts of the Cleveland Metroparks, Ohio & Erie Canal Reservation may be best known for its mountain biking experiences. Rest assured there's plenty to see on foot here as well.

DESCRIPTION

When CanalWay Center opened in 1999, naturalists told a three-part story explaining how the park embodies nature at work, people at work, and systems at work. It's still an apt description, but today plenty of people find the park a good place to play too.

For starters, there are the biking enthusiasts. Because the Ohio & Erie Canal Towpath Trail connects the southern suburbs to downtown Cleveland, the reservation has long been a pit stop for Towpath cyclists and long-distance runners. The more recently added mountain bike trails and pump track have made it a popular destination with mountain bikers of all skill levels.

Families looking for a day in the park or a group outing can take advantage of reservable picnic grounds with playgrounds, and the indoor nature and visitor center is a draw year-round, for all ages. CanalWay Center is arguably the most interactive of any nature center in the Cleveland Metroparks. Inside, visitors can step aboard a realistic canal boat and get their hands on other displays highlighting the

81

DISTANCE & CONFIGURATION: 2.8-mile loop on Towpath Trail with optional 2.2 miles on mountain bike trails

DIFFICULTY: Easy

SCENERY: River and canal views, active railroad trestle, pollinator garden, live animals in the nature center, a historic pump house, and petroleum tanks (yes, petroleum tanks)

EXPOSURE: Mostly exposed

TRAFFIC: Moderate; Towpath Trail and mountain bike trails are well traveled on warm weekends.

TRAIL SURFACE: Towpath Trail, mostly paved; some natural (dirt) trails

HIKING TIME: 2 hours, plus time to explore the visitor center

DRIVING DISTANCE: 4 miles from I-77/I-480 exchange

ACCESS: Daily, 6 a.m.–11 p.m. Nature center: Daily, 9:30 a.m.–5 p.m.; check website for closures on major holidays.

MAPS: USGS *Cleveland South;* also at nature center and park website

FACILITIES: Restrooms, phone, and water at nature center; restrooms on Towpath Trail near the Lower 40 Loop Trail, plus two playgrounds

WHEELCHAIR ACCESS: Towpath Trail, yes; other trails, no

CONTACT: 216-206-1000, clevelandmetroparks.com/parks/visit/parks/ohio-erie-canal-reservation

LOCATION: 4524 E. 49th St., Cuyahoga Heights

area's cultural history as well as the city's industrial base. There's also a bird-viewing area and wildlife display with live animals inside.

But this is a hiking guide! What will you see on the trails at Ohio & Erie Canal Reservation? Scenery that will surprise you. Let's get started.

While you can reach the Towpath trailhead from either the front or back of CanalWay Center, I like to wander through the center, say hello to the turtles (and staff), and head out the back door of the center to enjoy the pollinator garden, with its larger-than-life-size sculptures of birds and insects.

Follow the steps down to the All Purpose Trail and turn left. Soon you'll see a sign inviting you to turn right to reach Blue Heron Boardwalk. Although it's just a 0.1-mile loop, don't be surprised if you can't complete it, as the boardwalk can be submerged after heavy rains. It's an active wetland, after all, and nature is working to keep it that way. Even when it's wet, it's worth making this little loop to two small viewing docks.

Returning to the All Purpose Trail, turn right to continue heading south. Very shortly, you'll notice an unsigned, paved trail off to your left. Avoid it for now, as it loops back toward the nature center, and to bike trails that aren't shared with hikers. Veer right instead—the scenery is about to get interesting!

When you spot a white, O-shaped metal ring inviting you off the path again, this time, go and enjoy the view of the very-active train tracks from below. When you return to the All Purpose Trail, cross over a short footbridge and turn left. You can follow the Towpath Trail 50 miles south to Canal Fulton (page 162) and beyond, but for this hike, turn back at a small earthen bridge where you can get a good look at a portion of the canal. It's also a popular fishing spot.

Once you turn back, now heading north on the Towpath Trail, you'll walk under a sewer pipe interceptor and then through a wooden covered bridge celebrating the

Ohio & Erie Canal Reservation

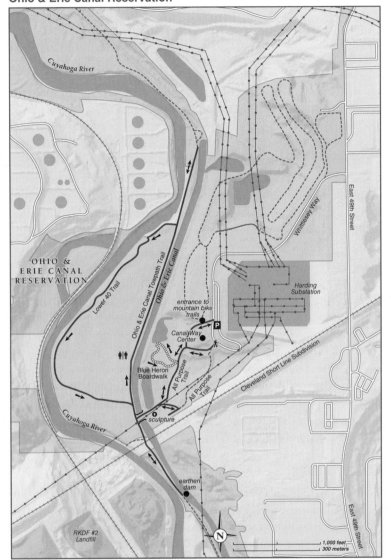

1907 two-track trestle (above you). Unusual for a hike? Maybe. It certainly serves to remind us that the canal and the river aren't the only things flowing here.

Continuing north on the Towpath Trail, you'll pass by the footbridge and soon have a clear view of industrial buildings straight ahead. That the narrow canal to your right—today a popular fishing spot—made so much industry possible may be hard to believe.

About 0.3 mile north of the O, you'll reach the Lower 40 Trailhead. You can turn left here to begin your loop back, but it's worth the time and short distance to continue north to get a better look at the pump house.

Although the canal closed for transportation in 1813, a long-term water usage rights agreement was in effect, and the pump house carried water to a steel plant on East 49th Street until 1997. With another history nugget in your collection, turn around to find the Lower 40 Trail again.

Turn right when you reach it, and just a few steps west of the Towpath, you'll find yourself in a very large circle. The interpretive spot approximates the circumference of one of the petroleum storage tanks that you can see to the north of the trail. In case you're wondering, a typical tank can hold up to 400 million gallons of petroleum products.

As you continue south on the Lower 40 Trail, you'll have several opportunities to watch the river as it makes its way to Lake Erie. Oaks and a variety of maples shade the trail, and mayapples spring up along the river too. (A handful of dogwoods, with their unmistakable spring blooms, can be seen closer to the nature center.)

Speaking of CanalWay Center, to return, simply turn right on the Towpath, then left to retrace your steps back over the footbridge to the center. While CanalWay Center celebrates much of Cleveland's history, this park is very much a current lesson in how many of the city's resources come together to support modern life in northeastern Ohio. And yes, modern life includes mountain biking!

While hikers are permitted on the mountain bike trails here—and they are interesting, providing a different look at the valley—if you choose to hike on them be aware that they are narrow, and you may have to scramble quickly to get out of the way. On these and any shared mountain bike trails, to avoid a biker/hiker collision, hikers are strongly encouraged to stay off the trails during busy mountain bike times. At all times, it's a smart practice for hikers to walk in the opposite direction of the bike flow.

After you've seen the interesting, industrial scenery here, you might be looking for a more serene natural setting—two suggestions that fill the bill are included below.

NEARBY ACTIVITIES

The Towpath Trail running through this park will take you north all the way to Cleveland's flats, so if you want more miles, you can get them here. Enjoy mountain biking? You may want to try the trails here, which include a beginner-friendly track that opened in 2022. For a more urban hike, consider Cleveland West Side Wanderings (page 31) or Downtown Cleveland Highlights (page 36). Prefer more natural or shadier trails? Brecksville Reservation (page 23) or Frazee House to Linda Falls (page 45)—both about a 15-minute drive from here—might be to your liking.

• •

TRAILHEAD GPS COORDINATES: N41.43350° W81.65879°

DIRECTIONS From I-77/I-480, take I-77 N to Exit 158 (Grant Avenue) and turn left onto Grant. Turn left onto E. 49th Street, then right onto Whittlesey Way to enter the reservation.

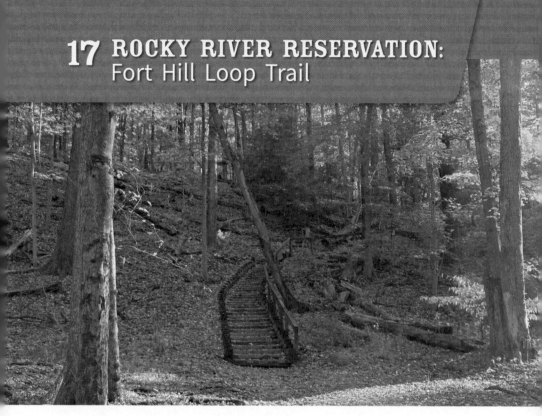

Rest assured the beautiful views will take your mind off the (many, many) stairs.

WHILE THE INITIAL climb might make your legs wobble, this hike rewards with some spectacular views. Steps not for you? There's plenty for natural history fans, too, inside the nice, flat nature center, including a "terrible fish" and ancient Indigenous ceremonial grounds.

DESCRIPTION

The earthworks on the Fort Hill Loop Trail are considerably less impressive than the better-known mounds of southern Ohio. But what these ridges lack in size, they make up for in location. To reach the earthworks, you'll have to do some climbing—up 155 steps, to be precise—but the views that await will make you forget about all of them.

However, before experiencing the climb and the view, you might find yourself a bit breathless in front of the nature center. There, approximately where a welcome mat should be, you'll face the "terrible fish" known as *Dunkleosteus terrelli*. The huge hunter swam the oceans that covered Ohio millions of years ago, probably terrorizing other ancient sea critters. A well-preserved specimen was discovered nearby, in the shale cliffs above the riverbed, making it difficult to retrieve. The fossil remains were moved to the Cleveland Museum of Natural History, but you'll find more information about the beast, including another terrifying replica, inside the nature center.

Before beginning your hike from the back of the nature center, you can relax for a moment by watching for birds in the feeding area to your left and around West

DISTANCE & CONFIGURATION: 1.2-mile loop

DIFFICULTY: Moderately difficult, with lots of stairs to climb

SCENERY: River views, earthworks, natural displays inside nature center

EXPOSURE: Mostly shaded

TRAFFIC: Can be busy, especially on warm weekends

TRAIL SURFACE: Dirt trail, wooden boardwalk, and stairs

HIKING TIME: 45 minutes for Fort Hill and Channel Pond Loops; add an hour for optional trails

DRIVING DISTANCE: 15 miles from I-77/I-480 exchange

ACCESS: Daily, 6 a.m.–11 p.m. Nature center: Daily, 9:30 a.m.–5 p.m.; closed January 1, Easter, Thanksgiving, and December 25. The steps leading to Fort Hill Earthworks are closed when icy; if in doubt, call ahead to check on weather conditions.

MAPS: USGS *North Olmsted;* also at nature center and park website

FACILITIES: Restrooms, phone, and water at nature center

WHEELCHAIR ACCESS: No

CONTACT: 440-734-6660, clevelandmetroparks .com/parks/visit/parks/rocky-river-reservation

LOCATION: Valley Pkwy., North Olmsted

Channel Pond on your right. From here, you may choose to follow two dirt paths: West Channel Pond Loop or the Wildlife Management Loop. But the biggest bang for your buck—and the best views in my opinion—await at the top of the stairs to your left. So go there first—and return to West Channel Pond later, if you like.

After you've scaled the stairs leading to the main trail, you'll find yourself almost 100 feet higher, likely taking another deep breath. There a sign explains what researchers understand about the earthworks in front of you. Some 2,000 years ago, Indigenous peoples formed these earthworks, probably for ceremonial purposes.

The earthworks' ridges lie like mussed-up blankets under the shade of pin oaks, and frankly, they're difficult to discern. The mounds here are small, but the mystery is great: Who were these people? Why did they select this spot—and for what? Inside the nature center, there are some answers, but still more questions, about these Indigenous peoples and the earthworks they left behind.

Here, you can walk on both sides of the earthworks. After pondering the mounds and their builders, be sure to return to the main path to enjoy more breathtaking views of the river below. Then follow the bright-yellow markers of the Fort Hill Loop Trail.

Along the way, interpretive signs describe how the river has changed, and continues to change, the landscape. Approximately 360 million years ago, all but the southeast portion of Ohio was under ocean. While the ocean is long gone, the Rocky River continues to cut away at the land. It's obvious, as you look at the trees clinging to the cliff sides, that much of the soil that once supported them has eroded and washed into the river below. The soil and other sediment have formed islands in the river, and the trees that grow there—sycamores, cottonwoods, and willows—are ones that can survive the silt and changing water levels.

The dirt path leaves the ridge and curves clockwise, descending slowly into thick woods. Wildflowers and a variety of trees, including hemlocks, are sprinkled along this portion of the trail.

Rocky River Reservation: Fort Hill Loop Trail

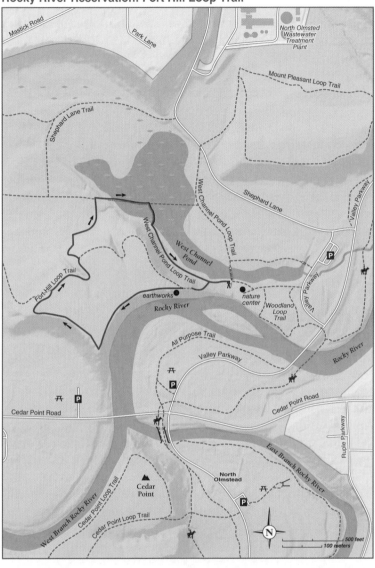

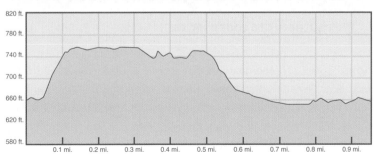

As you bottom out near the northern edge of West Channel Pond, complete the loop by taking the boardwalk in a counterclockwise direction back to the nature center.

Now it's time to decide how much more exploring you want to do. Just east of the nature center you can connect to little Woodland Loop Trail (0.25 mile). If you follow it to the All Purpose Trail and turn right, you'll be heading south. You'll soon cross the river via the pedestrian bridge on Cedar Point Road.

The historic Cedar Point Road (automobile) bridge was built in 1929 and underwent an extensive restoration and widening project starting in 2021. In addition to its age, it was deemed historically significant because of the use of local Berea sandstone in its construction, as well as an emphasis on aesthetics. With luck, you'll be able to enjoy those (restored) aesthetics by the time this book is published. Once across the river, turn left onto the bridle trail to follow it northeast.

The bridle trail crosses through the river again right before intersecting with the All Purpose Trail and connecting with the Woodland Loop again. This optional trek—which returns you to the nature center at the south end of West Channel Pond—adds another 1.5 miles to your total today.

NEARBY ACTIVITIES

Don't leave the park without a look inside the nature center, filled with fun, educational displays, including a water feature with fish and turtles. Then explore the rest of the reservation. The northern half is home to several ballfields and to the Emerald Necklace Marina. A park concession at 1500 Scenic Park Drive in Lakewood rents kayaks for river paddling. For more information, call 866-529-2541 or visit 41° North Coastal Adventures at 41n.com.

With a little planning, you can also visit the Frostville Museum, located in the park about a mile west of the nature center. The museum honors the history of the local area from the 1800s. There are tours of the restored buildings, including a church, barn, several homes, a general store, and an outhouse. For more information about the museum and tour schedules, see clevelandmetroparks.com/parks/visit /parks/rocky-river-reservation/frostville-museum or call 440-779-0280.

• •

TRAILHEAD GPS COORDINATES: N41.40930° W81.88418°

DIRECTIONS From I-77/I-480, take I-480 W to Exit 7 (Clague Road). Turn left off the ramp, and follow Clague south 0.3 mile, where it ends at Mastick Road. Turn right, heading west 0.4 mile to Rocky River Reservation. Turn left onto Shephard Lane and follow it 0.6 mile to Valley Parkway. Turn right on Valley Parkway and go 0.2 mile; park in the nature center lot, on the right at 24000 Valley Parkway.

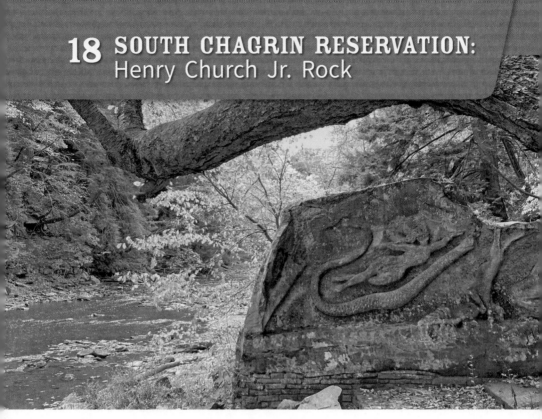

Henry Church carved images on this rock by lantern light.

A ROCKY RAVINE, gentle rapids, and a bit of a mystery are waiting for you in the Cleveland Metroparks South Chagrin Reservation. While you're there, you can enjoy a shady stretch of the Buckeye Trail and views of the scenic Chagrin River. Good hiking boots are highly recommended for this hike.

DESCRIPTION

Follow signs for the Henry Church Jr. Rock Trail at the southeastern edge of the parking lot. Taking the trail south in a counterclockwise direction is the quickest way to the namesake attraction. The path is paved along here, but don't worry, it gets more interesting soon enough. You'll also see the blue blazes of the Buckeye Trail at this point.

You'll catch a few glimpses of the Chagrin River below, to your left, and pass a connector trail leading to the Forest Loop; shortly thereafter, the Buckeye Trail veers off to your right. Keep straight, going over a small bridge, to reach the Henry Church Jr. Rock overlook, where you can see the trail below. The lower portion of the trail is not for everyone, with a steep descent on uneven stairs. (This portion is closed during icy conditions.)

Past the overlook, the trail becomes more rustic and rocky; you'll soon turn left to take the stairs down to the river and the rock. Take your time; the trail warrants it, and the views are worth it. There's easy access to a shallow stretch of the Chagrin

DISTANCE & CONFIGURATION: 2-mile figure eight, with options for 2-plus additional miles

DIFFICULTY: Moderate; Henry Church Jr. Rock Trail is steep with uneven stairs; Forest Loop is a flat, dirt trail.

SCENERY: Curious old carvings, a waterfall, river ravine overlooks, thick forest

EXPOSURE: Almost entirely shaded

TRAFFIC: Moderate on Henry Church Jr. Rock Trail

TRAIL SURFACE: Henry Church Jr. Rock Trail, rocky and stone steps; Forest Loop, dirt and roots

HIKING TIME: 1 hour

DRIVING DISTANCE: 15 miles from I-77/I-480 exchange

ACCESS: Daily, 6 a.m.–11 p.m.; parking lots that close at sunset are clearly posted. Steps to Henry Church Jr. Rock are closed when icy.

MAPS: USGS *Chagrin Falls;* also at park website

FACILITIES: Restrooms at Henry Church Jr. Rock Picnic Area; public phone at the sledding hill parking lot south of Miles Road

WHEELCHAIR ACCESS: No

CONTACT: 440-247-7075, clevelandmetroparks.com/parks/visit/parks/south-chagrin-reservation

LOCATION: Hawthorn Pkwy., Bentleyville

River at the bottom of the stairs, and you might want to skip stones or splash about a bit on a warm day—but most people come here to gaze upon and wonder about the rock, just a few feet to the north.

The rectangular sandstone rock is about 10 feet high. On its south face are several carvings, including a bird in flight, a bundle of quivers, a tomahawk, an Indigenous maiden, a rattlesnake, and an infant. Henry Church Jr. carved the images in 1885. Born and raised in Chagrin Falls, about 2 miles east of here, Church was a blacksmith by trade. He also enjoyed painting and sculpting. Though his art was considered unusual at the time, in 1980 (72 years after his death), his work was featured in a special exhibit at the Whitney Museum of American Art in New York City.

Church reportedly walked from his home to the rock every night to carve by lantern light. He quit when his neighbors found out what he was doing. On the east face of the rock are unfinished carvings of a log cabin and the U.S. Capitol. What Church intended by the carvings is unknown. Some speculate that the collage is a celebration of American history; others believe that it was meant to be an artistic condemnation of our government's policies in the late 1800s. This much we know: His work continues to lure many people to this trail.

When you've contemplated all you want, step back onto the path, again heading north. The trail is narrow, and slightly banked in places, but don't let that stop you from looking around. The river is lovely in all seasons, and it's easy to forget you're hiking in a long-developed suburban community. The hemlocks above grow right to the very edge of the trail above, and after a good rain, you'll appreciate a couple of thin waterfalls tumbling over the shale cliffs. A bit farther north, you'll climb a set of wooden stairs that take you back to the paved path and close to the parking lot.

At the top, you can turn right to return to the parking lot if you're done for the day. Although you may be winded from climbing the steps, you've covered less than a mile so far. Turn left if you want to keep going, on flatter terrain.

South Chagrin Reservation: Henry Church Jr. Rock

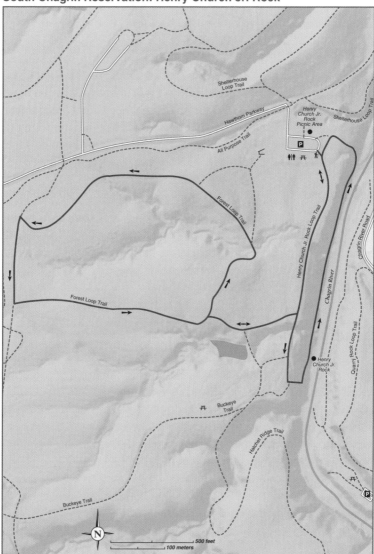

To reach the Forest Loop, follow the paved path south again, then turn right onto the connector trail to the Forest Loop. It's a shady trail, as its name implies, and it winds its way generally east from here to reach a small arboretum showcasing the reservation's deciduous trees.

Following the Forest Loop in a counterclockwise direction, you'll hear and occasionally catch a glimpse of traffic on the All Purpose Trail and Hawthorn Parkway to the north. The trail can be quite wet during the early-spring thaw or any time after a good rain, so if you wore sturdy boots for the rockier loop, they could come in handy here too. The trail veers left (south) to abut the bridle trail and soon delivers you to the arboretum, located in the Arbor Picnic Area.

Once you've memorized all the arbor info you can, return by crossing the bridle trail (heading east) and follow the bridle trail and the Forest Loop until the Forest Loop turns sharply left, splitting from the bridle trail to head east through the woods. About 0.2 mile from the bridle trail split, the Forest Loop curves left, where—just a few feet past the turn—you'll see the connector trail back to the Buckeye Trail and the top of the Henry Church Jr. Rock Trail. Turn left again to return to the trailhead and your starting point.

YOU HAVE OPTIONS

If you want to add another 2 (or more) miles to your route, from the arboretum, follow the bridle trail (which is also the Buckeye Trail at this point). As it heads south from the arboretum, where it splits, turn left to head east and then north to meet up with the All Purpose Trail. You can keep going at that point, of course, or turn right onto the All Purpose Trail to return to the Henry Church Jr. Rock Picnic Area parking lot where you started.

NEARBY ACTIVITIES

If you'd rather seek wildflowers than gawk at a carved rock, try Sulphur Springs Loop; at just over 1 mile, it offers a wealth of spring blooms. If you like parks with recreational amenities, South Chagrin Reservation delivers, with a sledding hill at the south end of Sulphur Springs Drive, multiple picnic areas, and more than 7 miles of All Purpose Trail. Fishing is allowed at Shadow Lake, and Look About Lodge, just north of the sledding hill, hosts a wide variety of programs throughout the year. Check the park website for upcoming events.

To visit Church's hometown, the quaint village of Chagrin Falls, travel about 2 miles east on Miles Road. There's a waterfall on the western side of Main Street, as well as numerous shops and restaurants that are worth a visit.

• •

TRAILHEAD GPS COORDINATES: N41.41645° W81.41518°

DIRECTIONS Take I-480 E until it ends at I-271/US 422 and exit right onto US 422 E. Follow US 422 E for 3.8 miles and exit onto OH 91 (toward Solon). Turn left onto OH 91 N/ SOM Center Road. In 1.5 miles, turn right onto Hawthorn Parkway. Follow Hawthorn east about 1.5 miles. The road ends at the bottom of the hill; Henry Church Jr. Rock Picnic Area and parking is on your right.

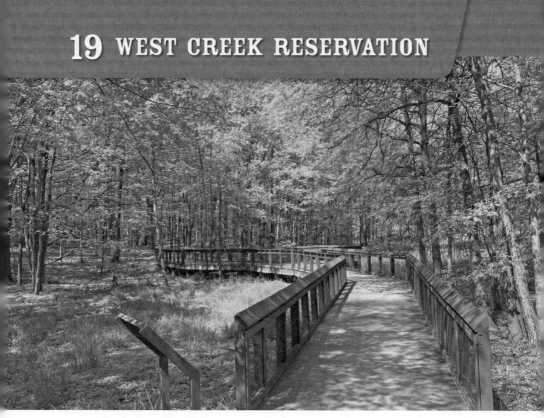

The Cleveland Hiking Club donated considerable time and resources to build Skyline Overlook Trail. The trail was dedicated on April 20, 2019, commemorating the club's centennial.

COME FOR A short climb and a peek at Cleveland's skyline; stay for an education in watershed management.

DESCRIPTION

West Creek runs through a densely developed residential area, but the 326-acre reservation set amid the neighborhoods protects pretty forest views and provides much-needed wetlands. As a bonus, this natural escape from urban life offers a glimpse of Cleveland's skyline—and enough of a climb to get your heart pumping.

Entering off West Ridgewood Drive, you'll find ample parking at the Keystone Shelter along Kordiak Drive and at the Keystone Loop Trailhead on the east side of the parkway. To reach the Skyline Overlook from the Keystone shelter parking area, cross the road and turn right onto the All Purpose Trail (APT). Shortly, you'll spot the Keystone Loop Trailhead sign and turn left onto Keystone Loop. Almost as soon as you start out on the hard-packed sand-and-gravel trail, you'll find yourself twisting through a thick forest. The path has been designed to mitigate your climb, so at first you may not notice the elevation change. Rest assured, however, you are ascending toward that overlook!

DISTANCE & CONFIGURATION: 2.6-mile figure eight

DIFFICULTY: Easy–moderate

SCENERY: Forested ravines, wetlands, and a glimpse of the Cleveland skyline

EXPOSURE: Mostly shaded

TRAFFIC: Moderate

TRAIL SURFACE: Keystone Loop and Skyline Trail, hard-packed limestone and gravel; All Purpose Trail, paved

HIKING TIME: 1.5 hours, plus time at nature center

DRIVING DISTANCE: 4 miles from I-480/I-77 interchange

ACCESS: Daily, 6 a.m.–11 p.m.; Watershed Stewardship Center: daily, 9:30 a.m.–5 p.m., closed major holidays

MAPS: USGS *Cleveland South*

FACILITIES: Restrooms at Skyline Overlook Trailhead parking area and Keystone Shelter; water and restrooms at Watershed Stewardship Center

WHEELCHAIR ACCESS: Keystone Loop and Skyline Trail, no; All Purpose Trail and Watershed Stewardship Center, yes

CONTACT: 440-887-1968, clevelandmetroparks .com/parks/visit/parks/west-creek-reservation

LOCATION: 2277 W. Ridgewood Dr., Parma

In spring, you'll enjoy great wildflower displays through here; look for mayapples and jack-in-the-pulpits. Seasonal blooms vary, but you can usually see them from late April to mid-May. In the warmer months, the Keystone Loop provides welcome shade.

Shortly after stepping onto the trail, you'll have the option to short-cut the loop by heading left. Don't do it—you'll miss the skyline view! Continue straight on Keystone Loop, passing a connection to Bluebird Trail. Just about 0.1 mile past the junction with Bluebird Trail, you'll take a sharp right onto the Skyline Trail and find the climb gets steeper as you head south, then north, and south again to the overlook.

While on the Keystone Loop—with its undeniable forest vibes—you probably also heard car traffic along West Ridgewood Drive. As you head south on Skyline Trail, most of the road noise falls away. However, while sounds from the road fade as you approach the skyline viewing deck, you're likely to hear more air traffic above, as Parma is directly in most flight paths from Cleveland-Hopkins Airport. That this is an oasis in an otherwise densely developed suburb is undeniable—that, and the importance of this land, will be even more obvious when you visit the Watershed Management Center.

Continue on Skyline Trail and step onto the viewing platform. Looking north, there's no mistaking the city's silhouette. After taking in the view from this ridge in the (suburban) forest, retrace your steps north and turn right to continue counterclockwise, still on Skyline Trail. You'll cross some small footbridges, which upon inspection are really drainage devices protecting the trail as much as your boots. Soon you'll meet the Keystone Loop and join it again as it descends gradually and edges closer to the park's boundary on Ridgewood Drive. As you approach the APT near the end of Keystone Loop, a large interpretive sign appropriately recognizes the Cleveland Hiking Club. Its members have done an incredible amount of work for the area's parks and trails, for more than 100 years. Their dedication is impressive, and all Greater Clevelanders reap the rewards of their efforts. (Thank you, CHC members!)

West Creek Reservation

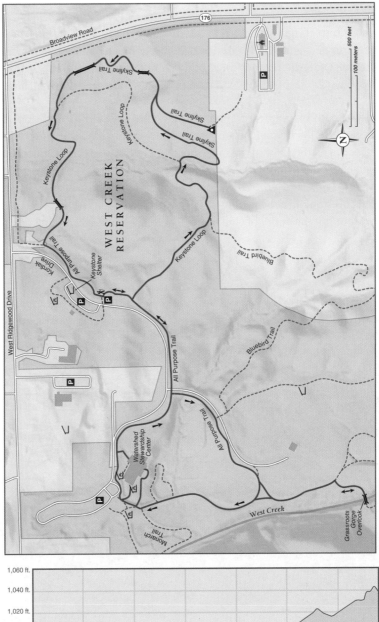

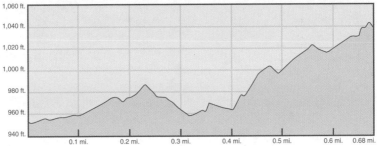

YOU HAVE OPTIONS

Once you return to the APT, turn left and head back to your parking spot. From there, you can decide to call it a day; you've just completed a pretty hilly, mile-plus hike, after all! Or, if you're ready for another couple of miles, continue on the APT to the Grassroots Gorge Overlook, and then on to the Watershed Stewardship Center.

To continue your exploration here, follow the APT southwest. Along the way you'll notice the low-lying land on either side of the parkway is often filled with water. This is a feature of water management and one way to protect our roads—and our basements—from flooding.

About 0.2 mile along the APT, you'll turn left to reach Grassroots Gorge Overlook. This overlook may be less impressive than Skyline Overlook, with its incredible city view, but the depth of Grassroots Gorge Overlook will remind you that this

The Watershed Stewardship Center at West Creek Reservation

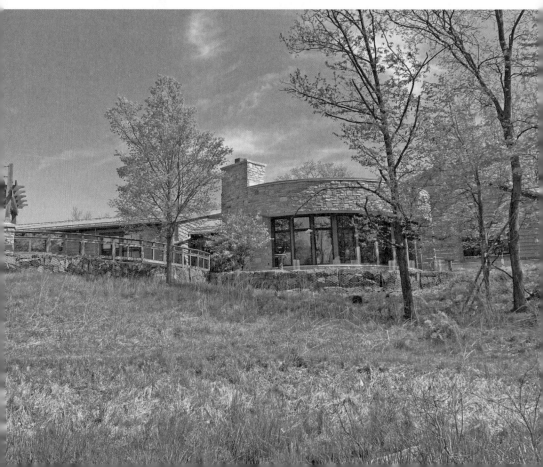

land does a lot of heavy lifting after storms, channeling water safely to treatment facilities and away from our homes and businesses.

For this hike, Grassroots Gorge Overlook is your turnaround point, and you'll head to the Watershed Stewardship Center from here. But note that the overlook is also a trailhead for the 0.7-mile Gateway Trail, a shared-used trail for hikers and mountain bikers.

Retrace your steps from the Grassroots Gorge Overlook and bear left on the APT to reach the back entrance of the nature center, or more formally, the Watershed Stewardship Center.

Inside the center, you'll find educational displays offering a practical, everyday perspective on water. If you've ever driven through a puddle that was too deep for your car's tires—or worried about water in your basement—you might be interested in how communities can improve stormwater management. The development of West Creek Reservation itself highlights new techniques in watershed management. The Metroparks management intends for the center to serve as a living laboratory, demonstrating real-world solutions for better stormwater and pollution control.

After checking out the displays inside, explore the rest of the nature center, including a few aquatic native animals and a gift shop.

To wrap up this trek as depicted on the map, exit the nature center from the front entrance, turn right on the APT, and head east to return to the Keystone Loop Trailhead parking area. Because more connections from this park to nearby neighborhoods and other park properties are in the works, if longer distances (or more mountain bike trails) are to your liking, you'll almost certainly want to plan a return trip here.

NEARBY ACTIVITIES

Mountain bike trails, which can be accessed from the southwest end of the nature center, are also fun. See the Cleveland Metroparks website for the most current mountain bike trail maps and trail conditions. Of course, if you work up an appetite, Parma is *the* place to get pierogis, with several shops still making and selling the Polish-style dumplings around town. Also nearby: Cleveland Metroparks Zoo is about a 15-minute drive north of here, and CanalWay Center, another relatively new nature center, is about 15 minutes northeast of here by car (page 81).

• •

TRAILHEAD GPS COORDINATES: N41.39015° W81.69159°

DIRECTIONS From I-480, take I-77 S to Rockside Road. Head west to Crossview Road and turn left (south). Follow Crossview Road to East Ridgewood Drive and turn right (west). Follow Ridgewood Drive for about 1 mile to the park entrance, on your left.

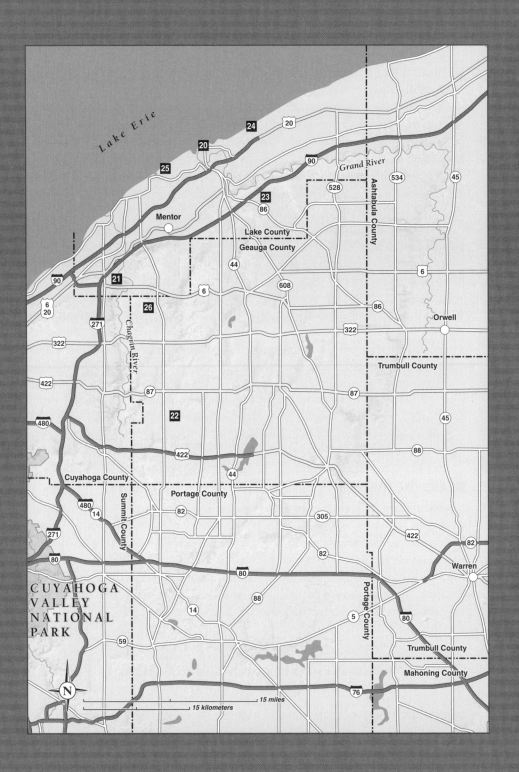

Lake Erie

24
20

20

25
90

Grand River

534
45

528

Mentor

23
86

Ashtabula County
6

21

Lake County

Geauga County

44

6

608

Chagrin River

26

86

Orwell

322

322

Trumbull County

87

87

45

22

88

422

44

Cuyahoga County

Portage County

82

305

480

14

82

422

82

271

80

CUYAHOGA
VALLEY
NATIONAL
PARK

Summit County

88

14

5

Portage County

Warren

80

Trumbull County

59

Mahoning County

N

76

15 miles

15 kilometers

GEAUGA & LAKE COUNTIES

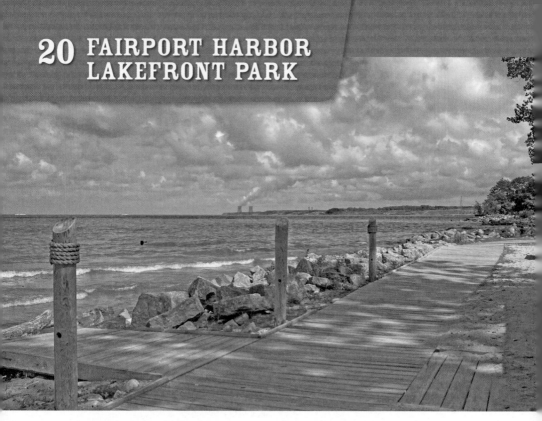

20 FAIRPORT HARBOR LAKEFRONT PARK

Fairport Harbor's beach boardwalk is wheelchair-accessible and stroller-friendly.

SUMMER IS TOO precious in northeastern Ohio. Visit Fairport Harbor to enjoy its postcard-worthy vistas, tour a lighthouse, and frolic on the beach to create memories you can relish when winter's dreariness descends.

DESCRIPTION

At the top of the town stands a small stone lighthouse, originally built in 1825. Behind the lighthouse sits the keeper's house, now the Fairport Harbor Marine Museum, packed with nautical exhibits as well as a mummified cat. But, of course, there's more to that tail. Er, tale.

In fact, the lighthouse harbors many tales. Step inside the museum (open seasonally) to begin your hike, tour, and history lesson.

Samuel Butler was the first lighthouse keeper and an abolitionist. Under his watch, the lighthouse was a stop on the Underground Railroad, offering a new life for many escaped enslaved people who were able to reach Canada via Lake Erie. Later, Civil War veteran Joseph Babcock became keeper of the lighthouse, which had been newly rebuilt in 1871. He and his wife, Mary, had three children, two of whom were born in the keeper's house. Unfortunately, their youngest son, Robbie, died of illness at the age of 5, and Mary spent several years afterward in bed due to sickness, depression, or both.

DISTANCE & CONFIGURATION: 1-mile loop, plus optional lighthouse stairs

DIFFICULTY: Easy beach stroll; lighthouse requires some stair climbing

SCENERY: Lake Erie, lighthouse, beach, stacks of Perry Nuclear Power Plant

EXPOSURE: Almost entirely exposed

TRAFFIC: Moderately heavy, especially on warm weekends

TRAIL SURFACE: Pavement, sidewalks, beach

HIKING TIME: 45–50 minutes

DRIVING DISTANCE: 39 miles from I-77/I-480 exchange

ACCESS: Fairport Harbor Marine Museum and Lighthouse: May–October, call for hours; adults, $13; children age 17 and under, $7; Park: Daily, 6 a.m.–11 p.m.; $3 parking fee ($2 for Lake County residents)

MAPS: USGS *Mentor OE N*

FACILITIES: Restrooms, water fountains, and concessions (seasonally) at park

WHEELCHAIR ACCESS: Sidewalks in town are accessible to the pier; parking lot and boardwalk access to concessions and beach sections

CONTACT: Lake Metroparks: 440-639-7275, lakemetroparks.com/parks-trails/fairport-harbor-lakefront-park; Fairport Harbor Marine Museum and Lighthouse: 440-354-4825, fairportharborlighthouse.org

LOCATION: Huntington Beach Dr., Fairport Harbor

Reportedly, Mary loved cats and had several, including a gray one. After Mary died, numerous people reported seeing a ghost cat playing in the kitchen and elsewhere on the lighthouse grounds. When HVAC repair workers found the mummified body of a cat inside a crawl space, it seemed to confirm the stories. Today, tales of the feline apparition live on.

After a new lighthouse was constructed in Lake Erie in 1925, the original lighthouse was ordered to be demolished. Fortunately, locals managed to save it, and today volunteers continue to maintain the lighthouse and operate the popular museum.

If you come here during the summer on a day the lighthouse is open, pay the small fee that grants access to the historic building and museum. Inside you can climb the 69 steps of the spiral staircase to reach the top of the light and look upon Lake Erie, where you will see the newer Fairport Harbor West Breakwater Lighthouse.

The oft-photographed red-and-white building sits on the breakwater, where it was operated and maintained by the U.S. Coast Guard until 2011. An individual has since purchased the property and restored it into what may be the coolest residence on the lake. (Very occasionally, the owner hosts an open house for the public. Information is shared on the Fairport Harbor West Breakwater Lighthouse page on Facebook.)

While the beachfront offers a pretty panorama, below the lake's surface, a busy salt mining operation provides the road salt that drivers are so dependent on during the winter months. In the summertime, it's easy to forget about that, especially as you watch boaters and swimmers enjoying the lake.

Once you've returned to the sidewalk, follow High Street downhill toward the lake. As the sidewalk curves down to the right, you'll probably spot beach umbrellas and families enjoying the lake well before you reach the official entrance to Fairport Harbor Lakefront Park. Stroll on the sand or take off your shoes and wade into the

Fairport Harbor Lakefront Park

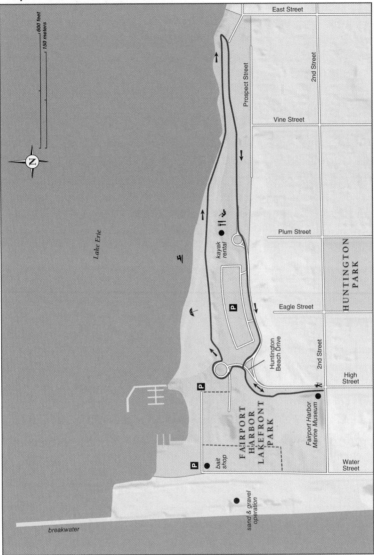

shallowest of the Great Lakes. The park offers very little shade, but the beach is dotted with all the amenities that make a visit, well, a day at the beach. Two small playgrounds, food concessions, kayak rentals, volleyball courts, and several picnic tables are sprinkled on the south side of the park.

You can walk about 0.3 mile along the beach before you reach the end of the park, all the while eyeing the two thick, silent stacks of the Perry Nuclear Power Plant perched on the horizon. Standing in odd juxtaposition to this picturesque landscape, they're quiet and easy to ignore but, at the same time, hard to resist snapping with your camera. Turn around and walk on the beach to the western edge of the park, where you can access the fishing pier for another look at the lake—and most likely, some large commercial and private boats in action.

Once you've soaked up some sun and stored a few images in your mind, camera, or both, return to the top of the village of Fairport Harbor, where your visit began.

NEARBY ACTIVITIES

During the summer months, there's plenty to do right here. Besides swimming, active visitors can rent kayaks at the park to enjoy Lake Erie's waves. While there's no admission fee for visitors walking on the beach, there is a parking fee. A surf chair, or all-terrain wheelchair, is available for visitors with physical disabilities; call 440-639-9972 for more information. Dogs are allowed only on the paved parking lot and in the designated dog swim area, and all dogs must be leashed. In town, history buffs can visit the Finnish Heritage Museum, just down the street from the lighthouse (440-352-8301; finnishheritagemuseum.org). If you'd like to explore another part of Erie's shore, consider Mentor Lagoons Nature Preserve (page 121) or Headlands Beach State Park, both less than 10 miles from Fairport Harbor.

• •

TRAILHEAD GPS COORDINATES: N41.75683° W81.27721°

DIRECTIONS Take I-77 N to Exit 163 and merge onto I-90 E, following signs to Erie, Pennsylvania. Go 10.9 miles to Exit 185 and merge onto OH 2. Go 15.6 miles, following signs to Painesville, and exit at OH 283/OH 535/Richmond Street toward Fairport Harbor. Turn right (northwest) on Richmond and then continue straight on Fairport Road/High Street. Continue following the road for a total of 2.2 miles. The lighthouse is at the corner of High and Second Streets; the park is down the hill, where High Street becomes Huntington Beach Drive.

Fairport Harbor beach boardwalk

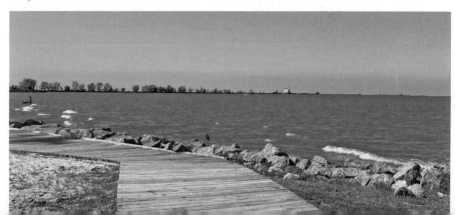

21 HACH-OTIS SANCTUARY STATE NATURE PRESERVE

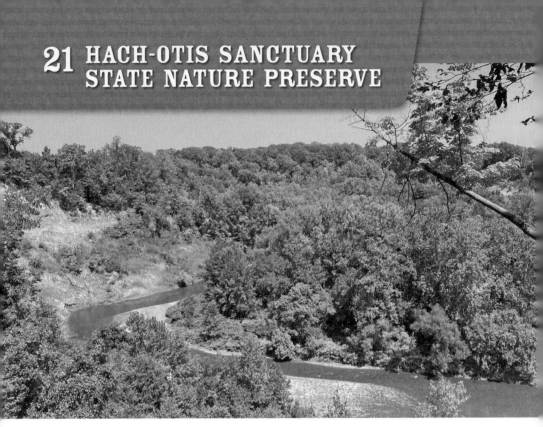

The Chagrin River snakes through Lake County.

THE SOUTHERN EDGE of this shady preserve offers great views of the Chagrin River, but it may feel precarious to anyone with a fear of heights. Warnings aside, this shady spot offers great bird-watching, a little slice of solitude, and some of the most breathtaking views in northeast Ohio.

DESCRIPTION

Since 1944, Hach-Otis Sanctuary State Nature Preserve has been protected as a bird sanctuary. The Hach, Otis, and Clark families who are primarily responsible for its preservation should be commended—their foresight and generosity have benefited not only the wildlife but also countless people who enjoy the land's remarkable scenery. Thanks to continued efforts by the state, local communities, and volunteers, adjoining properties have been added to the original preserve, and Hach-Otis now protects 130 acres. The trail system has not been expanded, making it even more of a harbor for birds and other wildlife in this otherwise very-developed corner of Lake County.

The parking lot is completely shaded, thanks to a thick beech-maple-oak canopy. The boardwalk trail is adjacent to a kiosk, where a trail map is posted. An unmarked (but oft-used) dirt path meanders north and tempts you to step off the boardwalk— but don't. While it meets up with the official trail in about 0.25 mile, the footing and

DISTANCE & CONFIGURATION: 1.2-mile figure eight

DIFFICULTY: Easy, with one staircase, a hill, and some very precarious edges

SCENERY: Forest, ravine, stunning river views

EXPOSURE: Mostly shaded

TRAFFIC: Light

TRAIL SURFACE: Dirt, grass

HIKING TIME: 1 hour

DRIVING DISTANCE: 28 miles from I-77/I-480 exchange

ACCESS: Daily, 8 a.m.–4 p.m.

MAPS: USGS *Mayfield Heights;* also at trailhead and park website

FACILITIES: None

WHEELCHAIR ACCESS: No

CONTACT: Audubon Society of Greater Cleveland: 216-556-5441, clevelandaudubon.org; Ohio Department of Natural Resources: ohiodnr.gov/go-and-do/plan-a-visit/find-a-property/hachotis-state-nature-preserve

LOCATION: Skyline Dr., Willoughby Hills

scenery are better on the sanctioned path. Even if your curiosity is piqued, hiking etiquette and legitimate concerns about erosion should keep you on the right track.

To complete the loops in a clockwise fashion, follow the wooden boardwalk, where you have hardwood trees for company; soon after the boardwalk ends, you'll meet a few hemlocks. As you continue on a dirt trail, veering left onto the North Loop, you'll start to notice how busy this corridor is with a variety of birds. You may catch a glimpse of a pretty little gully on the property's northern border. You will almost certainly encounter some of the many birds that crisscross the woods. Pileated woodpeckers, aptly named bank swallows, and owls are often sighted here; sometimes turkeys surprise visitors too. As you continue following the trail northeast, you can appreciate the rustic nature of the preserve in general and this trail in particular. Several tree falls have been cut away to allow you to pass, and the woods are thick. (You'd be smart to wear bug spray when you visit.)

While the trail is rustic, it is relatively level and easy to follow. It's almost like a bit of teasing—the calm before the storm—as it leads you to the edge of the preserve. And let's be clear: The emphasis belongs on *edge*.

About 0.5 mile from the trailhead, you'll reach the periphery of the preserve, turning right to appreciate its stunning view of the Chagrin River, about 150 feet below. As fantastic as the view is, hikers must not lose themselves in the moment—the edge is quite obviously eroding, day by day, minute by minute. (You'll see evidence for yourself shortly.) I recommend allowing a safety zone of 4–5 feet away from the edge; let common sense prevail.

Along this picturesque portion of the preserve, mind the trail map—although some unofficial paths are apparent, the sanctioned trail continues northeast and approaches a gully. If you find yourself precariously close to the edge, you've probably strayed, so turn away from the rim, look south and into the woods again, and you'll find the intended path. Follow it, and soon daylight bleeds through the canopy; you'll emerge from the woods and stand overlooking the Chagrin River again.

Hach-Otis Sanctuary State Nature Preserve

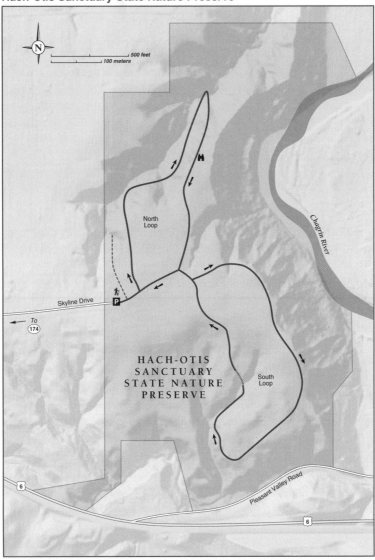

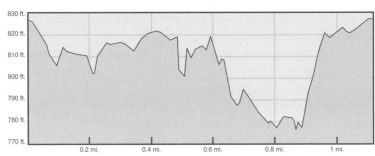

From this point, stop and turn to consider the northernmost overlook you just left. The erosion on the banks, probably where you were just standing, will likely convince you that staying away from the brink is the right thing to do.

The lesson is important, but don't let it overshadow the beauty here. I believe that this is the most picturesque spot on the trail—if not for pure scenery, then for its sweeping view. Even though directly west you can see OH 91 in the distance, to the east, you can appreciate just how high you are above the fields and homes on the other side of the river.

As the trail bends southwest, you follow it within spitting distance of the edge again. Notice the ravine that defines the southern portion of the trail and the preserve. Soon you return to the boardwalk trail, just a couple hundred feet from the parking lot. You can end your visit here, of course, if you're very time-pressed. But keep going, and you'll see a different side of this preserve.

Continue on the South Loop of the boardwalk trail, veering left (east). This portion of the boardwalk isn't long either. After you step onto the dirt trail, the path takes you once again to a narrow overlook area, where common sense is your best friend—there is no fence rail or other warning signs. Because of the primitive nature of this trail, I strongly recommend that you bring your better judgment on this hike and leave dogs and young children at home for this outing.

Now and again, your feet will find the boardwalk trail, likely put in where needed to help hikers across softer spots on the path. As the loop fans out to the east, you'll

Hach-Otis is a sanctuary for birds and people.

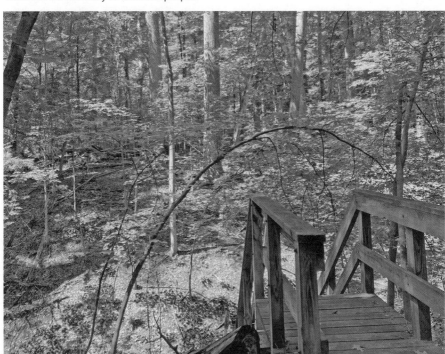

start to see that you're circling around a gully, also eroding, but shored up by a variety of plants, including several types of ferns and a thicker population of hemlocks.

On the South Loop, too, it's hard to stay on the trail, but obvious clues help guide you. In some areas, trees have noticeably been cleared away with the help of chainsaws and volunteers.

Because the woods are insulating, even in the hottest months, I recommend long pants and long sleeves on this hike—it's cool and very buggy. Hey, you may not like the bugs, but they're a big draw for the many birds you probably came to see.

Also because of the cool, shady nature of this area, you're likely to spot mayapples along the trail, long after their season is over on other trails.

With so many warnings in this description, why did I include these trails? There are several reasons. The dense bird population, wildflowers, and stunning scenery certainly earn high marks. Yet Hach-Otis offers even more. While the North Loop features fantastic views, the South Loop's less-dramatic ravine gives hikers a chance to feel as if they are immersed in nature, even though they are actually still within earshot of passing cars on OH 91 and I-271.

In short, we need to be able to let nature take our breath away, and to get away, in the middle of it all. You can do that here.

As the trail curves to the north, you're heading once again to the parking lot, your car, and your cares. But first you have to cross that gully you've been flirting with since you first saw it from the North Loop. A rustic but lovely set of stairs leads down, into, and across the gully.

Once across, you're out of stairs. A series of about a dozen railroad ties—the most strenuous and demanding part of the trail—helps you climb back up and out. If you need a distraction from your exertion, don't worry; the birds will likely be entertaining you all the while, as they're even more active on the south side of Hach-Otis than they seem to be on the north. Soon, you return again to the boardwalk, leading you back to the parking lot, likely more enthused than exhausted by the ground you've just covered.

• •

TRAILHEAD GPS COORDINATES: N41.59143° W81.41156°

DIRECTIONS Take I-480 E to Exit 26 and merge onto I-271 N. Go about 13 miles, continuing on I-90 E, and take Exit 189 to OH 91/SOM Center Road in Willoughby Hills. Follow OH 91 south about 1 mile, then turn left (east) onto US 6/Chardon Road. In 1.2 miles, turn left (north) onto OH 174/River Road, and then make an immediate right (east) onto Skyline Drive to the preserve parking lot.

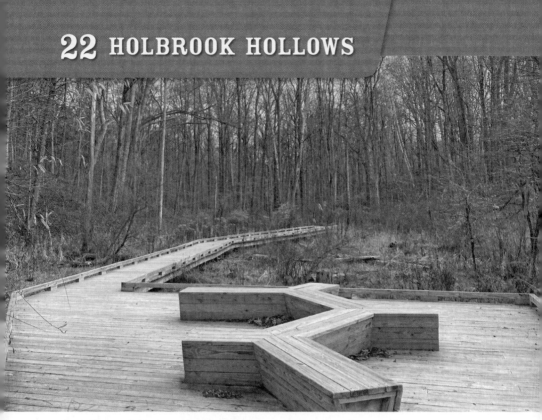

Relax as long as you like . . . but don't miss the ravine views!

ALMOST EVERYONE IN your hiking group will find a special spot here: There's a nature play space for the younger set, and trail surfaces vary from paved to (easy) creek crossings. A spacious seating area on the boardwalk is the perfect place for lunch, long chats, or just lounging.

DESCRIPTION

If you want to take the kids to a cool nature play space and then go for a hike, this is a great choice. The play space sits between the main parking area and the lodge, so it's hard to miss. The good news is there's no age limit for this play space—so everyone in your group can have some fun before your hike. Just save a little energy for the trail's gentle hills.

When you're ready to start your hike, from the southwest side of the parking lot, follow the signs for White Pine Way. Its paved surface wanders through the trees—yes, pines, but also beech and sugar maples—before it turns and begins to head south. At that point, about 0.4 mile in, turn left onto Old Ironsides Run, which hikers share with equestrians.

Note: For those with mobility limitations, White Pine Way is a completely accessible loop that returns to the parking lot. Winding its way through the wooded

DISTANCE & CONFIGURATION: 2.2 mile out-and-back with 3 loops

DIFFICULTY: Easy, with some gentle hills

SCENERY: Forest, ravine, creek crossing

EXPOSURE: Mostly shaded

TRAFFIC: Light

TRAIL SURFACE: Pavement, dirt, crushed limestone

HIKING TIME: 1 hour

DRIVING DISTANCE: 17 miles from the I-77/I-480 exchange

ACCESS: Daily, 6 a.m.–11 p.m.

MAPS: USGS *Chagrin Falls;* also at trailhead and park website

FACILITIES: Restrooms and water at trailhead

WHEELCHAIR ACCESS: White Pine Way, yes; nature trails, no

CONTACT: geaugaparkdistrict.org/park /holbrook-hollows

LOCATION: Country Lane, Chagrin Falls

scenery for a total of 0.5 mile, it makes a nice, mostly shaded excursion for visitors in wheelchairs, strollers, and anyone who appreciates flat surfaces.

Old Ironsides' hard-packed dirt-and-gravel trail leads you down a stairway and across a tributary of the Aurora Branch of the Chagrin River, then over a footbridge. (Horses have an alternate path over the creek here.)

As the trail veers left, you'll pass an entrance to Timber Ridge Trail—and soon after, another entrance to the short loop trail. You can follow Timber Ridge on your return trip—for now, stay on Old Ironsides. The path rolls gently along, almost fully shaded when the trees are leafed out.

Soon after you cross over another tributary, you'll turn right to pick up the primitive Bucktail Trail. Don't let the "primitive" designation concern you; while the trail narrows and is more dirt than hard-packed sand and stone, it's not a difficult trek. (A good pair of sneakers can carry you through.) Bucktail's narrow, less-traveled, more heavily wooded 0.6 mile may give you a sense of *really* being in the woods for a time, but shortly after Bucktail intersects with Old Ironsides again, your scenery really changes.

Turn right when you meet up with Old Ironsides, and walk up a gentle slope to a broad boardwalk with a spacious geometric-designed seating area. Pause, pose, or play here as you see fit, then continue north on Old Ironsides.

When you reach a covered viewing platform, you can turn around to complete the hike as described. The trail doesn't stop here, though—if you follow Old Ironsides north from here, you will find it ends at the Cleveland Metroparks' Bridle Trail, where you can head west to reach South Chagrin Reservation. Or, just a little farther north on Old Ironsides, you can opt to add 0.5 mile to your total mileage by taking the short, exposed Marsh Trail, which leads to the park's smaller entrance, off Franklin Street.

But that's not part of today's hike! Once you've soaked up the meadow and wetland view from the platform, follow Old Ironsides south, past Bucktail Trail; just after your second stream crossing, turn left onto Timber Ridge Trail.

Timber Ridge is aptly named, as you'll have a good look at the ravine and the river's tributaries below. Like the Bucktail Trail, Timber Ridge feels a little more

Holbrook Hollows

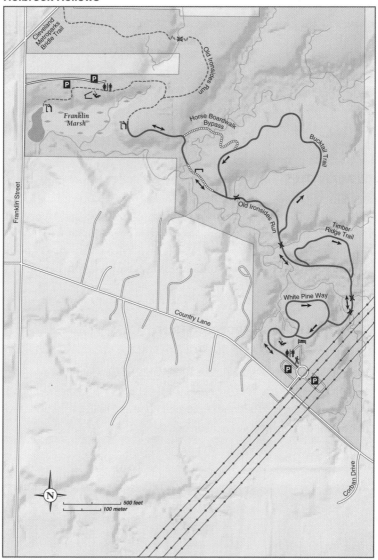

primitive. You'll see a few oaks mixed in with the fairly young beech and maple trees through here. When Timber Ridge ends at Old Ironsides, turn left again onto Old Ironsides, which you'll follow back to White Pine Way. Hold onto those feelings you had of being immersed in the woods because the next bit of scenery you'll encounter is a little different.

After turning left onto White Pine Way to complete that loop, you'll walk under power lines for a short time. Don't despair—we all like electricity and the conveniences it brings, right? Besides, it's a good reminder that if we don't plan ahead to preserve some land, we may run out of woodlands to walk through.

Speaking of conveniences, before returning to the parking lot, check out the reservable lodge, which opened in 2019. If it looks like a good place for a party, you're right. The back garage door opens fully to allow access to a tiered deck with a fire pit. And, unlike many park shelters, alcohol is permitted here when the lodge has been reserved. *Note:* Alcohol cannot be carried out into other park areas, such as on the trails or playground.

NEARBY ACTIVITIES

Feel like a different kind of hike? Liberty Ledges (page 260), with its cool rock formations, is about a 15-minute drive from Holbrook Hollows, and Henry Church Jr. Rock, at South Chagrin Reservation, is also nearby (page 89). Looking for lunch and perhaps a more urban stroll? The center of Chagrin Falls, with a variety of shops and its small, namesake falls, is also just about a 15-minute drive from here.

• •

TRAILHEAD GPS COORDINATES: N41.40408° W81.38351°

DIRECTIONS Take I-480 E to I-422 to Exit 18 for OH 91/SOM Center Road. Take a sharp left onto Solon Road and go about 1.7 miles. Turn right onto Chagrin River Road and follow it for about 0.4 mile. Turn left onto Holbrook Road and follow it for about 0.8 mile to reach Country Lane (the park entrance) on your left.

Viewing platform at Holbrook Hollows

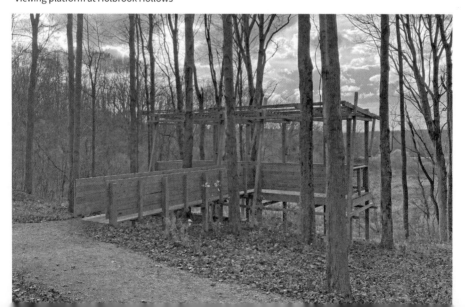

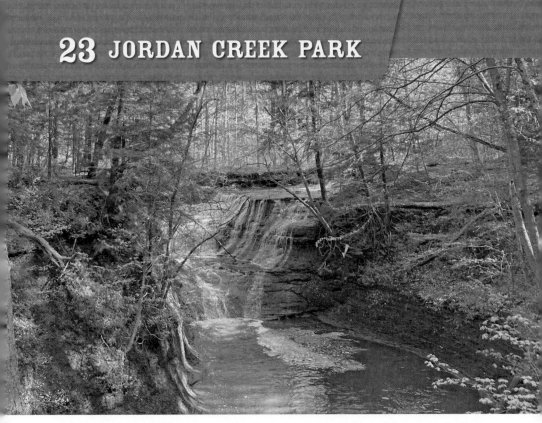

With a drop of almost 30 feet, Chair Factory Falls is just a short distance from the Greenway Corridor.

LIKE THREE PARKS in one, Jordan Creek offers a nature-themed playground for nimble adventurers, a sprawling nature education center, and forested trails that lead to quiet streams and a waterfall that wows.

DESCRIPTION

After parking in the upper lot by the Environmental Learning Center, it's almost impossible to ignore the Adventure Play area. Designed for kids ages 7 and up, the area includes a climbing wall, a 30-foot-long rope bridge, a zip line, and other activities that challenge balance and confidence. It's a great place to start and finish your hiking exploration—and the same can be said for the Environmental Learning Center.

Built as the main hall for a church camp that previously owned the property, the sprawling building is now a welcome center and educational hub. While there's plenty to see inside, if you're here for a hike, head outside. From the south end of the Environmental Learning Center, step onto Jordan Creek Crossing Trail and follow it as it wends down to the creek, for a short time sharing the path with the Buckeye Trail. Catch your breath as you cross over the wide bridge and enjoy a view of the creek (and a small falls) for the first time because you'll soon be heading uphill.

At the top of the rise, you're at the intersection of Ridge and Research Station Loop Trails. Turn left and take a quick excursion down a set of stairs to reach the edge

113

DISTANCE & CONFIGURATION: A balloon and an out-and back for a combined total of 3 miles

DIFFICULTY: Easy–moderate

SCENERY: Beech-maple forests, vibrant stream, and 30-foot-high waterfall

EXPOSURE: Mostly shaded

TRAFFIC: Moderate

TRAIL SURFACE: Crushed gravel, dirt, and pavement

HIKING TIME: 2+ hours

DRIVING DISTANCE: 36 miles from I-77/I-480 exchange

ACCESS: Daily, 6 a.m.–11 p.m.

MAPS: USGS *Perry;* also at trailhead and park website

FACILITIES: Restrooms, water, and reservable picnic shelter

WHEELCHAIR ACCESS: Only Learning Loop Trail, around the environmental center, is accessible.

CONTACT: Lake Metroparks: 440-358-7275, lakemetroparks.com/parks-trails/jordan-creek -park; Jordan Creek Park Environmental Education Center: 440-256-2118

LOCATION: Alexander Road, Painesville

of Jordan Creek, which you'll otherwise see mostly from a distance. Up close, Jordan Creek seems to sparkle on a sunny day. The serene view from the edge of the creek hardly suggests it could have been powerful enough to sustain industries, but it was.

Climbing back up to the trail intersection, you'll note several yurts that serve as the Remote Research Station. While you can hike any or all of the woodland trails from this point, to follow the map and description here, veer left to take Ridge Trail to Tulip Tree Trail for a counterclockwise loop.

You'll start up a slight grade. While these trails are rated "easy," some visitors may disagree. The level, hard-packed limestone surface makes for stable footing, but there are hills. Fortunately, there's plenty to see in the young woods on both sides of you, so pause to enjoy the scenery. In the spring, you'll spot wild violets, mayapples, and jack-in-the-pulpit, along with blossoms from the namesake tulip trees.

YOU HAVE OPTIONS

When you reach the intersection of the Ridge and Tulip Tree Trails, consider how long you want to spend on the nature trails. In this hike description, I turned right onto Tulip Tree, looped back to Ridge, then turned left onto Ridge to follow it back to the Environmental Learning Center so I could get to Chair Factory Falls before sunset. That route totaled 1.7 miles. However, if you combine Tulip Tree, Ridge, and Research Station Loop, you can log almost 3 miles on the nature trails before returning to the Environmental Learning Center the way you came, via the short Jordan Creek Crossing Trail. The Learning Loop Trail, just behind the Environmental Learning Center, offers another 0.4 mile, dotted with interpretive signage, and leads to the amazing playground area.

Whatever combination of trails you take—they're all fully shaded in summer, with lovely colors in fall—I recommend allowing time to visit Chair Factory Falls. If time (or daylight) is running short, you might even opt to just take a short hike to the falls.

Jordan Creek Park

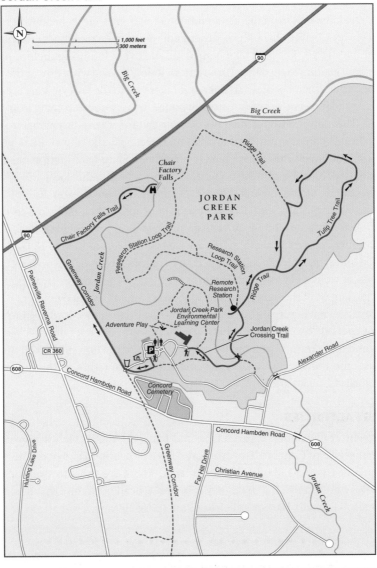

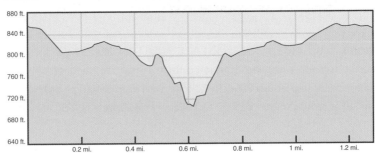

To reach the falls from the Environmental Learning Center, head west to access the Greenway Corridor from the southern end of the main parking lot, turning right onto the paved trail. The path takes you uphill and over a footbridge before you reach the dirt trail leading to the falls. Turn right to follow it as it twists down; the descent is gentle at first, then becomes steeper as it takes you to the falls viewing area.

Along the way, you'll almost certainly notice freeway noises coming from I-90, on your left. The traffic noise and the trail's twisting nature serve as distractions, so that the sight of the falls comes almost as a surprise. At 30 feet high, the falls were a popular spot for hikers, who snuck onto private land to view them. Since Lake Metroparks acquired the falls and additional land in 2010, you don't have to sneak in. But locals are still discovering these trails, so you might feel like you've stumbled onto a secret. Enjoy it, despite the road noise; ironically, the falls had a part in creating this well-trafficked corridor.

While it may seem strange to be in nature, gazing at a waterfall while listening to freeway noise, remember that the falls are well named. From 1846 to 1893, these falls powered industry, which included the manufacturing of not only wooden chairs but also beds, as well as hay and manure forks. The waterwheel driven by these falls was one of the largest in the area, standing 5 feet wide and 32 feet in diameter.

From the viewing area, you're still several dozen feet above Jordan Creek, which may not roar but certainly has proven itself a powerhouse over time. When you've had a good look, retrace your steps back to the top of the limestone path, then turn left back onto the Greenway Corridor and left again to return to the main parking area at Jordan Creek Park.

NEARBY ACTIVITIES

The Greenway Corridor is a paved hike-and-bike path that stretches almost 5 miles from Painesville to Concord Township, and from its southern end, it connects to the Geauga Park District's Maple Highlands Trail. There are spots to stop for refreshments along both trails. If a beach day is in order, head north on I-90 about 20 minutes to reach Fairport Harbor Lakefront Park (page 100).

• •

TRAILHEAD GPS COORDINATES: N41.78858° W81.17428°

DIRECTIONS Take I-480 E to I-271 N to I-90 E. From I-90, take Exit 200 for OH 44, heading toward Chardon/Painesville. Turn left onto Auburn Road, then left again onto Crile Road, which becomes Auburn Road. In 0.2 mile, turn right onto Concord Hamden Road, and then left onto Alexander Road. The park entrance address is 7250 Alexander Road.

24 LAKE ERIE BLUFFS

Lake Erie Bluffs is a good place to spot eagles.

HIKE IN THE company of various shorebirds, climb up the observation tower to gaze across Lake Erie, and stick your toes in the water, if you wish, at this Lake County Metropark.

DESCRIPTION

In 2012, 139 acres on Lake Erie's shore—tucked behind established industrial and residential developments, yet relatively unspoiled—were officially opened to the public. Later, this Lake County Metropark was expanded to 600 acres, and it's been growing in popularity ever since. In addition to nearly 3 miles of hiking trails, Lake Erie Bluffs boasts several scenic overlooks, two primitive campgrounds, a natural beach, fishing, and fantastic birding opportunities. The land mix includes coastal marshes and prairies.

Although kayaks may enter and exit the lake from the beach, there are no launch ramps, so boaters must carry all equipment to and from the parking lot. (And it's a tough slog.) The beach access here is chiefly that: access, so we can soak up and savor the lake at its natural best. In fact, Lake Erie Bluffs has been named one of the best beaches to hike! So where should you start? The stunning overlook beckoning from the east end of the parking lot seems like a good place.

Climb up the 50-foot-tall observation tower, and when you reach the top, go ahead and stare. The lake is the main attraction here and deserves your attention.

DISTANCE & CONFIGURATION: 3.2-mile figure eight

DIFFICULTY: Easy–moderate

SCENERY: Lake Erie's shore, natural bluff habitat

EXPOSURE: Mostly exposed

TRAFFIC: Moderate

TRAIL SURFACE: Crushed gravel, dirt, and sand

HIKING TIME: 1 hour

DRIVING DISTANCE: 47 miles from I-77/I-480 exchange

ACCESS: Daily, 6 a.m.–11 p.m.

MAPS: USGS *Perry;* also at trailhead and park website

FACILITIES: Restrooms, water, and reservable picnic shelter

WHEELCHAIR ACCESS: Yes, partially: Bluff Loop and Eagle View Trails are densely packed gravel; Shoreline and Forest Edge Trails, no.

CONTACT INFORMATION: Lake Metroparks: 440-358-7275, lakemetroparks.com/parks-trails /lake-erie-bluffs

LOCATION: Clark Road, Perry

From here you can also get an overview of the property: to the east, there's the mostly shaded Eagle View Loop Trail; to the west, Bluff Loop Trail; and in between, the Lakeview and Shoreline Trails deliver exactly what their names suggest.

When you are ready to climb down, turn left from the bottom of the tower to follow Eagle View Loop Trail as it rolls east over several small hills. You really could see an eagle here, as active adults are in the area. Of course, you are also likely to see (and hear) several varieties of shorebirds on this short loop. A handful of benches dot the trail, so you can stop and see who swoops in to take a look at you.

When you return to the parking lot trailhead, continue straight and follow Lakeview Trail about 0.25 mile west to Bluff Loop Trail. Both trails offer views of the lake and its habitat from a vantage point atop the bluffs. They are also bike-, wheelchair-, and stroller-friendly. However, Shoreline Trail isn't, so plan accordingly. (If you plan to ride, bring a lock, too, so you can leave your bike behind to enjoy a sandy stroll.)

Walking (or rolling) along these flat trails, in addition to the natural scenery, you'll see the entrance to one of the park's two primitive campsites, as well as a stairway leading to a lakeside observation deck. Take those steps down to access Shoreline Trail, and turn right to head east on the beach.

As you start on Shoreline Trail, you'll traipse downhill under the shade of mature trees, probably hearing the lake before you see it. Once you arrive on the thick silvery sand, you may have to step over large branches and driftwood as you pick your way across a fairly wide expanse of beach. While the point of this trail (and the park itself) is to allow us to enjoy our Great Lake, this particular spot is not especially inviting for swimming, and park rules prohibit it. You might dip your toes in the water, so you can say you did; then continue your walk on shore. Don't be surprised if you find yourself slowing down here, and not just to enjoy the scenery. The sand can be thick, meaning every step requires a bit more effort. As in the rest of the park, birding opportunities abound here. And on this trek, you'll see something else that is distinctly Erie.

When you reach the eastern end of the beach trail, you can't help but notice the stacks of Perry Nuclear Power Plant. Of the 61 nuclear power plants in the United

Lake Erie Bluffs

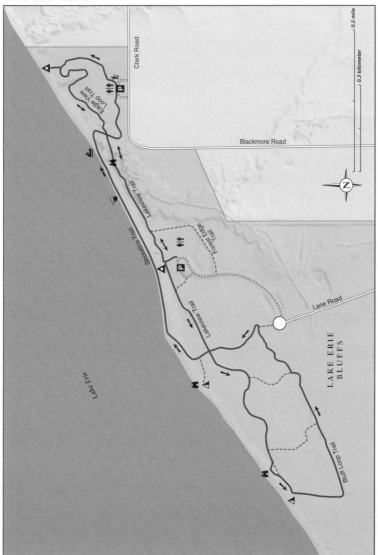

States, 2 sit on the Lake Erie shore: Perry, here, and Davis-Besse, in Oak Harbor. Although Perry's plant was scheduled to close in 2019, as of this writing, it remains in operation. Even if smoke isn't billowing from the stacks, the structures are awesome, if unnatural, sites along the shore, adding interest to the overall picture. They are a reminder that we certainly leave our mark here, sometimes intentionally, sometimes absentmindedly.

Speaking of absentmindedness, as you walk along the beach, with its colorful assortment of rocks and driftwood and pretty, fragile white shells, unfortunately, you'll also notice a few items your fellow humans have left behind. A gentle nudge: It doesn't have to be Earth Day to carry a small trash bag and pick up debris from the trail. Future generations will appreciate it, even if they don't know your name. To return to the parking lot, climb back up to meet the Eagle View Loop Trail.

NEARBY ACTIVITIES

Even more so than other parts of the very green and lush Lake County, Perry is dotted with nurseries and greenhouses. If you're seeking a specific tree or plant, or advice on growing almost anything, you're likely to find what you're looking for within a mile or two of Lake Erie Bluffs. And if your return trip takes you west along OH 2, you'll be very close to Fairport Harbor, where you can swim, tour the lighthouse, or visit a museum (page 100).

• •

TRAILHEAD GPS COORDINATES: N41.78863° W81.17409°

DIRECTIONS Take I-77 N to Exit 163, and merge onto I-90 E, following signs to Erie, Pennsylvania. Go 10.9 miles to Exit 185, and merge onto OH 2. Continue on OH 2 E for 19.7 miles, when it ends and becomes US 20. Follow US 20 for 1.1 miles to Blackmore Road in Perry township. Turn left (north) and follow Blackmore 1.3 miles until it ends. Turn right (east) onto Clark Road. The park entrance will be on the left (north). Note that there are two entrances to the park; for easiest trail access, use the entrance at 2901 Clark Road.

One of many spots to enjoy a view from the bluffs

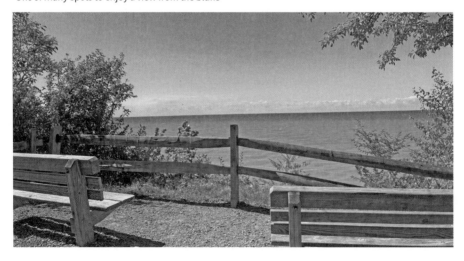

25 MENTOR LAGOONS NATURE PRESERVE

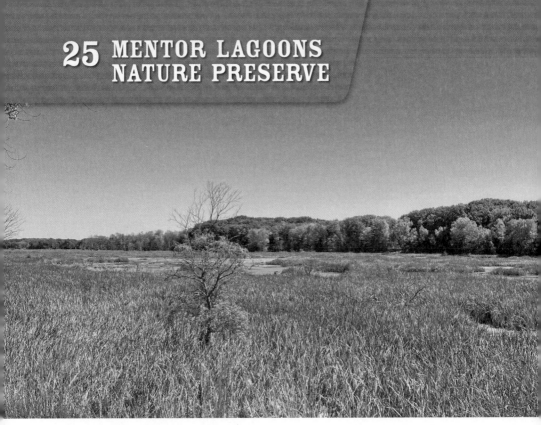

Hike, bike, kayak, or just relax at Mentor Lagoons.

THIS GREAT PRESERVE protects the largest unbroken bluff forest in northeast Ohio and one of the finest coastal dune communities in the state. Rare plants and more than 150 species of birds can be found here—along with some solitude.

DESCRIPTION

Purchased by the city of Mentor in 1997, the 450-acre Mentor Lagoons Nature Preserve protects one of the few riverine marshes still surviving along Lake Erie's shore. (And more than 800 acres of similar marshland is preserved at Mentor Marsh State Nature Preserve, on the east side of Mentor Lagoons.) On the west side of this city preserve is Mentor's marina, dedicated to recreation, not preservation, which isn't necessarily a bad thing—after all, enjoying our natural resources makes us more likely to want to protect them.

With that in mind, you have options on how to enjoy this preserve. The city offers kayak rentals in season; call ahead to reserve if you want to paddle when you visit. (*Note:* Swimming is prohibited here.)

With six different trails, you have hiking options too.

The Marsh Rim Trail is the most primitive of the trails here, and it's worth trekking. To maximize your distance, follow Marsh Rim, then join back up with

DISTANCE & CONFIGURATION: 4- or 5-mile loop

DIFFICULTY: Easy

SCENERY: Lake Erie shore, riverine marshes, woodlands, wildflowers

EXPOSURE: Mostly exposed, except for Marsh Rim Trail, which is mostly shaded

TRAFFIC: Moderate

TRAIL SURFACE: Hard-packed limestone, dirt, soft sand

HIKING TIME: 2–3 hours for all trails

DRIVING DISTANCE: 33 miles from I-77/I-480 exchange

ACCESS: Daily, sunrise–sunset

MAPS: USGS *Mentor;* also at trailhead, marina office, and cityofmentor.com/wp-content/uploads/Mentor-Lagoons-Marina-Trifold-2019-web.pdf

FACILITIES: Restrooms by marina office

WHEELCHAIR ACCESS: Overlook and Marina View Trails are accessible via electric carts; call 440-205-3625 prior to visit to reserve a cart. Other trails are not accessible.

CONTACT: Parks, Recreation & Public Facilities Department: 440-974-5720, cityofmentor.com/departments/parks-recreation; marina phone: 440-205-3625

LOCATION: Harbor Dr., Mentor

Overlook Trail, for a total of almost 5 miles. If you forgot your bug spray or good trail shoes, or if you're not sure you have time or daylight to complete Marsh Rim, opt instead to take the Overlook Trail to where it ends, then return on Overlook, making an optional loop out of White Pine and Salamander Trails. This outing will give you almost 4 miles. Both options can be seen on the map.

For the longer route, head northeast from the trailhead parking lot on Overlook Trail, then turn right onto Marsh Rim Trail. The Cleveland Museum of Natural History works with the city here sometimes, and you may find some portions of the trail restricted while they conduct research and conservation projects. (Visitors must abide by all posted notifications.)

As you follow the shady trail northeast about 0.5 mile, it will feel quite primitive in places, even though—engulfed in the woods—you're likely to hear some boats on the lake. While the trail is narrow and vegetation can overtake the path, there are signs. Still, keep your eyes peeled for the sharp left, heading north, taking you back to Overlook Trail. Tangles of grapevines along the trail offer atmosphere for you, as well as shelter for many small animals. Speaking of animals, while leashed dogs are permitted on several trails, they're not allowed on Marsh Rim Trail.

After traipsing about 1 mile through the woods, you'll emerge to find a bench perched high above the lake. You'll also find your feet on the limestone of Overlook Trail. If you turn right, the trail continues northeast to a gated residential area immediately west of Mentor Marsh. Instead, head west–southwest for about a mile along this completely exposed section of Overlook Trail, walking high enough above the water to enjoy a great view of wildflowers growing amid tall marsh grasses. This is a great place for bird-watching, and because you're not far from Lost Nation Airport, don't be surprised if a big bird (a small plane) buzzes by too.

About 2 miles into your hike, you'll reach a cart turnaround. Here, by a rocky outcrop, a narrow unmarked path and stairs lead down to a very narrow beach,

Mentor Lagoons Nature Preserve

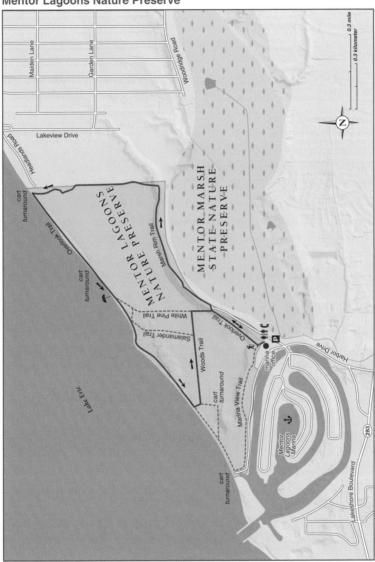

which is not much wider than a hiking boot. If you're willing to take the narrow path, walk down to the shore and follow along the beach for the next 0.5 mile. Otherwise, you can continue along Overlook Trail and turn left onto Woods Trail.

The shore of Lake Erie is interesting. Whether you follow the beachfront or upper trail, you'll probably spot a working rig or two on the lake; when you look east, you can see the east pier light near the Port of Cleveland. On the coarse sand, driftwood as soft as a baby's skin rests among stones worn smooth and ringed with various pastel colors. Rough-looking, rocky outcrops and ceaseless wind make the area seem especially wild; at times you can imagine that it is too big to be tamed. At the same time, you can't forget that you're surrounded by the civilization of a large industrial center, thanks to the eclectic collection of manufactured items also found here on the beach. The odd pieces of debris mingle on the beach next to the driftwood and sea oats. Gulls perch on antique machine parts; castaway tires embedded in the sand hold back erosion. On my first visit here, I found a button that was threaded by a small vine. It's something of a compromise, this use and abuse of our unique landscape.

As you continue southwest along the shore, about 2.5 miles from your starting point, you'll see two sets of wooden stairs leading up to the Woods Trail on your left. True to its name, the trail is entirely shaded. If you're looking for a cooler, greener trail, head in. It will take you east, and back to the inland portion of Overlook Trail, with access to Salamander and White Pine Trails along the way. (They join in the middle, so whether you follow either as an out-and-back or follow both to form a loop back to Woods Trail, you'll cover about the same distance.)

NEARBY ACTIVITIES

There's plenty to do right here! Bring your bike, if you like—cyclists are allowed on both Woods and Overlook Trails but are prohibited elsewhere in the park. During spring and summer, you can rent kayaks to explore the preserve from both sides of the shore. (Contact the marina at 440-205-3625.) Mentor hosts a handful of concerts here during the summer as well; see the city's website or Facebook page for the seasonal schedule.

For a look at a different sort of shoreline habitat, plan a visit to the lagoon's next-door neighbor, Mentor Marsh State Nature Preserve. The entrance is at 5185 Corduroy Road in Mentor. The nature center there, managed by the Cleveland Museum of Natural History, is open April–October, Saturday–Sunday, and November–March, the first Sunday of each month. For more information and a schedule of events, see cmnh.org/Mentor-Marsh.

• •

TRAILHEAD GPS COORDINATES: N41.72686° W81.33873°

DIRECTIONS Take I-77 N to Exit 163, and merge onto I-90 E, following signs to Erie, Pennsylvania. Go 10.9 miles to Exit 185, and merge onto OH 2. Continue on OH 2 E for 9.8 miles, and exit at OH 615/Center Street. Turn left (north) and follow Center Street as it becomes Hopkins Road. In 2.5 miles, turn right onto Lakeshore Boulevard and make an immediate left onto Harbor Drive. In 0.4 mile you will reach the trailhead parking, to the east of the docks and marina office.

26 ORCHARD HILLS PARK

There are several spots to reflect along the McIntosh Trail.

ROLLING OVER 237 acres, Orchard Hills Park is a unique place in Chester township. Operated as a golf course until 2007, today the property situated immediately west of the Patterson Fruit Farm invites nature lovers to enjoy its forest and meadow views; dramatic hills; and, nearby, a panoramic view of Lake Erie.

DESCRIPTION

Orchard Hills opened to the public as a golf course in 1962. The course saw its last tee time in 2007, when Geauga Park District, with grants from the Ohio and US EPA, began to restore the land. Today, the hills offer visiting hikers both a challenge and a reward. You may feel a bit of a burn as you walk the "course," but you'll also enjoy a great view and wonderful perspective on many facets of this versatile land.

With several intersecting loops, this park has options for you to take a shorter trek or complete all the trails for a total of 3 miles. The route described here gives a good overview of the property on a counterclockwise circuit.

Start from the northern parking lot, by the sledding shelter. Head west on the paved (accessible) Cricket Trail to connect to the McIntosh Trail. Turn right onto McIntosh, and you'll soon appreciate the rolling landscape.

The park district has successfully encouraged many native plants to return along the now-abandoned fairway, and you'll notice their work as soon as you step onto any

DISTANCE & CONFIGURATION: 2 miles with options to shorten or lengthen via connected loops

DIFFICULTY: Easy, with only a few rolling hills

SCENERY: Pine stands, orchard, meadows, wetlands, and a glimpse of Lake Erie nearby

EXPOSURE: Mostly exposed

TRAFFIC: Moderately heavy on weekends and evenings, particularly in the fall

TRAIL SURFACE: Crushed limestone, some dirt trails, short paved sections

HIKING TIME: Allow 90 minutes or more

DRIVING DISTANCE: 30 miles from I-77/I-480 exchange

ACCESS: Daily, 6 a.m.–11 p.m.

MAPS: USGS *Chesterland*; also at trailhead and park website

FACILITIES: None

WHEELCHAIR ACCESS: Sedge and Cricket Trails only

CONTACT: Geauga Park District: 440-286-9516, geaugaparkdistrict.org/parks/orchard-hills-park

LOCATION: Caves Road, Chesterland

trail—if you didn't know it was a former golf course, you probably wouldn't suspect it. In order for this property to become the idyllic hiking destination that it is, the Patterson family worked closely with the Western Reserve Land Conservancy and Geauga Park District. They arranged to have a conservation easement placed on the former golf course property, stating that the land would be used as a passive-use public park.

In this case, *passive* is a legal term; those who visit Orchard Hills Park can enjoy a variety of activities. Speaking of passive: Throughout the park, benches are strategically placed, making ideal spots to stop and consider the changes that this land has seen in a relatively short span of time. The natural rolling hills in this part of Geauga County lend themselves to cross-country skiing, and all of the trails are open for skiing when conditions are right. Though the trail sections generally follow paths that were originally paved for golf cart traffic, today McIntosh Trail has a mix of hard-packed gravel and natural surfaces.

Some remnants of the golf course design remain: The wide clearings that were necessary for long drives have also made this piece of land a favorite haunt of hawks and other birds of prey; watch for them as you wander Orchard Hills's paths.

After about 0.25 mile on the McIntosh Trail, Pine Warbler Trail juts off to the left. If you follow this short (0.2-mile) trail, you'll rejoin McIntosh and, if you turn left, you'll skip some of the hills and enjoy a lovely view of the pine stands, native forest, and wetlands.

To follow the hike mapped here, though, stay on McIntosh Trail and enjoy those hills! Shortly after passing a footbridge, you'll reach the western end of Pine Warbler Trail, then McIntosh rolls up and down a few more (smaller) hills and crosses another footbridge to intersect with White Pine Trail. Continue on McIntosh as it approaches the pond and intersects again with White Pine Trail, past the pond shelter. Soon, turn left on the paved Cricket Trail to make your way back to the parking lot for the sledding hill.

Orchard Hills Park

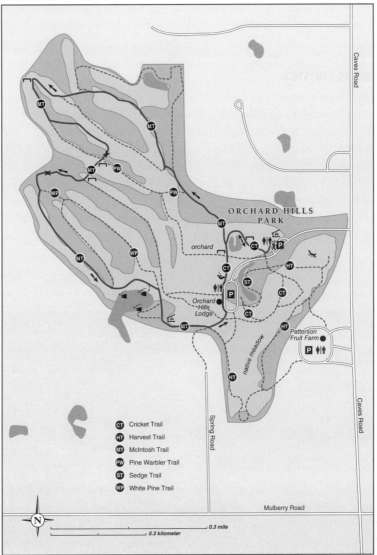

As you follow the Cricket Trail back to the lot, you'll walk along the edge of an apple orchard. The orchard is a sweet reminder of the annual treasure to be found here. But it won't be the first reminder you'll have—throughout the property, it's almost impossible to miss apples, as the fruit and their seeds have been scattered here for years by a variety of critters. (*Note:* Please don't pick the apples! The orchard here is still maintained by the Patterson family.)

Visitors who want a few more steps can explore the paved Sedge Trail and the natural-surface Harvest Trail, which make a great, easy introduction to hiking for toddlers.

NEARBY ACTIVITIES

Obviously, there's more to do right here. When the snow flies, the sledding hill just west of Caves Road is a popular destination with families. The supersmart design of the indoor-outdoor lodge gives visitors a nice place to warm up during the winter months or enjoy the sweet smell of the orchard during the warmer months. The park is popular year-round because the trails are groomed for cross-country skiing and the sledding hill is lighted for after-dark runs. Contact the Geauga Park District for sledding condition updates.

Next door, Patterson Fruit Farm is definitely worth a visit. On Caves Road just south of the park entrance, the popular market is open year-round, offering fresh

Even on a cloudy day, you can see Lake Erie from here.

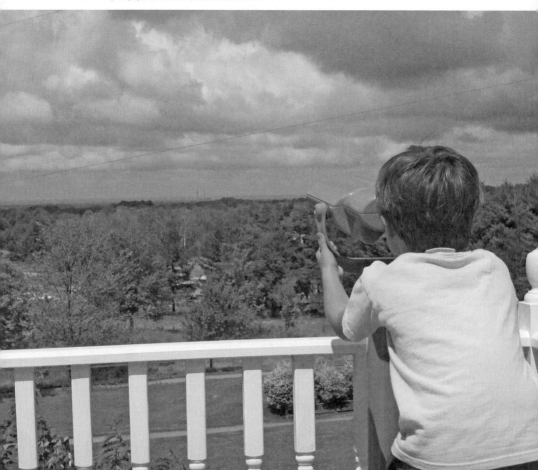

produce and baked goods. From a deck behind the market that overlooks Orchard Hills Park, visitors can enjoy a sweeping vista to the north, which includes a view of Lake Erie. It's one of the few spots in Geauga County offering a view of the lake.

Even on an overcast day, you can spot a layer of deep blue gray on the horizon. (Admittedly, binoculars help.) If it's more hiking that you're after, head east on Chardon Road/US 6 from here to find North Chagrin Reservation (page 77) or Hach-Otis Sanctuary State Nature Preserve (page 104).

• •

TRAILHEAD GPS COORDINATES: N41.56120° W81.36716°

DIRECTIONS Take I-480 E to Exit 26 (I-271 N). Once on I-271 N, go 7.3 miles to Exit 34 (US 322 E/Mayfield Road). Turn right (east) onto US 322 E/Mayfield Road, and go 4.6 miles. Turn left (north) onto Caves Road, and go 1.4 miles. The park entrance will be on your left.

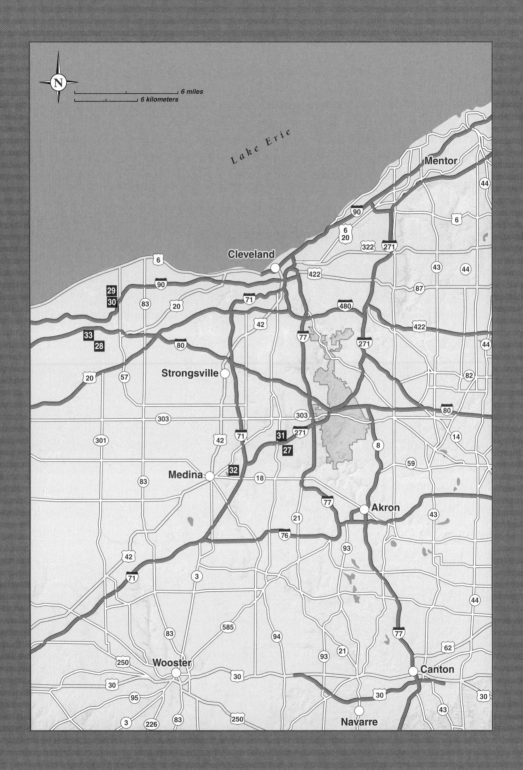

LORAIN & MEDINA COUNTIES

27 ALLARDALE PARK

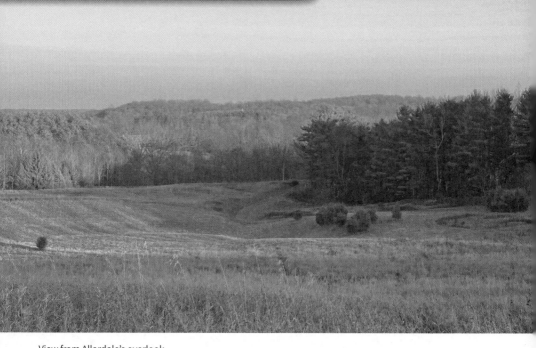

View from Allardale's overlook

WITH A VARIETY of habitats, wide and well-maintained trails, easy creek crossings, and marvelous vistas, Allardale Park is a joy to explore. Look a little closer and you'll find clues to the property's rich history.

DESCRIPTION

When Esther and Stan Allard donated their property to the Medina County Park District in 1992, they guaranteed that the land they loved would remain, for the most part, beautifully undeveloped. Just as beautiful was the guarantee that it would be shared with countless thousands for decades to come.

What the Allards did with the land before they gave it away is almost as impressive as their generosity. In the 1930s, they were among the first to practice soil-saving techniques such as contour strip farming and erosion control, using pine and spruce plantings on the steep hillsides here. The property was recognized several times as an outstanding example of forestry and land conservation.

As you roam the trails, you'll learn a bit about the Allards' legacy. And if you're just here for a great vista, you're in luck: on the western edge of the trails, there's one that's really worth the trek.

Where to start? Three natural-surface hiking trails and a paved, 0.5-mile accessible trail form interconnecting loops here. In this description, you'll follow the

DISTANCE & CONFIGURATION: 2.3-mile loop with shorter and longer options

DIFFICULTY: Easy–moderate

SCENERY: Rolling woodlands, stream, great sunset view

EXPOSURE: About half shaded

TRAFFIC: Busy

TRAIL SURFACE: Dirt and gravel

HIKING TIME: Allow an hour or more

DRIVING DISTANCE: 20 miles from I-77/I-480 exchange

ACCESS: Daily, 6 a.m.–dark (one hour after sunset)

MAPS: USGS *West Richfield;* also posted at trailhead and on website

FACILITIES: Restrooms and water at trailhead

WHEELCHAIR ACCESS: No, but there is a 0.5-mile paved trail

CONTACT: Medina County Metroparks: 330-722-9364, medinacountyparks.com /parks/parks/allardale

LOCATION: Remsen Road, Medina

outermost ring in a counterclockwise direction for a 2-mile hike. Doing it that way, you get to enjoy the stunning overlook near the end of your loop. Along the way on both the pink and yellow trails, particularly in the spring, you will find some nice wildflower displays.

From the trailhead sign, turn right and follow the blue hexagon sign markers. The trail is paved as it heads down a steep, short hill. Where the pavement ends, the trail veers left to lead you over a short footbridge. White pines and Norway spruce stand to your left; on your right you'll have a good view of the reservable lodge and the park's popular sledding hill.

Leave the blue trail, following the pink trail (oval markers) up a set of stairs. The pink trail—the most strenuous of those here— takes you up a hill, on the trail and stairs, with a view of the pines and ravine below.

After crossing a footbridge (and another nice view), you'll soon reach the yellow trail, then another footbridge. There the path splits briefly into two, so you can choose the drier one. Where they rejoin, you'll have the option to continue south to cut through the midsection of the park along the stream restoration corridor. If you do that, you'll miss the overlook—so unless you have to hurry home, stay on the yellow trail with its square markers, heading east to the lovely Scotch pine planting. The trail meanders south, then veers left (east) a bit to rejoin the blue trail. Again, you can choose to cut short your visit here—but don't!

Follow the blue trail as it takes you through a thick forest scene, then to a planting of black walnuts. As you creep uphill, you'll arrive at the magnificent overlook. The uphill portion on the blue trail is paved as you approach the overlook. Several benches along the trail offer a chance to slow your heart rate and enjoy the view.

The climb is rewarding, even if you don't stop to soak it all in. But I suspect the Allards—and the park planners—were hoping you'd do just that.

Speaking of the park planners, they did a great job. While some early tree identification tags remain (and add greatly to a visit), the newer interpretive signs offer

Allardale Park

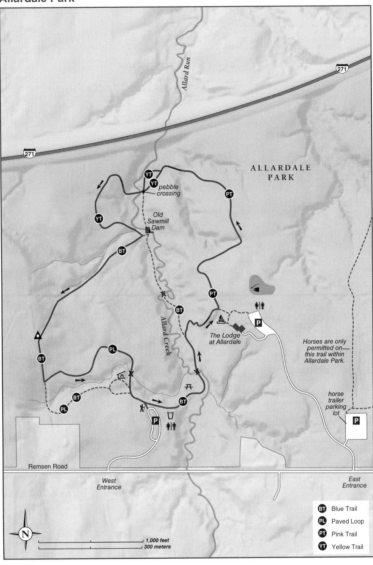

Legend:
- BT Blue Trail
- PL Paved Loop
- PT Pink Trail
- YT Yellow Trail

Allard Run

271

ALLARDALE
PARK

YT pebble crossing

Old Sawmill Dam

YT

BT

PT

PT

Allard Creek

The Lodge at Allardale

Horses are only permitted on this trail within Allardale Park.

horse trailer parking lot

Remsen Road

West Entrance

East Entrance

1,000 feet
300 meters

N

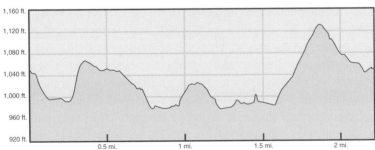

enough education to answer your basic questions, and perhaps to further pique your interest in the native and introduced species here.

As you head downhill on the nature trail, it soon offers up another playscapes area, then joins up in two spots with the fully paved loop. You can continue south on the blue nature trail or the paved portion—from this point, all trails lead back to the parking lot (and your starting point).

Thanks to three separate nature playscapes on the short, paved loop, it's very popular with families. The way things came together to create this gem in the Medina County Park District, I think it's worth a visit for hikers and nature lovers of all ages and abilities. Check out the "You Have Options" section below for some thoughts on how to make these trails a good fit for you.

YOU HAVE OPTIONS

If you turn left from the trailhead, heading west, you can follow the paved loop less than a quarter of a mile, then continue north onto the natural-surface blue trail another 0.2 mile to reach the overlook. This might be a good compromise for new hikers just testing their legs. Trail runners or others looking to maximize their hill work can create a figure eight by starting on the blue trail north through the center of the park, continuing on the yellow nature trail, then heading east to pick up the pink trail. Where the pink trail intersects the blue trail, head north again to complete a figure eight by following the blue trail west back to the parking lot.

NEARBY ACTIVITIES

Did you bring your horse? From the east entrance to the park, there's a nearly 2-mile bridle trail here.

If you're hiking on two legs and want to explore some nearby trails with very different scenery, you're in luck. Worden's Ledges at Hinckley Reservation is just about a 5-minute drive from Allardale (page 148), and Bath Nature Preserve, in neighboring Summit County, is just about 5 miles west of here (page 216).

• •

TRAILHEAD GPS COORDINATES: N41.19000° W81.69868°

DIRECTIONS Follow I-77 S to OH 176 (Exit 143) toward I-271/Richfield. Turn right onto OH 176 N, then left onto Brecksville Road. At Everett Road, turn right, then turn left onto North Medina Line Road, which becomes Remsen Road. Note that there are two entrances on Remsen Road. Use 401 Remsen Road as a street address to reach the trail entrance (west entrance); the other (east) entrance goes to the lodge parking lot.

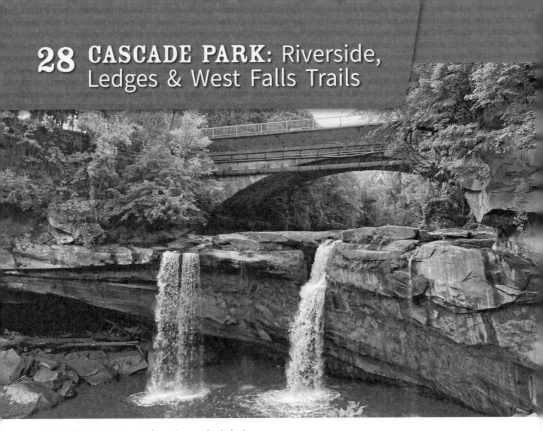

28 CASCADE PARK: Riverside, Ledges & West Falls Trails

Two Falls Bridge, as seen from the overlook deck

CASCADE PARK IS a lovely little surprise tucked below the city of Elyria, with a small nature center; paved trails along the river; and some rockier, hilly paths that lead to two scenic waterfalls.

DESCRIPTION

It's a good thing that Cascade Park has a large parking lot: between the playground, nature center, sledding hill, and easy access to the North Coast Inland Trail, it's popular for many reasons. Just want to relax? Several benches dot the riverside. But you're here to hike, so let's get started.

The hike described here starts from the southern end of the playground. Follow Riverside Trail, which is paved and then a sidewalk surface, as it heads uphill. A sign to your left indicates your entrance to Ledges Loop and the West Falls Trail. Follow the still-paved path into the woods. Although several sections of this paved path are quite steep, bicycles are permitted here, so if you find you're sharing the trail with cyclists, give them plenty of room to maneuver.

Shortly after stepping onto the Ledges Loop, you'll see a short path to your left leading to a small overlook deck. After a look-see, return to the paved portion of the trail, turning left to continue south. The pavement gives way to a sandier, rocky path as you head toward the river.

DISTANCE & CONFIGURATION: 1-mile loop

DIFFICULTY: Moderate due to rocky, uneven surfaces

SCENERY: Waterfall, ledges, river view

EXPOSURE: Roughly half shaded, half exposed

TRAFFIC: Busy

TRAIL SURFACE: Pavement, grass, dirt, and loose stone

HIKING TIME: 1–1.5 hours

DRIVING DISTANCE: 30 miles from I-77/I-480 exchange

ACCESS: Daily, 8 a.m.–sunset

MAPS: USGS *Lorain;* park map posted at trailhead

FACILITIES: Restrooms by trailhead parking lot

WHEELCHAIR ACCESS: No—while a long stretch of trail is paved, most of these trails are uneven and rocky.

CONTACT: 440-865-8786, loraincountymetroparks.com/cascade-park

LOCATION: 387 Furnace St., Elyria

Moving among Berea Sandstone formations, it's easy to imagine how this land and the all-important river have supported a variety of industrial and recreational uses over the years. Look a little closer and you'll notice that the small tributaries feeding the river are still instrumental in the environment, supporting northern species like hemlocks, numerous deciduous trees, and dozens of bird species that make their homes in them.

As you approach the southernmost point in your hike, you'll hear the falls before you can see them. Just about at the half-mile mark, you'll take the short West Falls Connector trail to reach an overlook deck with a stunning view of the 35-foot West Falls.

From the deck, you can also see Two Falls Bridge, constructed in 2007. Just south of here, where the East and West branches converge at Cascade Falls, is where the Black River officially begins. It runs just over 15 miles before emptying into Lake Erie in the city of Lorain.

Unfortunately, because the land on both sides of the river has shifted (the forces that shaped this area are still at work!), Two Falls Bridge was closed in 2019. As of this writing, it was unclear whether the bridge could be returned to service safely. In the meantime, enjoy the view from this deck . . . and when you're ready, retrace your steps to the paved trail, turning right to continue to the river's edge.

Follow the mostly paved trail as it heads down a short-but-steep hill. When the path curves left and approaches the river, the wide asphalt trail transitions to concrete. It's almost as if slabs of a sidewalk escaped the city to hang out by the riverside. A wide, flat area at the edge of the river serves as an unofficial splash pad. While you can't see the falls from here, you can still hear the rushing water behind you.

YOU HAVE OPTIONS

If you prefer to stay on sidewalks or pavement, you can trace your footsteps back up to the paved portion of the West Falls Trail to make this an out-and-back. The hike as mapped is a loop. Both options are approximately the same total distance.

Cascade Park: Riverside, Ledges & West Falls Trails

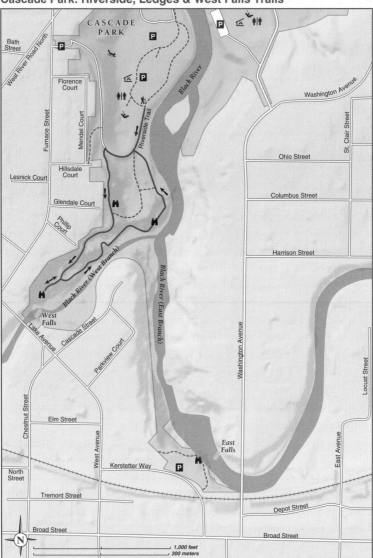

Once you've enjoyed the view from the river's edge, it's time to head uphill to the natural-surface portion of the Ledges Loop. Follow a short stairway up to the trail, the river still in view.

This portion of Ledges Loop is more primitive, and while it's unmarked in places, it's still fairly easy to follow. When in doubt, remember that you're following the trail along the river to complete the loop in a counterclockwise fashion from where you began. Explore the rock formations as you make your way back toward the parking lot.

Even this somewhat-wild portion of the trail is popular with many local hikers, so you'll almost certainly meet other people while you're on Ledges Loop. Almost too soon, the trees thin and the trail emerges at a set of stairs across from the playground and your starting point.

NEARBY ACTIVITIES

Bring your bike if you like to pedal. The North Coast Inland Trail rolls 25-plus miles along a paved path through Cascade Park, crosses the Black River, and is routed through neighborhoods where the dedicated hike/bike trail isn't yet completed. Tram rides are scheduled at Cascade Park and several other Lorain County properties throughout the year; watch the website for dates and times.

Like waterfalls? The East Falls viewing area, off Kerstetter Way, just a short drive from here, offers paved, easy access to see the falls.

Before leaving Elyria, stop at the beautiful downtown square, which features an impressive fountain and several historic markers.

Want to visit the beach? It's not far: Lakewood Beach Park (3801 East Lake Road, Sheffield Lake) is popular with local families.

• •

TRAILHEAD GPS COORDINATES: N41.37657° W82.10900°

DIRECTIONS Follow I-480 W to OH 10 W, then take OH 20 W, toward Carlisle Township. Exit at Grafton Road and turn right. Continue onto East Avenue, turning left onto Broad Street. Turn right onto West Avenue, continuing onto Lake Avenue. Turn right onto Furnace Street, then right again onto Cascade Street to enter the park. Park in the lot by the playground.

The Black River flows through Cascade Park.

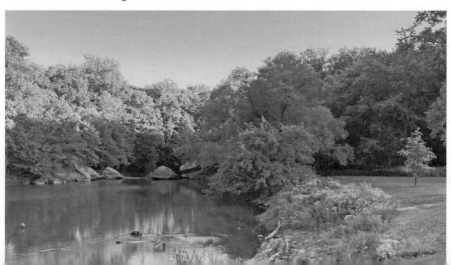

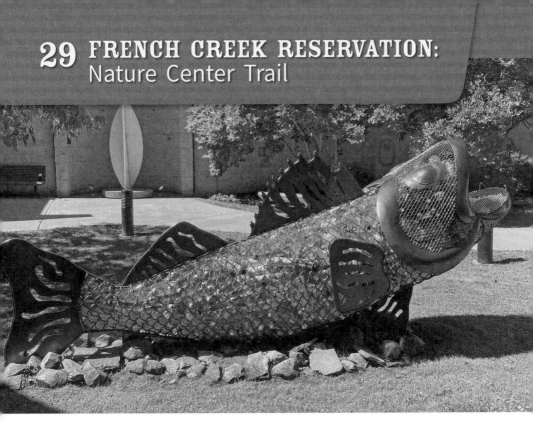

This fish sculpture delivers a message about recycling.

ENJOY A SHORT-BUT-HILLY out-and-back hike on what are said to be "the most forested trails in Lorain County."

DESCRIPTION

Note that there are two entrances to French Creek Reservation. For this hike, start at the nature center (4530 Colorado Avenue, Sheffield), not the Pine Tree Picnic Area. Although trails from both properties connect, here they're mapped out for two different hikes. See the "You Have Options" section for more information.

While the trails here are lovely, going into the nature center makes a visit even lovelier. Inside, live animal exhibits and other displays appeal to all ages. For this hike, if you time it right, you can start from the southwest corner of the parking lot and pick up the trail behind the nature center, then linger inside after and ask questions of the naturalists.

From the parking lot, follow the asphalt connector trail that leads south to the back of the nature center. Even before you reach the gravel Nature Center Trail, you'll want to venture to the edge for your first good peek at French Creek.

Yellow trail markers indicate a left turn to pick up the Nature Center Trail. Soon you'll be heading downhill to more creek and ravine views. Along the way you'll find a bench and, soon, a lovely footbridge.

DISTANCE & CONFIGURATION: 1.2-mile out-and back; loop through the nature center for indoor fun

DIFFICULTY: Easy, but some steep sections

SCENERY: Creek corridor, forest wildflowers spring through fall, sandy ravine cliffs

EXPOSURE: Almost entirely shaded

TRAFFIC: Moderate–heavy

TRAIL SURFACE: Dirt and other natural surfaces

HIKING TIME: Allow an hour for hiking and lingering by the creek

DRIVING DISTANCE: 30 miles from I-77/I-480 exchange

ACCESS: Daily, 8 a.m.–sunset

MAPS: USGS *Lorain;* also posted at trailhead

FACILITIES: Restrooms and water inside the nature center

WHEELCHAIR ACCESS: No

CONTACT: Lorain County Metroparks: 440-949-5200, loraincountymetroparks.com /french-creek-reservation

LOCATION: Colorado Ave., Sheffield

Like most metroparks, this one isn't far from the bustle of automobile traffic. For the most part, however, sounds of nature overpower the sounds of traffic on nearby Colorado Avenue.

Roughly following the creek, veer left again to stay on the trail. Be aware that a number of active but unofficial trails lead down to the water's edge here, and avoid them as best you can. (Extra foot traffic only speeds up erosion.)

Follow the wide, well-grated gravel path to another bridge and overlook, with eastern hemlocks on both sides of the creek. Just past the second bridge you will come to a hill that's steep enough to increase your heart rate. This is the steepest point of your trek, and if you're completing the trail as an out-and back, it's your turnaround point.

YOU HAVE OPTIONS

Here, where the Nature Center Trail and Big Woods Trail intersect, you can continue on the Big Woods Trail to add another 1.5 miles to your outing. If you continue on Big Woods from here, you can expect a flatter but still shady nature trail—sans creek views. (Big Woods Trail is described in the next hike description.) As this is the end of the Nature Center Trail, most people turn around and retrace their steps to complete a pretty and challenging 1.2-mile track.

Full disclosure: I prefer a loop trail to an out-and-back, but the configuration has grown on me over the years. An out-and-back offers an opportunity—well, forces you, really—to see the same trail from a different perspective. The Nature Center Trail here has enough varied scenery and elevation change to provide a good workout and great views, going both ways.

As you return, heading north, you have another chance to soak up the views of sandstone and rocky cliffs and enjoy the sounds of French Creek trickling quietly toward the Black River.

French Creek Reservation: Nature Center Trail

If you started your hike from the parking area (outside the nature center), watch for a stone stairway before you reach the asphalt trail connector to visit the center now. The stairway leads to the nature center's back entrance, and the 30 steps offer a little extra cardio too.

Inside the nature center you'll find a play space, displays of live turtles and native fish, and a large indoor wildlife-viewing area. If the center is closed when you visit, don't despair—a few informational displays outside, near the front entrance, are worth a stop.

NEARBY ACTIVITIES

A flatter, 1.5-mile loop through the woods awaits at French Creek Reservation's Pine Tree Picnic Area. Got a kayak? French Creek boat launch and bike trail is close by, on Old Colorado Avenue, off Colorado Avenue, just west of East River Road. (Boat launch coordinates are N41.46017° W82.11269°).

• •

TRAILHEAD GPS COORDINATES: N41.46075° W82.09984°

DIRECTIONS Follow I-480 W to I-90 W, exiting at OH 611 W (Colorado Avenue) in Avon. Turn right onto OH 611 and follow it about 2.5 miles to the French Creek Reservation Nature Center entrance. Use street address 4530 Colorado Avenue, Sheffield, for trailhead parking.

Visitors can enjoy the park's namesake French Creek from several points on the trail.

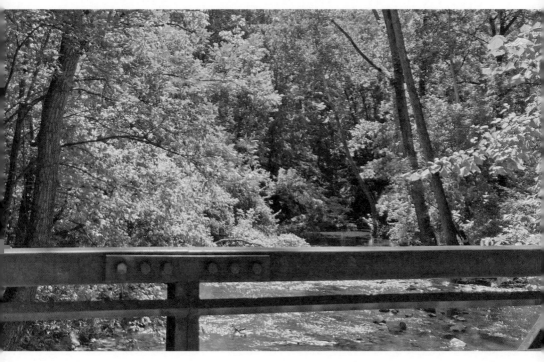

30 FRENCH CREEK RESERVATION:
Pine Tree Area & Big Woods Trail

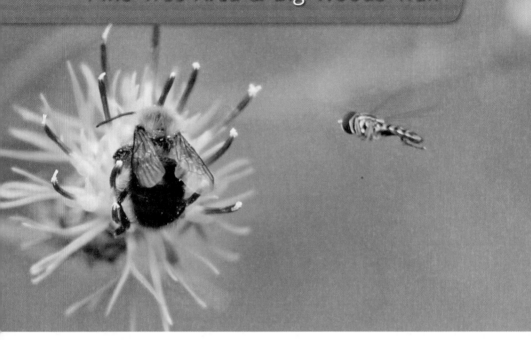

Most insects you'll find outside are more fascinating than fearsome.

THE "WILDER" OF the two French Creek Reservation properties, Pine Tree Picnic Area features a large playground and a quiet but well-traveled, shady loop trail.

DESCRIPTION

From French Creek Road, follow the park's long, shaded driveway until it ends. There you'll find a large playground, a covered reservable shelter, a restroom, and the primary entrance to the Big Woods Trail. At first glance, this trail doesn't seem very exciting, but it's extremely popular with locals and sees a surprising amount of traffic, even during the week. Maybe it's not all that surprising—myriad studies have proven that we are nature-deprived, nationwide, and it's probably true of the entire human race. So here, in this inviting-but-not-obviously-exciting trail, is a testament to the fact that a woodsy loop trail appeals to a wide audience. Especially one that's flat and easy to negotiate.

So go ahead and step onto the hard-packed gravel trail. While you're sure to see other hikers on this loop, bicycles are permitted here, too, so be aware that you may share the trail with folks out for a relatively easy trail ride. The surface is easy for most strollers to negotiate, and possibly even for some wheelchairs. (The park district has designated it an accessible trail, but some of the surfaces could be difficult for those who rarely use their wheelchairs outdoors.)

DISTANCE & CONFIGURATION: 1.5-mile loop

DIFFICULTY: Easy

SCENERY: Woods and wildlife

EXPOSURE: Almost completely shaded

TRAFFIC: Busy

TRAIL SURFACE: Hard-packed gravel trail with some dirt sections

HIKING TIME: 30–45 minutes

DRIVING DISTANCE: 30 miles from I-77/I-480 exchange

ACCESS: Daily, 8 a.m.–sunset

MAPS: USGS *Lorain;* also posted at trailhead

FACILITIES: Restrooms at trailhead

WHEELCHAIR ACCESS: Yes

CONTACT: Lorain County Metroparks: 440-949-5200, loraincountymetroparks.com /french-creek-reservation

LOCATION: French Creek Road, Sheffield

From this entrance, the wide crushed-limestone trail meanders directly into the woods, but soon you'll find that it's not entirely shaded. Even in the exposed areas, thanks to the mostly hardwood forested landscape of this and the adjoining French Creek Reservation property, you'll enjoy a fine natural insulation from wind and noise on the Big Woods Trail. While it lacks the scenic creek crossings of the Nature Center Trail immediately north of here, you'll probably notice fewer traffic noises as you wander along.

Speaking of the Nature Center Trail, about 0.3 mile into the Big Woods Loop, a sign to your left invites you to head downhill on a sandier path toward the ravine scenery on the Nature Center Trail. To complete this hike, stay on the Big Woods Trail.

As you continue east, you'll see a few narrow, unmarked paths jutting off the trail, but the wide, mostly crushed-limestone path is easily identified as the intended route. Soon, you'll have a chance to dive deeper into the woods on an official trail. After covering about 0.7 mile, a sign indicating the Big Woods Primitive Trail beckons you onto a narrow dirt path.

YOU HAVE OPTIONS

This description follows the primary trail clockwise for just 1.5 miles; however, if you follow the Big Woods Primitive Trail offshoot, you'll add about half a mile to your distance for a 2-mile total loop. (*Pro tip:* You'll need insect repellent on the primitive trail almost anytime in the summer!) From here, when you follow the primitive portion of the trail, you'll continue east about 0.2 mile before turning right (south) and joining up with the main Big Woods Trail to return to the trailhead.

Another option, mentioned above, is to take the Nature Center Trail as an out-and-back to French Creek's nature center. Doing so adds some hills and creek views, plus a chance to visit the nature center. The combined distance of both trails, including the addition of the Big Woods Primitive Trail, is about 3.5 miles.

Shortly after the second junction with the primitive trail, Big Woods Trail crosses over the park roadway. Although most drivers are looking for hikers at this

French Creek Reservation: Pine Tree Area & Big Woods Trail

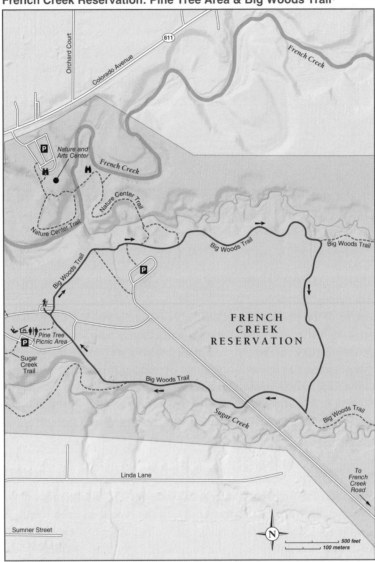

point, encourage young hikers or bikers in your party to stop and look both ways before crossing over the roadway.

On the home stretch of your clockwise loop, you'll catch sight of the playground, then dart back into the woods for a glimpse of little Sugar Creek, one of the two tributaries in addition to French Creek that all feed the Black River.

Soon you'll find yourself back at the picnic shelter and parking lot. If you'd like to see a bit more of Sugar Creek, head to the western edge of the parking lot to pick up Sugar Creek Trail. The 0.5-mile path has a soft woodchip surface and drains well. In fact, if you're just getting back into hiking, hoping to hook the next generation on nature, or looking for a shorter loop for any reason, it's a great place to start.

NEARBY ACTIVITIES

Just 2 miles away, at the "other" French Creek Reservation, you'll find a nature center with an indoor play space and wildlife observatory, along with the French Creek Theatre, which offers seasonal productions. If you're looking for another flat loop trail, see Rowland Nature Preserve in Elyria, about a 15-minute drive from here.

• •

TRAILHEAD GPS COORDINATES: N41.45706° W82.09971°

DIRECTIONS Follow I-480 W to I-90 W, exiting at OH 611 W (Colorado Avenue) in Avon. Turn right onto OH 611, following it about 1 mile before turning left onto Abbe Road N. Follow Abbe Road about 1.2 miles to French Creek Road, and turn right. Use street address 4540 French Creek Road, Sheffield, for the Pine Tree Picnic Area entrance.

You're likely to find a big hollow tree in the big woods—and it's likely to be home to a critter or two.

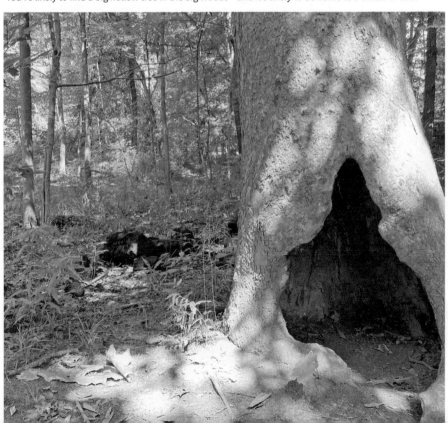

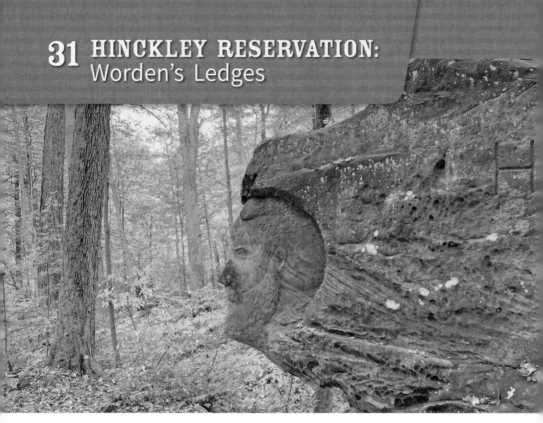

Noble Stuart left at least nine carvings on the land now known as Worden's Ledges.

LESSER KNOWN AND less crowded than other trails in Hinckley Reservation, Worden's Ledges Loop Trail packs a fascinating variety of natural and human-made scenery into a short-but-rewarding hike. Swimming and boating draw many to the park's lakes in the summer, but fall may be this trail's best season.

DESCRIPTION

Fans of Henry Church Jr.'s carvings in South Chagrin Reservation, meet Noble Stuart. In the 1940s, Stuart took to carving the large sandstone conglomerate rocks tucked behind his in-laws' family home. On this short, pretty wooded loop, you'll get to see them—but first, a bit of backstory is in order.

Before Stuart lived here, the land belonged to Hiram Worden. Worden was a tombstone and statuary carver who built a home here in 1860 for himself, wife Melissa, and their four children. After the couple died, their daughter Nettie inherited the estate. When she was 80, she married her third husband, the 64-year-old Stuart. A year later, she died, leaving the estate to Stuart.

Shortly thereafter, he began creating large carvings and smaller reliefs in the stones in the woods behind the house. His subjects varied, from presidents (Washington and Jefferson) to icons (Ty Cobb, a sphinx) to more personal symbols (a cross, a Bible, and Nettie's name in a pretty script).

DISTANCE & CONFIGURATION: 1-mile balloon with options to do 3–6 or more miles

DIFFICULTY: Easy

SCENERY: Woods, hills, ledges, historic carvings, and lakes (on optional loops)

EXPOSURE: Almost completely shaded

TRAFFIC: Moderate

TRAIL SURFACE: Dirt with some rocky sections

HIKING TIME: 30-45 minutes for Worden's loop

DRIVING DISTANCE: 20 miles from I-77/I-480 exchange

ACCESS: Daily, 6 a.m.–11 p.m.

MAPS: USGS *West Richfield;* also posted at trailhead and on website

FACILITIES: Parking only (for cars and horse trailers) at trailhead

WHEELCHAIR ACCESS: No

CONTACT: Cleveland Metroparks: 330-278-2160, clevelandmetroparks.com/parks /visit/parks/hinckley-reservation

LOCATION: 895 Ledge Road, Hinckley

The home stood until 2017, when it was demolished due to maintenance expenses. The parking area and trail are named Worden's Ledges because it was their estate, although Stuart arguably left the more permanent impression. Head onto the trail to see his handiwork.

Find the trailhead kiosk and map by a picnic table in the Worden's Ledges parking lot. From there, head north and descend into the woods, parallel to and just a bit east of the bridle trail. Thick maples shade the trail most of the year.

Although the trail is classified as easy, because it is narrow and uneven in places, it is not accessible, even for most rugged strollers.

After rolling down a gentle slope, the trail eventually splits; turn left to follow the loop portion, signed with white markers, clockwise. On the westernmost edge of the loop, you'll merge with the (yellow) bridle trail for a short time.

Going clockwise, you won't approach the ledges until you turn right, leaving the bridle trail. At that point you'll probably notice that, as is typical of ledge trails, it feels a little cooler between these big rocks. While ledge trails can be difficult to follow as intended, this one is well marked, with easier footing than at Nelson's Ledges and the nearby Whipp's Ledges, making it a good "starter" ledge trail for kids and new nature hikers.

As you search the rocks for Stuart's carvings—there are nine, or more, depending on how you classify a single work—you'll notice that, more recently, some graffiti artists have added their marks to these ledges. Art is art, you might say— but it is worth noting that when Mr. Stuart carved these rocks, he had the deed to the property.

The trail rolls and dips a bit before it turns west again and rejoins the out-and-back portion of the trail. Turn left, heading south, to return to the trailhead. Ready for more? There's quite a bit to explore at Hinckley Reservation, either on foot from here, or from another trailhead nearby.

Hinckley Reservation: Worden's Ledges

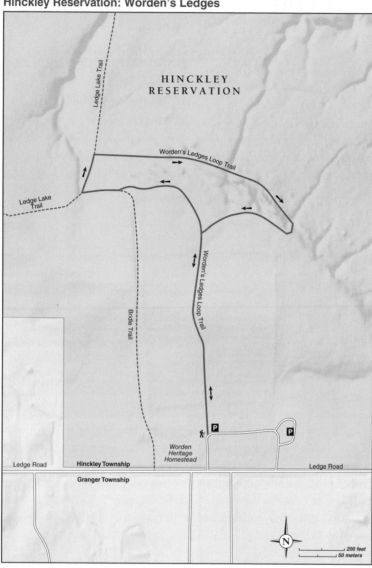

YOU HAVE OPTIONS

From here, you can follow the bridle trail, which connects to Ledge Lake Trail and Carriage Trail for a 2-mile loop, returning here, to Worden's Trailhead parking. For more miles, continue on Ledge Lake Trail, then follow the Buckeye Trail north where it joins with the 3.1-mile Hinckley Lake Loop. Staying close to the lake's edge, this trail can be muddy during a wet spell, in which case, you might want to take the (paved) All Purpose Trail that loops the lake for 3.3 miles. It offers much of the same scenery, with less squish. To enjoy Whipp's Ledges, park at either Whipp's Ledges Picnic Area or Top O'Ledges Picnic Area.

NEARBY ACTIVITIES

If you've enjoyed the ledges in Portage and Summit County, you'll want to visit Whipp's Ledges—they're well known for a reason. The stunning rock formations are just a short drive north and can be accessed off State Road. Hinckley Reservation's lakes are full of visitors who enjoy swimming and boating during the summer, and the crowds come back in the fall for the fabulous colors. In other words, there's no shortage of things to do right here. For more rustic trails nearby, try those at Richfield Heritage Park (page 273).

• •

TRAILHEAD GPS COORDINATES: N41.20269° W81.71824°

DIRECTIONS Follow I-77 and I-271 S, taking Exit 3 off I-271 toward Wadsworth/North Royalton. Turn right onto OH 94, and in about half a mile, turn right onto Ledge Road. Turn left into the Worden's Ledges parking lot. Use street address 895 Ledge Road for directions.

The Hinckley spillway dam will be 100 years old in 2027. A rehab project is expected to be completed in 2026.

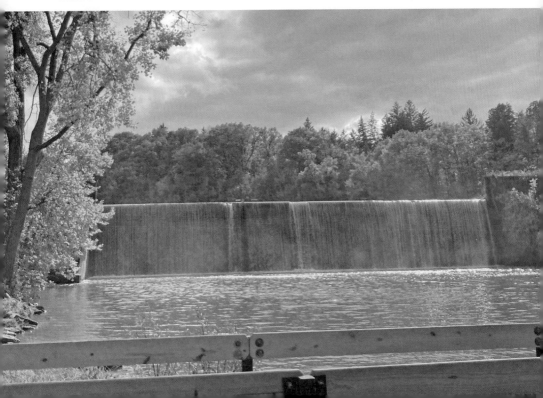

32 LAKE MEDINA

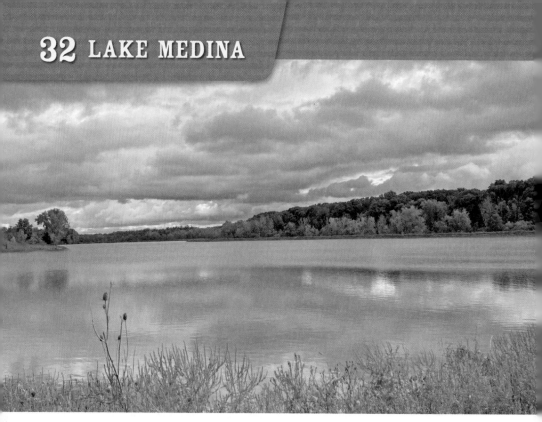

The hiking is easy here—and the park is growing.

THIS EASY LOOP overlooking expansive Lake Medina is flat and popular with dog walkers and joggers. Get here at sunrise for a real treat.

DESCRIPTION

Bordered by busy OH 18 to the south and Granger Road to the north, and situated just west of I-71, Lake Medina is an extremely accessible property. Between that and the fact that the park supports a wide range of activities, including hiking, fishing, biking, canoeing, and cross-country skiing, it can be a pretty busy place.

So here's a tip: If you want the place mostly to yourself, get up early and head over before sunrise. Not only is Lake Medina positioned for easy driving access, it's also a fine spot to watch the sun come up.

While you're unlikely to find any solitude here—especially on sunny afternoons—thanks to the wide trail and expansive views, it also never quite feels crowded.

Before you leave for this scenic lake loop trail, note that there are two entrances to the park. For this description, you'll start in a counterclockwise direction from the OH 18 lot trailhead, but as it's a straightforward trail, it would be as easy to follow from either direction or start from the northern entrance off Granger Road.

DISTANCE & CONFIGURATION: 2.5-mile loop

DIFFICULTY: Easy

SCENERY: Sprawling views of 105-acre lake ringed by trees

EXPOSURE: Almost completely exposed; partially shaded on summer and fall afternoons

TRAFFIC: Busy

TRAIL SURFACE: Hard-packed gravel with some dirt sections

HIKING TIME: 30–45 minutes

DRIVING DISTANCE: 26 miles from I-77/I-480 exchange

ACCESS: Daily, 6 a.m.–dark (1 hour after sunset)

MAPS: USGS *Medina;* also posted at trailhead

FACILITIES: Restrooms at trailhead

WHEELCHAIR ACCESS: No

CONTACT: Medina County Park District: 330-722-9364, medinacountyparks.com/parks/parks/lake-medina

LOCATION: 3749 Medina Road, Medina

The trail is paved at the trailhead, where it comprises part of the Greenway Trail. A few steps north of there, turn right toward a long staircase to get a good look at the namesake lake.

In the 1960s, wanting to supplement its water supply, the city built an earthen levy and pumped water from the west branch of the Rocky River to flood a portion of the valley. For several decades, the concrete pump house on the north side of the lake pumped water into the lake daily to be used for the city water supply.

In the early 2000s, when the city began to get its water from Lake Erie, the city and park district began planning for the artificial lake to become a recreational destination. It is—and not just for the area's human residents. Today Lake Medina is a migratory stop for a wide selection of waterfowl, including loons, grebes, and a variety of ducks, geese, and swans. Throughout the year, visitors report eagles, ospreys, and other birds of prey hunting for fish.

Buckeye Trail section- and through-hikers are also sometimes spotted here, as the Lake Medina and Greenway Trails overlap portions of the Medina section of the Buckeye Trail. Although there are no camping facilities here, trail amenities like restrooms and water—and being close to local restaurants—make for popular stops.

Like other waterfront trails with broad, shimmering views, and with no noticeable elevation changes, twists, or turns to distract your gaze, the distance here can be deceptive. If you let it, a walk on this narrow loop trail can be somewhat mesmerizing or meditative. Just don't zone out—you wouldn't want to miss a call from a passing jogger, cyclist, or dog walker!

Once you reach the northern turnaround point and return on the westernmost side of the loop trail, you will have some shade, at least during the summer months.

Starting in 2025, you will notice some construction activity, mostly concentrated on the northern end of the park. A local family's donation of more than 17 acres enabled the park system to plan, with the help of the family, an outdoor amphitheater, an indoor space for public programs, more trails, and an observation tower. Short story: visit now, then be sure to return. There will be more to see!

Lake Medina

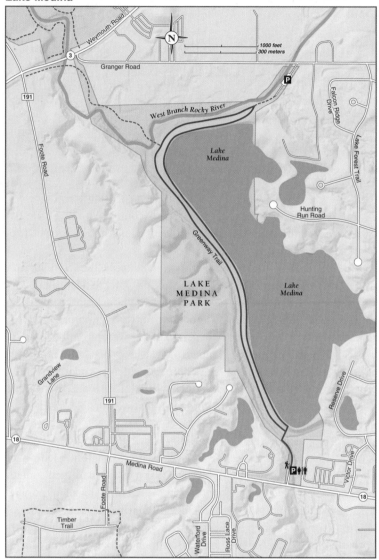

YOU HAVE OPTIONS

This is a pretty basic loop, so there's not much room for creative trail configurations here. However, if you bring your bike, you could choose to take the Greenway Trail north to Granger Road, where you can pick up the city's bike trails and pedal about 4 miles to reach the historic Medina Public Square. (The bikeway is a combination of bike-only trails and markings along city streets and therefore is not recommended for foot traffic.) It's also worth noting that for folks who are working their way up to longer distances, Lake Medina's two parking areas offer the option of hiking with a friend and leaving a shuttle vehicle at one entrance, so you can hike the length of the lake, but just once, for a distance of a little over 1 mile.

NEARBY ACTIVITIES

Fishing, cross-country skiing, and bicycling are allowed here. If you'd like to follow your hike here with a more urban walk, head west on OH 18 to Medina's very pedestrian-friendly historic downtown, where you'll find many interesting shops and restaurants. Prefer a "wilder" walk? Visit the Alderfer-Chatfield Wildlife Sanctuary, where you'll find almost 4 miles of rustic trails and the sprawling Oenslager Nature Center. The nature center is typically open Tuesdays–Saturdays; check the Medina County Park District's website for current hours. Mountain biking enthusiasts should know that the city maintains 10 miles of trails in the nearby Huffman/Cunningham and Reagan Parks. CAMBA members designed the trails for riders of various abilities. For more information, see the city's website at medinaoh.org.

• •

TRAILHEAD GPS COORDINATES: N41.13774° W81.82251°

DIRECTIONS Follow I-77 S to Exit 144, merging onto I-271 S toward Columbus. Merge onto I-71 S, then take Exit 218 for OH 18 toward Akron/Medina. Turn right. The park entrance is about 1.5 miles west of the exit. Use the address 3749 Medina Road, Medina, for GPS driving directions.

Get your vitamin D here: the trail perched above Lake Medina is fully exposed.

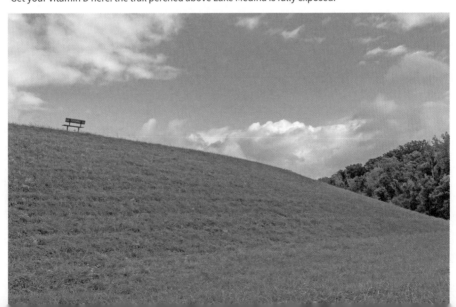

33 ROWLAND NATURE PRESERVE

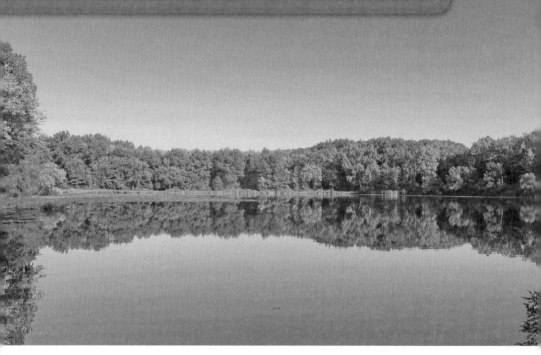

Rowland Nature Preserve's stocked lake is a popular spot to fish.

BIRDS AND OUTDOOR enthusiasts flock to this shady fishing pond surrounded by flat, wooded trails.

DESCRIPTION

While Rowland is a relatively small preserve, there's good reason to visit. More than 100 bird species have been noted here, and seasonal wildflower displays are no doubt of interest to the birds as well as the park's human visitors.

Before you even embark on the trails, children can burn off some energy on the small playground near the entrance, and visitors can contemplate our recent history at an area honoring those who perished in the attack on the World Trade Center. The memorial includes a piece of steel from one of the towers.

When you step on the trails, you'll find they're lined with deciduous trees, so the interconnecting loops are shaded during the summer months. They're flat, too, making them inviting for leisurely walks as well as trail running. While traffic noise is never far away, the trails and 13-acre lake offer lovely scenery, although rarely solitude, as it's a popular local spot.

Starting from the parking lot, Chipmunk Trail leads you about 0.1 mile to Mallard Trail. The first time I visited, I found a lot to like here, but I think my favorite

DISTANCE & CONFIGURATION: 1.1-mile figure eight with shorter and longer options

DIFFICULTY: Easy

SCENERY: Woods and wildlife, fishing lake

EXPOSURE: Almost completely shaded

TRAFFIC: Busy

TRAIL SURFACE: Hard-packed dirt and grass

HIKING TIME: 30–45 minutes

DRIVING DISTANCE: 30 miles from I-77/I-480 exchange

ACCESS: 24/7

MAPS: USGS *Lorain;* also posted at trailhead

FACILITIES: Restrooms at trailhead

WHEELCHAIR ACCESS: No, but the Mallard Trail will accommodate most strollers.

CONTACT: Elyria Township: 440-324-9462, sites.google.com/view/elyriatownship/community/rowland-nature-preserve

LOCATION: Murray Ridge Road, Elyria

part was the signage. All of the trails are marked with street signs, which made me wonder, why aren't *all* trails marked like this? Besides the fact that they're easy to see and hard to steal, there's also a bit of whimsy in seeing SQUIRREL TRAIL on such serious signs. Kudos to the Elyria Township crews who planted them here!

Following the signs, turn left onto Mallard to loop around the lake in a clockwise fashion. The dirt-and-gravel trail is level and firm enough for most strollers.

You can take in most of the lake from Mallard Trail. A large deck sits on the south side of the lake; in the middle, a small windmill powers the aeration system to help keep the fish alive year-round.

To follow the path as the figure eight shown in the map, at the end of Mallard (just past the lake), turn left to follow Wolverine Trail a short distance, then turn right onto Squirrel Trail.

Just about 0.1 mile along Squirrel Trail, turn left onto Turkey Trail, and then turn left again to follow Redhawk Trail as it loops back to Wolverine Trail.

YOU HAVE OPTIONS

You can shorten your distance by turning right from Mallard onto Wolverine Trail to just loop around the lake. On the east side of the lake, you'll find several benches well positioned to catch a sunset.

If you want to add a bit to your hike, follow the 0.36-mile Squirrel Trail to its endpoint, where it connects the park to a neighborhood, then return to Turkey or another connecting trail.

As you continue south on Wolverine Trail, it intersects with Squirrel and Mallard Trails. Along the way you'll catch glimpses of the lake on your right. Several picnic tables and park benches make nice spots for a lunch or dinner in the fresh air.

Wolverine also intersects with Deer Trail, which skirts a residential development and reconnects with Mallard on the south side of the lake. (If you follow it, you'll add about 0.3 mile to your trek.) In the hike as mapped, you'll continue to the south end of the lake on Wolverine, then turn right, following Mallard Trail to Kerstetter Lane.

Rowland Nature Preserve

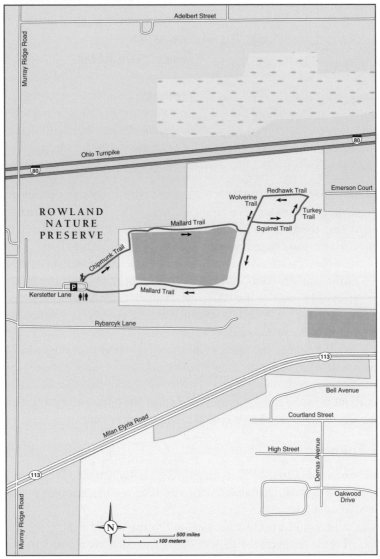

The lane was named to honor the Kerstetter family for its service to the community. In particular, it honors James L. Kerstetter, a longtime Elyria firefighter, and his son James "Jim" Kerstetter, a police officer killed in the line of duty in March of 2022.

From the intersection of Kerstetter and Mallard you can loop back to take one last look at the lake or follow Kerstetter back to the other end of the parking lot.

Rowland packs a lot of fresh air and greenery into a small space and otherwise developed Elyria Township, and it's clear the locals love it. Even if you have to drive a bit to visit, you'll be rewarded with its peaceful, easy hiking trails and scenery.

NEARBY ACTIVITIES

If you like to fish, bring a pole—you might get a bite from a largemouth bass, bluegill, crappie, or pumpkinseed sunfish. (Note that permits are required.) The lake is stocked by the Ohio Department of Natural Resources, and depth markers are posted around the perimeter of the lake. Looking for a hike with more hills? Try Cascade Park in Elyria (page 136).

• •

TRAILHEAD GPS COORDINATES: N41.387306° W82.149752°

DIRECTIONS Follow I-480 W to I-80 West to Elyria. Take Exit 145 to OH 57 N toward Lorain. Turn left onto Griswold Road and follow it about 1.7 miles, where it curves and turns into Murray Ridge Road. Follow Murray Ridge about 0.9 mile, then turn left into the entrance for the preserve.

Why aren't all trails signed like this?

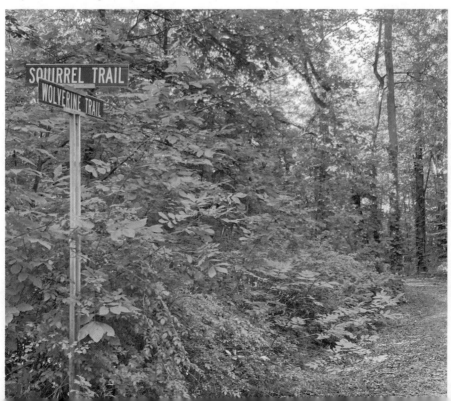

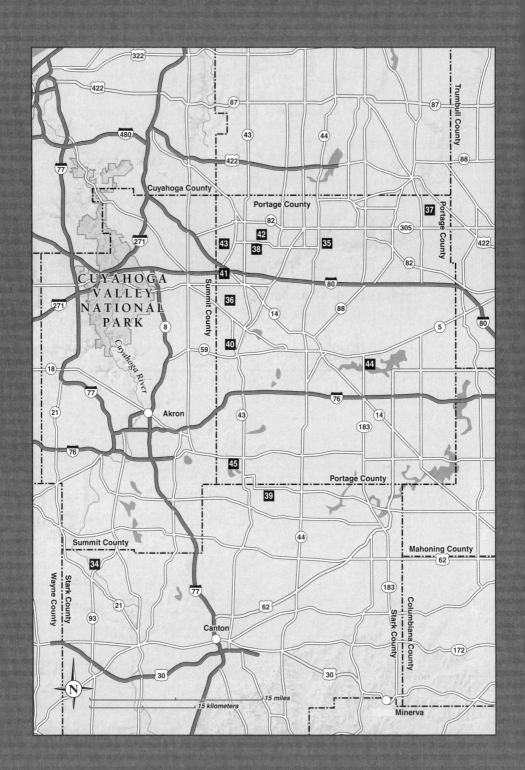

PORTAGE & STARK COUNTIES

34 CANAL FULTON: Ohio & Erie Canal Towpath & Olde Muskingum Trails

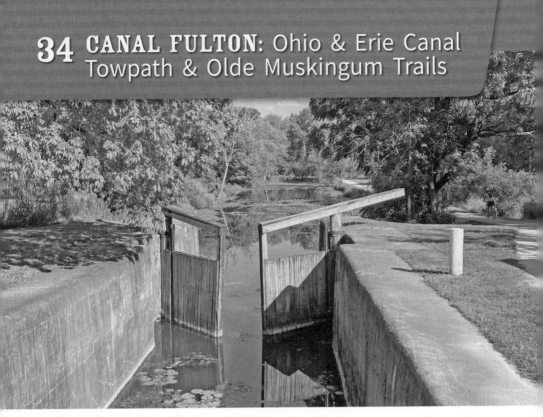
Time your hike right and you may get to see a working lock demonstration.

SETTLED IN THE early 1800s, Canal Fulton has maintained and celebrated its rich canal history. Following the Ohio & Erie Canal Towpath Trail on the eastern side of the Tuscarawas River and the Olde Muskingum Trail on the west, hikers and bikers can enjoy historical landmarks and scenic views on both sides of the river.

DESCRIPTION

Step up onto the Ohio & Erie Canal Towpath Trail in Canal Fulton during peak summer weekends, and you may plod alongside a couple of draft horses pulling the fully restored *St. Helena III* canalboat. Is this the land that time forgot? Well, not really, but for an afternoon, you can pretend that it is.

A large public parking area on the south side of Cherry Street is a good spot to begin. (Plus, it's conveniently located near shops selling ice cream and other necessities.) Even if the *St. Helena III* isn't running when you're here, a replica sits in the north end of the parking lot, making a good photo stop and a great interactive play spot for kids.

Cross over the footbridge on the east side of the parking lot, and step onto the crushed limestone of the Towpath Trail. There's really no chance you'll lose your way,

DISTANCE & CONFIGURATION: 5.9-mile point-to-point (with shuttle) or 10.5-mile loop

DIFFICULTY: Moderate

SCENERY: Historic town of Canal Fulton; Tuscarawas riverbed, wildflowers, and working canal lock

EXPOSURE: Mostly shaded during warm months; completely exposed when trees are bare

TRAFFIC: Busy, especially on warm weekend afternoons

TRAIL SURFACE: Ohio & Erie Canal Towpath Trail, crushed limestone; Olde Muskingum Trail, gravel and pavement

HIKING TIME: 2.5 hours with shuttle; 4.5–5 hours as loop

DRIVING DISTANCE: 39 miles from I-77/I-480 exchange

ACCESS: April–September: Daily, sunrise–9 p.m. October–March: Daily, sunrise–7 p.m.

MAPS: USGS *Canal Fulton* and *Massillon;* also at visitor center and trail websites

FACILITIES: Restrooms in visitor center and at some trailheads along Ohio & Erie Canal Towpath Trail

WHEELCHAIR ACCESS: The Towpath and Olde Muskingum Trail are hard-packed limestone, described as "basically flat and mostly ADA accessible." For more information about specific trailheads, see ohioanderiecanalway.com/explore/the-towpath-trail or call 330-477-3552

CONTACT: Ohio & Erie Canal Towpath Trail: 330-854-6835, ohioanderiecanalway.com/explore/the-towpath-trail; Olde Muskingum Trail: 330-477-3552, starkparks.com/parks/olde-muskingum-trail

LOCATION: Cherry St. W., Canal Fulton

so relax and enjoy the journey—as far as you like. The trail narrows a bit as you leave the welcome area behind, and about 1 mile south of your starting point, you'll find a canal lock that still works. Stop at Lock 4 to read the interpretive sign. There's also a bike tire pump here. While the Towpath here in Stark County is far less traveled than the miles running through Cuyahoga and Summit, it sees quite a few cyclists.

Continuing south, enjoying the view from about 10 feet above both the canal bed on your left and the river on your right, it's obvious that it's been a long time since canalboats passed through here. For the most part, the canal bed is overgrown with cattails and duckweed, providing a haven for birds, butterflies, and ducks. Pick a quiet evening for your trip and you're almost certain to see warblers, finches, robins, jays, and cardinals.

One mile south of the trailhead where you started, you'll come to the trailhead at Butterbridge Road. Immediately west of the trail, a private farm with a majestic red barn paints a scene typical of Stark County's beautiful farmland. (With restrooms, benches, and picnic tables, this trailhead is a good spot for a break.)

The Towpath is flat, wide, and often, but not always, busy. Strolling on the trail when it's less busy can be almost meditative. I've watched herons catch and enjoy their meals here many times. Their slow and careful hunting techniques are another reminder that hurrying can be overrated and under-rewarded.

A little more than 5 miles south of your start, you'll reach Crystal Springs Bridge, an obvious spot to rest and contemplate your next move. A couple of restaurants sit across the street to the northwest. If you'd like to extend your walk, continue on Towpath Trail less than a mile to Forty Corners Road. (There's a parking lot there,

Canal Fulton: Ohio & Erie Canal Towpath & Olde Muskingum Trails

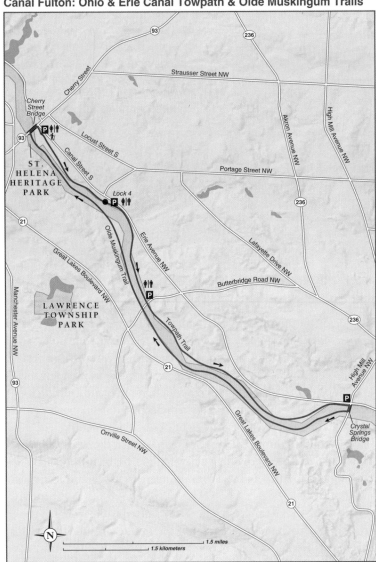

too, so if you'd prefer to complete this hike as a shuttle, you can.) Before going anywhere else, however, take a moment to learn more about the bridge.

Built in 1914, the bridge replaced one damaged in a flood. The slightly newer iron grid floor (added in the 1940s) has an almost lacy appearance. In 1996, the bridge was saved from demolition, and the area around it was designated Crystal Springs Bridge Park. This small park—no facilities are here other than a spot for the canoe livery to collect tired paddlers—closes the gap between the Olde Muskingum

Trail on the west and the Towpath Trail on the east bank of the river, creating an obvious loop for hikers who want to get two different perspectives on Canal Fulton's history. The route described here follows this loop, so turn right, crossing Crystal Springs Bridge, and then turn right again to travel north on the rail-trail.

(*Note:* The southern portion of the Little Loop of the Buckeye Trail is here, too, so you may notice blue blazes on nearby trees.)

If you've timed your hike just right, you'll be able to watch the sun begin to drop in the sky as you head back to Canal Fulton. Stretches of farmland reach out to the west; the panorama is quite pretty. Toads, rabbits, and deer will join you, bumping along this old railroad right-of-way. You may also share the road with horses, as equestrian traffic is allowed all along the Olde Muskingum Trail, which is managed by Stark County Parks. This is real farmland, by the way—you'll want to heed that CATTLE CROSSING sign.

After crossing to the north side of Butterbridge Road, the trail winds slightly to the right before depositing you onto Cherry Street. Turn right and cross over the bridge, heading east. Pause to look upstream, and perhaps to wave at a canoe as it drifts under the bridge on the river that has carried traffic through town for at least 200 years.

NEARBY ACTIVITIES

Canal Fulton was incorporated in 1814, and visitors can relish a sort of time warp feeling here, walking along brick streets lined with historical-looking street lamps. From May to September, the *St. Helena III* offers an authentic canalboat ride experience; call 330-854-6835 for a schedule and rates. Those who prefer to paddle down the river can rent canoes from a livery on Cherry Street.

Budding botanists may want to visit Jackson Bog, just 2 miles east of Crystal Springs Bridge. The bog is managed as a state nature preserve; more than 20 rare plants, some considered threatened or endangered by the state, can be viewed from its 1.5-mile boardwalk trail. Visit ohiodnr.gov/go-and-do/plan-a-visit/find-a-property /jackson-bog-state-nature-preserve for more information.

• •

TRAILHEAD GPS COORDINATES: N40.88778° W81.59698°

DIRECTIONS Follow I-77 S toward Akron and take Exit 136 (OH 21 S toward Massillon). Continue onto OH 21 S for 17.4 miles. Turn left onto Arcadia Street Northwest, which becomes Cherry Street West. Follow Cherry Street for 1 mile to Tuscarawas Street Northwest. Turn right into the parking area for Canalway Visitor Center and the *St. Helena III* boarding area.

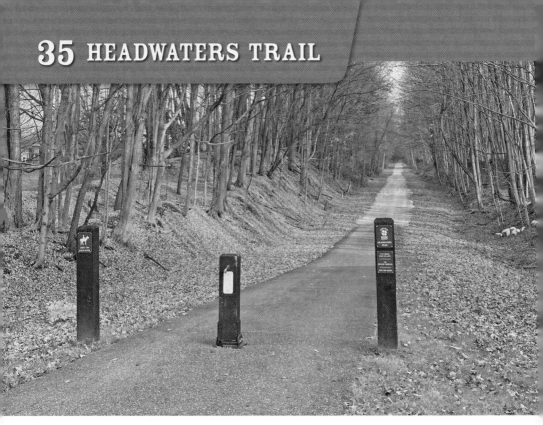

The Headwaters Trail abuts the Mantua Bog and Marsh Wetlands State Nature Preserve.

THIS RAIL-TRAIL IN Portage County makes for peaceful, easy walking (as well as jogging and biking). Running east–west between Mantua and Garrettsville, it offers a waterfall for scenery, two historic landmarks, and excellent bird-watching opportunities. The trail also crosses a watershed divide.

DESCRIPTION

From the trailhead parking lot just south of High Street, cross over OH 44 (Main Street) and onto the crushed limestone trail as you parallel Mill Street, heading east. In addition to Headwaters Trail signs, you'll also see markers for the Buckeye Trail. The flat trail offers broad views of this space between Portage County towns.

Soon, on your right (to the south of the trail) you'll see a sign for (but not an entrance to) the 152-acre Marsh Wetlands State Nature Preserve. As you approach Peck Road, you'll walk alongside a different kind of wetland: Mantua Bog is actually an alkaline fen. Both areas were designated as National Natural Landmarks in 1976 and as state nature preserves in 1990. Here in this wetland corridor, you can enjoy the migrating waterfowl as you stroll by the edge of these protected areas. You might also find a generously sized garter snake, or even a skunk that has wandered away from its protected habitat to gawk at the funny two-legged creatures plodding along the trail.

DISTANCE & CONFIGURATION: 4.5-mile point-to-point or 9-mile out-and-back with option for shorter or longer routes

DIFFICULTY: Easy

SCENERY: Beech forests, creek ravine, lots of waterfowl; Western Reserve architecture, historical markers

EXPOSURE: About half exposed

TRAFFIC: Moderate

TRAIL SURFACE: Crushed limestone

HIKING TIME: 2–4 hours

DRIVING DISTANCE: 32 miles from I-77/I-480 exchange

ACCESS: Daily, sunrise–sunset; pets must be leashed; note that horses (allowed only outside of village limits) and bikes frequent the trail.

MAPS: USGS *Mantua* and *Garrettsville*; also at park website

FACILITIES: Restrooms and water at trailheads at Gerald E. Buchert Memorial Park in Mantua and at OH 700.

WHEELCHAIR ACCESS: No

CONTACT: Portage Park District: 330-297-7728, portagecounty-oh.gov/portage-county-park-district/parks-maps/pages/headwaters-trail

LOCATION: E. High St., Mantua

Along this stretch you'll probably notice some sights indicative of the mixed-use nature of 21st-century trailways, such as a horse grazing on one side of the road and a mini-storage facility or a convenience store on the other. Keep going and be happy that the trail managed to cut a swath through this interesting place and time.

About a mile into the hike, the trail offers some gradual changes of scenery: shallow but pretty ravines, cornfields, and a mix of both old and new homesites.

As you pass Vaughn Avenue heading east, you'll soon cross the Lake Erie–Ohio River Drainage Divide. While it hardly marks a cosmic shift, trivia fans should note that water east of here flows into the Ohio River, while waters west of here make their way to Lake Erie. Watershed fans will want to know that the trail more or less follows Eagle Creek, a tributary of the Mahoning River, even though you won't see much of it from the trail. You needn't be a hydrology expert to notice, depending on the season, cattails, thistles, and other delicious butterfly food growing on either side of the trail. While Portage is still one of Ohio's more sparsely populated counties, it, too, is growing, so enjoy the relative space and quiet as you continue on the path.

This portion of the trail east of Limeridge Road is nestled between banks of tall trees, which may make your trek feel extra dark and quiet. It's easy to forget that this trail came about largely thanks to the railroad that came through here long ago. A reminder is coming up: On the south side of the path, a plaque on a large rock describes a deadly train accident that occurred in 1949. After reading the somber story, you'll head up an ever-so-gentle slope to reach a clearing and greet Asbury Road. Stop to enjoy a lovely vista.

As you continue east from there, you'll notice that the landscape changes on both sides of the trail rather quickly. Now, instead of being flanked by banks of trees, you can look into a ravine on either side of the path. A small but reliable waterfall along here reminds you that the trail is aptly named. Less than a mile farther down, you'll reach OH 700.

Headwaters Trail

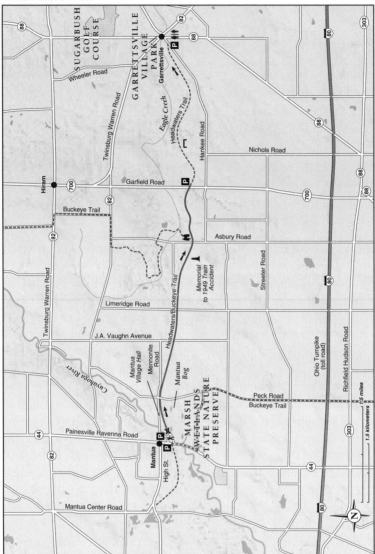

YOU HAVE OPTIONS

OH 700 is your turnaround point if you're following the map and description here, as well as the spot to park your shuttle vehicle if you want to make this a 4.5-mile hike. Alternatively, if you want to add miles, you can continue for about 3 miles east to reach Garrettsville Village Park, another spot where you can park a shuttle vehicle. Or, near Asbury Road, you can follow the Buckeye Trail as it winds north and west through Camp Asbury and beyond. (Compared with the Headwaters Trail, this section of the Buckeye Trail is primitive and almost always offers solitude.)

Whether you walk, ride, or drive back to Mantua, if you started your trek in the afternoon, you should enjoy great sunset views as you return to your starting point.

NEARBY ACTIVITIES

Interested in Western Reserve history? Continue eastward a bit to Garrettsville, which, like Hiram and Mantua, was settled in the early 1800s, just as Ohio gained statehood. All three towns conjure up visions of New England—including central village squares with imposing churches surrounded by large frame-style houses.

Garrettsville came into being when John Garrett III of Christiana Hundred, Delaware, purchased 300 acres of land in Nelson, obtaining Silver Creek waterpower rights so he could build a gristmill. Unfortunately, Garrett soon died of pneumonia, but his widow, Eleanor, managed the mill, and it and the town thrived. A clock reminiscent of the gristmill era chimes at the corner of High Street and Maple Avenue. And before you leave Garrettsville, you might want to pick up a pack of Life Savers. Clarence Crane invented the candy here in 1912.

More hiking can be found at Eagle Creek State Nature Preserve, heading east from the village by way of Center Street to Hopkins Road. The preserve is open 30 minutes before sunrise to 30 minutes after sunset year-round; see ohiodnr.gov/go-and-do/plan-a-visit/find-a-property/eagle-creek-state-nature-preserve for more information. (Note that pets are not allowed in the nature preserve.) Also nearby: rocky Nelson-Kennedy Ledges State Park (page 175).

• •

TRAILHEAD GPS COORDINATES: N41.28355° W81.21641°

DIRECTIONS From I-77, take Exit 156 and merge onto I-480, heading east. In 6.6 miles, take Exit 26 (US 422 E), following signs to Warren, and in 2 miles, continue to follow US 422 E. In 15.4 miles, exit and turn right (south) onto OH 44 toward Ravenna. Follow OH 44 approximately 7 miles, and then turn left (east) onto East High Street in Mantua, where trailhead parking is available on the south side of the road. Additional parking is available behind the McDonald's on OH 44 at Mill Street.

36 HERRICK FEN STATE NATURE PRESERVE

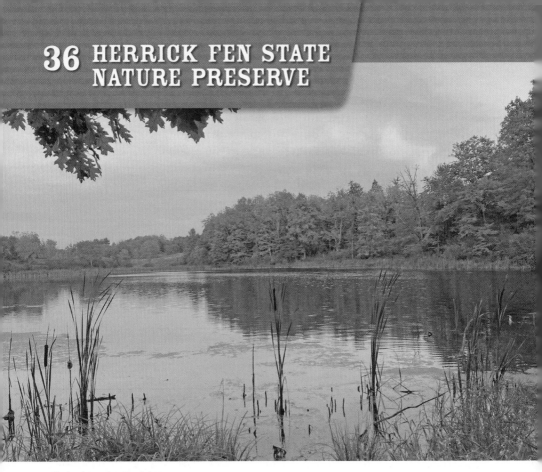

The back pond at Herrick Fen

NOTICE: HERRICK FEN CLOSED AT PRESS TIME

A storm damaged the bridge at the entrance to Herrick Fen, and the park is closed until a replacement or alternate access can be arranged. For the latest updates, visit nature.org/en-us/get-involved/how-to-help/places-we-protect/herrick-fen-nature -preserve. For information on other wetlands and trails close to Herrick Fen, see the "Nearby Activities" section at the end of this description.

WHO KNEW THAT carnivorous plants could be so cute? Who knew that beavers could cause such trouble? As pretty and peaceful as this place is, you may not notice battles raging all around you. This fen harbors the tiny insect-eating sundew plants, state-endangered bayberries, and rare sedges. While only careful observers will notice some of the many unusual species here, the tamarack trees are fairly easy to spot. Tamaracks, Ohio's only native deciduous conifer, are not evergreen. They have needles that turn bright yellow in autumn and then fall off. Visit in autumn to see the tamaracks' remarkable display; visit anytime to watch for birds and stay, perhaps, for a sunset.

170

DISTANCE & CONFIGURATION: 1.6-mile balloon

DIFFICULTY: Easy

SCENERY: Rare plants, herons, beavers, muskrats; good bird-watching

EXPOSURE: Mostly shaded

TRAFFIC: Moderate

TRAIL SURFACE: Wooden boardwalks, dirt trail

HIKING TIME: 45 minutes

DRIVING DISTANCE: 28 miles from I-77/I-480 exchange

ACCESS: Daily, sunrise–sunset; pets and bicycles prohibited

MAPS: USGS *Kent*

FACILITIES: None

WHEELCHAIR ACCESS: No

CONTACT: Nature Conservancy: 614-717-2770, tinyurl.com/herrickfen

LOCATION: Seasons Road, Streetsboro

DESCRIPTION

If you know the difference between a fen and a bog, you probably paid very close attention in biology class. (Unfortunately, I didn't.) While bogs, swamps, fens, and other wetlands have some commonalities, they're not the same.

So what is the difference between a bog and a fen? An overly simplified explanation is that a fen is alkaline and a bog is acidic. Both areas are ecologically important, too scarce these days, and generally damp. Bogs receive their water from above-ground sources (mostly rain and snow). Groundwater seeps and springs, usually coming out of glacial deposits, feed fens. Bogs are often isolated from groundwater—sometimes from impermeable soil conditions but frequently from an impermeable layer of compressed, humified peat. Peat is what really sets bogs and fens apart from other wetlands. Peat, combined with the continual wetness, causes and perpetuates extreme soil conditions. You don't have to be a science whiz to realize that different types of plants live in alkaline and acidic soils. But shades of gray exist in nature, and in the relative acidity of bogs and fens. Because bogs and fens are both generally wet, some plants exist in both, and some of those species cannot exist anywhere else. This concludes the science lesson; now it's time for a field trip. Well, make that a fen trip.

While the fen isn't well marked from the road, the narrow entrance drive can be found just east of a (privately owned) red barn. The barn sits on a small hill on the eastern end of the preserve. Keep driving, slowly, over a culvert, to reach the parking area and trailhead. From there, follow the wide gravel path east, past tall marsh grass and seasonal wildflowers. When the goldenrods explode under a sunny fall sky, the scene is as colorful and glossy as a still-wet painting. But behind the pretty picture, there is turmoil. Battles rage, quietly but constantly, among the fen's inhabitants.

About 0.2 mile from the trailhead, you'll come to a large stone recognizing the work of The Nature Conservancy and the Akron Garden Club in preserving this land. While it is an Ohio Department of Natural Resources property, this land is managed by a group of organizations and volunteers. Almost as soon as you step onto the boardwalk, you'll have a chance to stop at three wooden benches. These

Herrick Fen State Nature Preserve

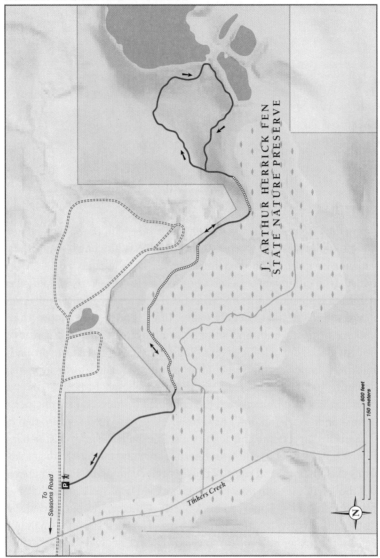

are good seats for watching the herons and marsh wrens that commonly appear here. These seats also offer a chance to observe a constantly changing landscape.

A few cattails appear here and there, almost like sentries on guard along the boardwalk. But are they here to protect or invade? The answer depends on whom you ask. Cattails provide high-energy food for migratory birds and butterflies; so birds and butterflies, and people who watch them, may root for the cattails. But the answer also depends on the type of cattails. Some are native and nonaggressive, content to enjoy their view of the fen without overtaking it. Other cattail species are invasive and quite aggressive, threatening some of the fen's indigenous plants.

What needs protection here? Bayberries, for one; they appear on the state's list of endangered plants. This fen is one of just three spots in Ohio where they grow. Unfortunately, the cattails and bayberries aren't the only species at odds in this preserve. The invasive cattails and reed canary grass threaten the open fen as a whole, driving out the sedge meadow and shrubby cinquefoils. Glossy buckthorns, small trees or large shrubs (distinguished by their shiny oval leaves and speckled bark), threaten the tamarack population as well as the bayberries. The skirmishes among the plants and animals here started long ago, and along the way, people have stepped in—for better or for worse.

The lakes and dam on this property—though on portions not open to the public—date to the 1950s, when the Frame family raised mink and muskrats here. J. Arthur Herrick bought the initial tract of land that would form the preserve in 1969; for some time after that, the area was known as Frame Lake Bog. The muskrats (who didn't care what the place was called) stayed, and beavers joined them. But beavers, like cattails, can be troublemakers. Beaver dams cause the water levels to rise, threatening the tamarack population. The tamaracks in this fen comprise one of the few reproducing populations of this tree in the state.

What can—and what should—be done to tip the balance in favor of the bayberries and the tamaracks? Again, the answers vary depending on whom you ask, and a resolution is not expected anytime soon. The good news is that the fen has been preserved, so the battles may continue. The Nature Conservancy sends aid in the form of volunteers who diligently thin the ranks of invaders in hopes that the natives can continue to fight for themselves. While some natives are under duress, the volunteers who visit typically report finding the battlegrounds overwhelmingly beautiful. So march on.

As you continue south on the boardwalk, tamarack trees line the trail; you may see or hear a catbird at this point. It's easy to spot the mayapples and skunk cabbages growing along the boardwalk. Skunk cabbage is probably most noticeable in the spring, thanks to its white flower that resembles a lily. In the fall, however, its fruit is worth a look. Waxy and dark brown, with a hint of purple, its shape might be described as somewhat reminiscent of a hand grenade (in keeping with the battlefield imagery).

Notice, too, the fen-loving shrubby cinquefoils, whose bright-yellow flowers bloom May–September. You'll have to look hard for the less common sundews, small but mighty carnivorous plants resembling a sunburst. When an insect lands on the plant's hairy, sticky leaves, it triggers an enzyme reaction that makes a leaf grow so quickly that it wraps up the insect like a burrito before absorbing the bug's nutrients.

Another unusual plant to look for is white turtlehead. It has waxy, dark-green stems and white flowers. Each bloom is about a half-inch long. When viewed from the side, with just a bit of imagination, the bloom indeed forms the outline of a turtle's head. Also look for poison sumac, cousin to the more common sumacs that occur only in fens. (Admire, but don't touch it!)

Just 0.4 mile into the trail, the boardwalk ends, and you'll step down onto a narrow, root-filled dirt trail that winds between the base of a wooded hill and the shrub swamp. Soon, the boardwalk begins again, curves to the left, and then redeposits you on the dirt trail.

The hard-packed dirt path bends left, leading up a small hill into a beech-maple wood that offers color-charged spring wildflower displays. Circling back down the hill, the path bends to the right and levels out, where you'll find two shallow lakes separated by a narrow dam. The water levels are dropping here, by design. Releasing the dams that created the artificial lakes allows more native wet meadow plants to return.

The trail loop rejoins the original path at this point; you will retrace your steps back to the boardwalk and return home from here. You probably won't have any war stories to tell when you return, but you should bring home some lovely pictures.

NEARBY ACTIVITIES

Herrick Fen sits just around the corner from the much-tamer Trail Lake Park, where you'll find a paved, 1.6-mile trail encircling an artificial lake. From there, you can glance east to appreciate the fen from a distance. Serious wetlands fans will want to visit two other properties: The Tom S. Cooperrider–Kent Bog on the south end of Kent preserves what is thought to be the southernmost stand of tamarack trees in the country. Triangle Lake Bog State Nature Preserve in Ravenna, while short on trails, is long on rare and beautiful bog-loving species, including a healthy population of pitcher plants. For more information about Triangle Lake Bog, see ohiodnr.gov /go-and-do/plan-a-visit/find-a-property/triangle-lake-bog-state-nature-preserve.

Interested in volunteering to protect Ohio's natives? Contact The Nature Conservancy at nature.org.

• •

TRAILHEAD GPS COORDINATES: N41.21398° W81.37113°

DIRECTIONS From I-77, take Exit 156 and merge onto I-480, heading east. In 6.6 miles, keep right to stay on I-480 East, and in another 5.5 miles, keep right again to stay on I-480. Continue on I-480 East another 10.6 miles to OH 14 in Streetsboro. Follow OH 14 E 1.7 miles, and turn right onto OH 43, following it 0.2 mile to Seasons Road. Turn right. Approximately 2 miles west of OH 43, Seasons Road curves sharply to the left and crosses a railroad track. Turn left into the gravel drive providing preserve access on the eastern side of Seasons. Follow the drive past a stream crossing to the small parking lot on the right.

37 NELSON-KENNEDY LEDGES STATE PARK

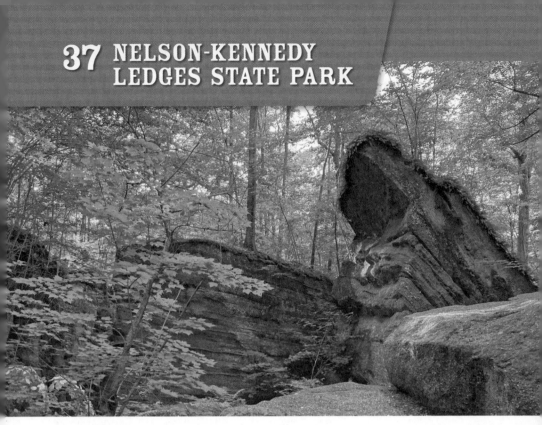

Shipwreck rock

SMALL AND SURPRISING, Nelson-Kennedy Ledges State Park offers one of the wildest 2-mile walks in the eastern United States. Don't let the short distance fool you; you could easily spend several hours here. Dramatic ledges and tight crevasses team up with two waterfalls and several small caves, creating striking beauty.

DESCRIPTION

With formation names such as Devil's Hole and The Squeeze, these trails may sound a little scary. To be clear, these ledges are made for sure-footed visitors; horseplay is discouraged. The rock formations that give this park its amazing beauty also make it dangerous, but by heeding the posted warnings, most visitors thoroughly enjoy the cliffs, caves, and crooked trails here on this little plot of land in Portage County.

Four trails run through the park with a combined length of about 2 miles. While the park's direction is STAY ON MARKED TRAILS ONLY, it's not always easy. Although the trails have seen significant improvements in recent years, they still dart in and out of huge rock formations. Since exploring is the whole point, and it's practically impossible to get lost here, why not step onto the first trail you see and look around?

Once you cross the road from the parking lot, you'll see the Blue Trail. Turn left and follow it south, with the namesake ledges clearly in view. About 0.3 mile along

175

DISTANCE & CONFIGURATION: 2-mile balloon

DIFFICULTY: Moderate–difficult

SCENERY: 60-foot cliffs, creek, caves, crevasses, and two waterfalls

EXPOSURE: Mostly shaded

TRAFFIC: Moderately heavy

TRAIL SURFACE: Rock surfaces, dirt, peat, leaves

HIKING TIME: 1–2 hours

DRIVING DISTANCE: 37 miles from I-77/I-480 exchange

ACCESS: Daily, 30 minutes before sunrise–30 minutes after sunset; cars in the lot 30 minutes after sunset are subject to towing. Do not attempt hiking here when icy conditions exist. Dogs are allowed on leashes; however, I don't recommend bringing them here.

MAPS: USGS *Garrettsville;* also at park website

FACILITIES: Restrooms at parking lot; picnic tables on both sides of OH 282

WHEELCHAIR ACCESS: No

CONTACT: 330-235-0030, ohiodnr.gov/go-and-do/plan-a-visit/find-a-property/nelsonkennedy-ledges-state-park

LOCATION: Nelson Ledge Road, Garrettsville

the trail, you'll approach a weathered footbridge and staircase. From there, you can turn right, cutting into the center of the park on the Red Trail, or continue on the Blue Trail a bit farther south. I like to crisscross the property on the trails as much as I can, so I opt to continue south on the Blue Trail, looping back through Devil's Icebox, picking up the Red Trail, and then turning left again onto the White Trail a little later.

By this point, you've probably noticed traffic passing by on OH 282, and you might hear music coming from the private campground on the southwest side of the park. Does it detract from the wildness of the place? Perhaps. Does it remind us how lucky we are to have a property like this both preserved and open to the public? Definitely.

The Red Trail offers a number of obstacles and a good introduction to the geology of the park. The top portion of the ledges seen here are primarily Sharon Conglomerate, from the Pennsylvanian period. Get close and you'll notice they're decorated with small, smooth quartz-like pebbles, which were polished before they were deposited into the sandstone around 320 million years ago.

The giant slabs of darker bluish-gray stones that you walk between on the lower portions of the trails are much older Meadville Shale. The 20-foot-long tunnel known as Fat Man's Peril is made of it, and, like it or not, the passage won't accommodate anyone wearing much larger than a size 44 belt.

After squeezing through (or going around) Fat Man's Peril, gaze up at Shipwreck Rock, then turn left, heading south on the White Trail.

The White Trail is a loop that offers a chance to look down on some of the other trails, affording a glimpse of Shipwreck Rock from above, among other things. Never mind that you may not be following the trails in a "logical" order—you're here to enjoy the journey.

With that in mind, however, don't miss Minnehaha Falls on the south end of the White Trail. While you may have to crane your neck to see it, the dramatic little waterfall tucked between the rocks is worth the effort.

Nelson-Kennedy Ledges State Park

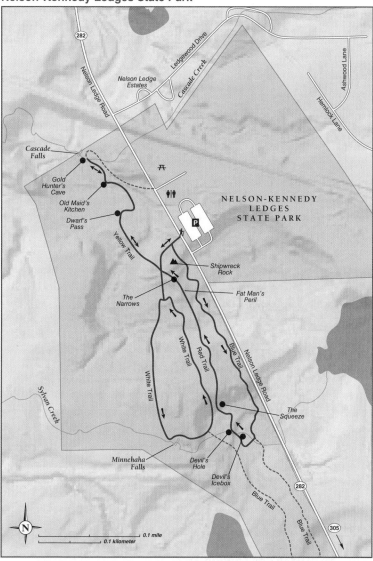

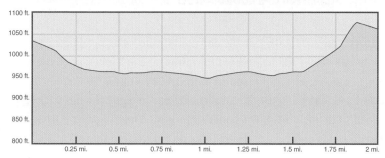

After looping around on the White Trail, you'll find yourself heading north and downhill, for the most part, and onto the Yellow Trail. You'll jog right and then left to pad along a sturdy wooden bridge into Old Maid's Kitchen. When you exit the dark and drafty "kitchen," it's nice to see the sky again! You can also see the parking lot across the road—but don't leave yet. Follow the trail as it juts west, turning left and heading along a wooden boardwalk to the bottom of Cascade Falls. The small stream that tumbles over a 40-foot drop enters the Grand River, eventually making its way to the St. Lawrence River. For trivia buffs: This park sits on a watershed divide. This stream, and water north of here, ultimately lands in the St. Lawrence River; Sylvan Creek, where Minnehaha Falls lands on the park's south side, eventually finds its way to the Mississippi River via the Mahoning and Ohio Rivers.

At the bottom of Cascade Falls, you can peer into Gold Hunter's Cave. Though the cave is not open to explorers, you can see inside from the wooden platform at the bottom of the falls. Alas, there was no gold in the cave; all that was found was pyrite, or fool's gold, but it did cause a bit of excitement for a short time in the 1800s. Retrace your steps on the Yellow Trail, then turn left on the White Trail to return to the trailhead, or simply cross OH 282 to the east to return to the parking lot. Or, maybe, you'll decide you need to see the whole thing again. Nelson-Kennedy Ledges is definitely worth a repeat trek and a return visit.

NEARBY ACTIVITIES

If the trails here are a bit much for hikers in your group, consider the rocky but easier trails at Liberty Park's Twinsburg Ledges (page 260) and come back here another time. If you're looking for lunch or dinner after your hike, try one of the local restaurants in Garrettsville on your way back. Or, if you visit during the late-summer or fall season, stop at one of the sunflower farms or corn mazes in rural Portage County, like Derthick's Corn Maze in Mantua. See derthickcornmaze.com for hours and admission information.

• •

TRAILHEAD GPS COORDINATES: N41.32843° W81.03896°

DIRECTIONS From I-77, take Exit 156 and merge onto I-480, heading east. In 6.6 miles, take Exit 26 (US 422 E), following signs to Warren, and in 2 miles, continue to follow US 422 E. In 19.5 miles, turn right (south) onto OH 700. Follow OH 700 for 5.3 miles into Hiram. Turn left (east) onto OH 305/Wakefield Road and go 5.7 miles to OH 282/Nelson Ledge Road. Turn left (north). The park entrance is 1.3 miles north of OH 305. Parking is on the eastern side of the road; the trails are on the western side of OH 282.

38 PADDOCK RIVER PRESERVE

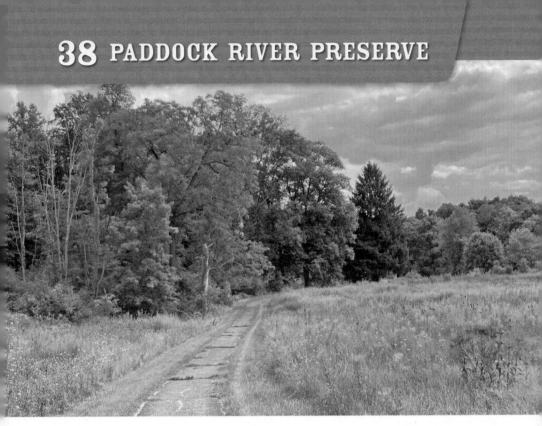

Nature is quickly reclaiming the golf cart paths here.

FOLLOW WINDING PATHS over hills and along the stream corridor through this former country club that is becoming a popular birding spot in northern Portage County.

DESCRIPTION

While the name may conjure up a horse farm, this 194-acre parcel of land was previously part of the Aurora Country Club. Paddock River Preserve is named for Harold "Pappy" Paddock, Sr., a prominent figure in the history of the property as both an early owner of the club and a well-known golf course architect.

Thanks to Paddock's stewardship, the property remained undivided from the early 1940s until 2012, when the City of Aurora bought the land. Falling as it does within the Chagrin River Watershed, and containing the Aurora Branch of the Chagrin River, this parcel is a vital piece of the local environment.

Recognizing its importance, the Ohio EPA helped fund the purchase, and the city worked with cooperating agencies, including the Northeast Ohio Regional Sewer District, to remove a dam, restore over 1.3 miles of the Aurora Branch of the Chagrin River and its headwater tributaries, and restore more than 17 acres of golf course to forested stream corridor and floodplain.

DISTANCE & CONFIGURATION: 2.5-mile loop

DIFFICULTY: Moderate

SCENERY: Woodlands, hills, watershed corridor

EXPOSURE: Mostly exposed

TRAFFIC: Light

TRAIL SURFACE: Dirt and gravel

HIKING TIME: 1–1.5 hours (more if you're a bird-watcher)

DRIVING DISTANCE: 24 miles from I-77/I-480 exchange

ACCESS: Sunrise–sunset

MAPS: USGS *Aurora, OH*

FACILITIES: Primitive restroom on south end of trail

WHEELCHAIR ACCESS: No

CONTACT: 330-562-4333, auroraoh.com /departments/parks___recreation/index.php

LOCATION: 129 Trails End, Aurora

As the area returns to a more natural state, human visitors can enjoy the hilly trails and many birding opportunities here. Like most former golf course properties, this one is evolving. While the trails here are mostly former golf cart paths, they are well on their way to being reclaimed by native grasses and wildflowers.

Starting from the trailhead at the southwest corner of the parking lot, follow the red trail, Cardinal Loop, as it ventures east. The path rolls over hills and across a small footbridge, carrying you over the Aurora Branch of the Chagrin River.

YOU HAVE OPTIONS

The frequently intersecting cart paths are a potential source of confusion, but they also offer several chances to cut your trek short. If the hilly nature of these trails proves a bit much, you can turn right on Blue Heron Pass and return to the trailhead, logging less than a mile. If you'd prefer to start off with a shorter, flatter hike, take the orange Oriole Trail (with some rolling hills) to the flat Hummingbird Path on the southwest edge of the property. This description generally follows the red, yellow, and orange trails in a clockwise fashion.

Once across the first footbridge on the Cardinal Loop, you'll pass the intersection with Blue Heron Pass, and then roll over a series of gentle (and some steep!) slopes, offering wide views of the river. With so much young brush and native wildflowers growing here now, the formerly manicured property is a haven for birds and insects.

As you continue east, you'll have an opportunity to take a grassy path into the Aurora Audubon Sanctuary. While the property, also known as Bretschneider Park, is lovely, stay on course here and continue on the Cardinal Loop, now heading downhill again. The surface varies as you go, from weathered cart path, to gravel, to grass, almost like a nudge from nature reminding us that change is constant. Roll with it!

You'll pass a pond and continue heading uphill to find a primitive restroom. (File under "need to know" because, as of this writing, it's the only one in the park.)

Paddock River Preserve

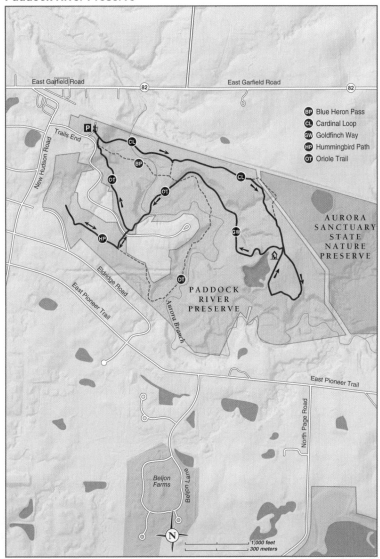

In late summer, you'll find milkweed along here. You could stay on the red Cardinal Loop here and return the way you came, but instead, take a sharp left and follow the yellow markers for Goldfinch Way.

Where the orange and yellow trails converge, you'll want to head southwest on the orange Oriole Trail, crossing over the river again and starting to see the end of the hills on today's hike.

Follow the orange markers for Oriole Trail to Hummingbird Path, which you can take as an out-and-back, or continue right on the Oriole Trail through the parkland to return to the parking lot.

Although from some places on the Oriole Trail and Hummingbird Path you will notice former golf club buildings and be able to see some private homes, wandering through this property provides a brief escape from suburbia, both for the plants and animals who can live here again, as well as for the enjoyment of visitors like you.

NEARBY ACTIVITIES

Hungry? Aurora's historic district has several locally owned eateries and bars. Want to do some more hiking to work up an appetite? You're close to Sunny Lake Park (page 197), with mostly paved trails, and also just a short drive from the more rustic (and much flatter) trails at Tinkers Creek State Nature Preserve (page 201). For a very different type of scenery, head east to Nelson-Kennedy Ledges State Park (page 175).

• •

TRAILHEAD GPS COORDINATES: N41.31545° W81.33165°

DIRECTIONS: Take I-480 E to US 422, and take Exit 23 to turn right onto OH 306. Follow OH 306 south almost 5 miles, then veer left onto OH 82 through historic Aurora. Turn right onto New Hudson Road and then left onto Trails End.

Thanks to the combined work of several organizations, this important stream corridor is being restored.

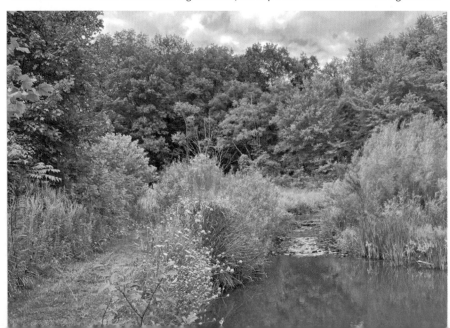

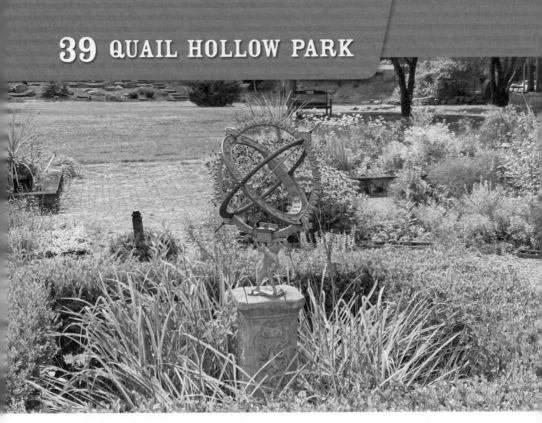

You can use the sundial to check your hiking time.

FROM THE HISTORIC, stately manor home with an herb garden and an iconic sundial to rough-and-tumble mountain bike trails—plus more than 7 miles of hiking trails—Quail Hollow's sprawling 700 acres will satisfy a wide range of interests.

DESCRIPTION

This park property can trace its roots back to a farmhouse, built—and then expanded—on the ridge of a hill by the Conrad Brumbaugh family in the mid-1800s. In the early 1900s, Harry Bartlett Stewart, then chief executive officer of the Akron Canton & Youngstown Railroad, began acquiring adjacent land, initially using it as a hunting camp, then later expanding and enlarging the home to what you see today. Three generations of the Stewart family lived here until 1975, when they offered the property to the state for half its appraised value. The 700 acres of marsh, woods, and rolling meadows were a state park from 1975 through 2015; in 2016, Stark Parks began managing the property.

While the lovely herb garden looks as if it could have been part of the Stewarts' private landscape, in fact it was established by the Quail Hollow Herbal Society in 1986. Featuring a rose arbor, native and introduced flower gardens, and a traditional sundial, it's a beautiful place to pause and reflect before or after hiking the grounds.

DISTANCE & CONFIGURATION: 2.1-mile loop

DIFFICULTY: Easy

SCENERY: Marsh and prairie, pine and deciduous forest, herb garden with sundial

EXPOSURE: Purple Trail, shaded; herb garden, exposed

TRAFFIC: Moderate

TRAIL SURFACE: Dirt, some pavement and grass

HIKING TIME: 1 hour

DRIVING DISTANCE: 47 miles from I-77/I-480 exchange

ACCESS: 24/7

MAPS: USGS *Hartville*; also posted at trailhead and on park website

FACILITIES: Restrooms and water by manor house and visitor center parking lot; restrooms, playground, and basketball courts at Pond Parking Area; picnic tables and grills throughout park

WHEELCHAIR ACCESS: Approximately 1,000 feet of the Purple Trail is paved from the herb garden north; the remainder of the trail is not accessible.

CONTACT: 330-477-3552, starkparks.com/parks /quail-hollow-park; ranger on duty: 330-353-2377

LOCATION: 13480 Congress Lake Ave., Hartville

You have many route options (see below) to explore more than 7 miles of hiking trails here, but for this hike, you'll stay on the easy Purple Trail in the northern section of the park. From the small, accessible parking lot on the west side of the manor house, head to the herb garden. Wander around or sit a spell—several benches and a gazebo in the herb garden provide shade to view what was the Stewart family's backyard.

Returning to the archway on the northwest end of the herb garden, turn right onto the paved trail. You'll see signs for the Buckeye Trail, as well as markers for the Purple Trail. Your path is paved (and carpeted with pine needles) until it diverges from the Buckeye Trail. But just a few hundred feet into your hike, you'll have a chance to veer off the outer loop by turning left onto a connector trail (at sign marker P4) to reach a unique feature: a wind phone.

A wind phone is intended to be a tool to help people deal with grief. The name suggests that a grieving person can talk to a lost loved one, and the wind will carry their words where they need to go. Wind phones are usually set in somewhat secluded, natural settings inside a phonebooth-like structure. The phones are not connected to any telephone lines.

According to mywindphone.com, the first wind phone was installed in 2010 in Japan, and there are at least six such phones in Ohio. The wind phone on the Purple Trail connector was installed in 2021. The project was proposed to the park system by two community members who had recently lost family members.

After visiting the wind phone, you could continue west to reach the western side of the Purple Trail loop, but if you did, you'd miss the north half of the trail. Instead, turn around and head east, then turn left to continue north on the Purple Trail. The pavement soon ends, and the rest of your trek is on natural surfaces.

Where the Buckeye Trail turns right into the deciduous forest, another trail connector veers left, and into the peat. Continue following the Purple Trail straight, on a hard dirt surface, still blanketed with pine needles. While the Purple Trail is relatively flat, there are quite a few roots to navigate.

Quail Hollow Park

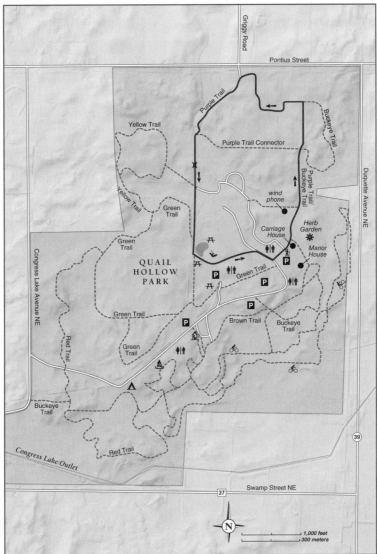

The Buckeye Trail rejoins the Purple Trail as it heads north and then west, skirting Pontius Street. The Buckeye Trail continues north on Griggy Road, but you'll continue on the Purple Trail as it heads southwest.

By now, the path has narrowed and you're walking amid a mix of young and old-growth hardwoods. A couple of short footbridges will carry you over spots that can stay soggy long after a rain. (The peat soil that's so good for farming can be hard on hiking shoes.)

Another intersection with the connector trail gives you the option to turn left and follow it east. If you do, you'll return to the spot where the Purple and Buckeye Trails diverge; there you can turn right and return, on pavement, to your starting point, shaving about 0.3 mile off the distance of the hike as mapped.

To complete the loop as described here, follow the Purple Trail straight as it intersects with the Yellow and Green Bridle Trails. Soon you'll emerge from the forest at a small pond; there is also a small playground and restroom there.

Hike around the perimeter of the pond to continue east, up a small grassy incline. Turn right at the edge of the meadow with a broad view of the manor house, where you'll be very close to your parking spot.

A wind phone can help people talk through grief.   Photo credit: Stark Parks

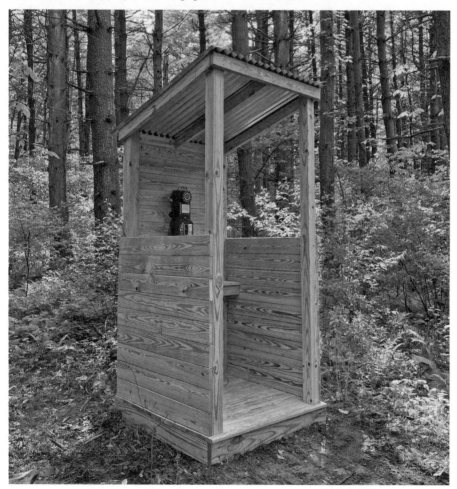

YOU HAVE OPTIONS

It's worth noting that a short loop trail behind the herb garden is paved and accessible by wheelchair and stroller, making it easily passable even when the muck-like soil is wet. If you're not quite done for the day when you return to your parking spot, you can cross the park road and follow the Brown Trail as an out-and-back, or make it a loop by taking a section of the Buckeye Trail that heads east, abutting the mountain bike trail, before rejoining the Brown Trail. Either way will add about a mile to your total.

NEARBY ACTIVITIES

The park offers a number of activities. You may want to bring a mountain bike, a fishing pole, or your horse to enjoy it all. The extensive bridle trails are also open to hikers (be smart about sharing the trail, please) and offer some delightful hills to give your legs a good workout. A portion of the Buckeye Trail also winds through the park.

Tours of the 40-room manor house are offered on select dates throughout the year—see the park website or call about available dates. The manor house and visitor center are maintained and staffed by the Quail Hollow Volunteer Association, and more help is always appreciated! Find out about opportunities at qhva.org, or contact the park office.

Once you've worked up an appetite, you won't have to go far to satisfy it. A handful of popular restaurants in Hartville, near the junction of OH 43 and OH 619, serve hearty meals in the Mennonite tradition, and several nearby wineries serve locally made wines and cheeses.

• •

TRAILHEAD GPS COORDINATES: N40.97976° W81.30456°

DIRECTIONS From Cleveland, follow I-77 S through Akron, and take Exit 129 (I-76 W). Follow I-76 W 1.7 miles to Exit 18 (I-277). Continue straight onto US 224, and go 9.5 miles, heading east past I-76 and turn right (south) onto Congress Lake Road. In 2.6 miles, the road turns left (east) and becomes Pontius Road. In 0.5 mile, turn right (south) onto Congress Lake Avenue NE. The park entrance will be on your left (east) in 0.7 mile at 13480 Congress Lake Avenue. Follow the long park driveway approximately 1 mile, following signs to the manor house on the park's eastern side.

Sincere thanks to Jared Shive, Community Engagement Coordinator at Stark Parks, for sharing his enthusiasm for the outdoors and for his review of this hike description.

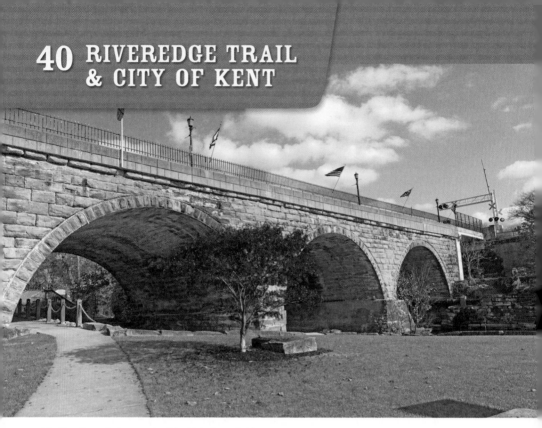

40 RIVEREDGE TRAIL & CITY OF KENT

The Kent Dam sits just south of the Main Street bridge.

THIS STROLL ALONG the Cuyahoga River and through the city of Kent highlights the town's history since the 1800s. It will lead you through a pioneer cemetery, by Ohio's oldest masonry dam, and by some of Kent's historical buildings, many of which are still in use. You'll also visit a large city park, filled with tall shade trees and fun playground areas.

DESCRIPTION

Legend has it that Captain Samuel Brady leapt across the Cuyahoga River to escape from Indigenous peoples in 1780. The river is narrow as it runs through Kent; still, it must have been a mighty leap. We'll never know just how far he jumped or how much credence to give the story. Nevertheless, Riveredge Trail in Kent is the setting for this and many other interesting tales in American history.

Start your hike at John Brown Tannery Park, where a paved path leads from the parking lot down a slight slope toward the river. Veer right and pick your way along the river's edge for a few hundred feet, where you'll find a wide, paved, shared trail.

Riveredge Trail is true to its name; it doesn't stray far from the Cuyahoga River. The river was the primary reason that Kent was a popular settlement in the early 1800s. At first, the town was named Franklin, for the son of the original landowner.

DISTANCE & CONFIGURATION: 3-mile figure eight

DIFFICULTY: Easy

SCENERY: Great variety—from a healthy river community to a vibrant, historic downtown

EXPOSURE: Mostly shaded, with a few exposed stretches

TRAFFIC: Moderate

TRAIL SURFACE: Dirt, pavement, wooden boardwalks, city sidewalks

HIKING TIME: Allow an hour

DRIVING DISTANCE: 31 miles from I-77/I-480 exchange

ACCESS: 24/7

MAPS: USGS *Kent;* advkeen.co/portagehike

FACILITIES: Restrooms at east end of Fred Fuller Park and at the Kramer ball fields

WHEELCHAIR ACCESS: No

CONTACT: 330-673-8897, kentparksandrec.com/parks

LOCATION: Summit St., Kent

In 1805 the Haymaker family moved to Kent and built a dam to power a gristmill. As other mills popped up, the town came to be known as Franklin Mills.

What was then Franklin Mills is now a busy university town, full of folks with flexible schedules, so the trail sees a fair share of traffic all week long.

But as you continue south, you'll find yourself feeling comfortably far away from the busy streets of the college town and enjoying the river's company.

After you pass the Harvey Redmond Bridge on your left, cross Stow Street to continue on Riveredge Trail. Here the trail is also known as The Portage, and the wide, paved trail that runs throughout the city (and university, and beyond) sees a lot of traffic.

YOU HAVE OPTIONS

If you continue southwest on The Portage here, you'll eventually reach the edge of the county, where the Summit Hike-Bike Trail (starting at the Freedom Trail trailhead) continues into Akron. From the Crain Avenue Bridge, on the north side of Kent, you can take The Portage northeast to Towner's Woods, where you can explore more than 5 miles of nature trails, or continue east on the rail-trail (also The Portage) to the city of Ravenna.

To complete the hike as described and shown in the map here, continue on the path alongside the river just about 0.5 mile south of Stow Street, then take a right up a steep, shady hill. At the top, you'll emerge at the southern end of Fred Fuller Park, Kent's largest city park. Restrooms and a playground are located here.

Turn right to follow the park road back toward town. Cars are permitted here, but traffic is light. You'll soon come to the park's reservable shelter house, then pass the park office to come to the historical Kent Jail.

The jail was built in 1869 by the order of Mayor John Thompson. It might easily have not existed, as Mayor Thompson won the office by just two votes. (Thompson

Riveredge Trail & City of Kent

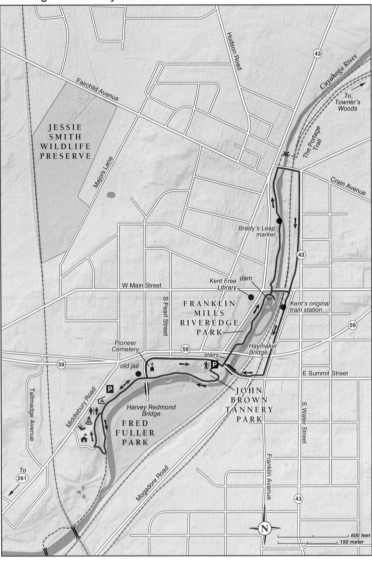

got 145 votes; runner-up Luther Parmelee had 143.) In 1999, the jail was moved to the park and completely renovated, though elements of the original building remain.

From the jail, head north down a steep, grassy hill dotted with a few swings, grills, and picnic tables. Continue west to cross Stow Street, and follow the sidewalk to find Kent's Pioneer Cemetery, dating to 1810.

Headstones here represent the families who figured prominently in Kent's history, including Haymaker, DePeyster, and Woodard. The cemetery gate is open sunrise–sunset.

Back on Stow Street, follow the sidewalk down to the John Brown Tannery Park parking lot, where you began. To complete your figure eight, cross Stow Street (again) to continue along the river trail. A sign here marks the entrance to Franklin Mills Riveredge Park. Head down a series of steps; at the bottom, you'll find yourself under the Haymaker Bridge.

Follow the path as it bends left; shallow river rapids gurgle to your right. This is the only part of the trail that's likely to be at all muddy, and it's a short stretch. (No boots needed!)

As you walk toward the city on wooden stairways and elevated boardwalks, you'll see some of Kent's historic industrial buildings on the left; the old downtown is on your right. From the top of a set of stairs, you'll get a good look at the Kent Dam, the oldest masonry dam in the state of Ohio. This area, including the Kent Dam (constructed circa 1836) and canal basin from the Main Street Bridge to the Stow Street Bridge, comprises the old industrial district that is listed on the National Register of Historic Places.

While other dams on the Cuyahoga have been removed, the dam here was spared demolition because of its historical significance. Instead, it was modified to allow the river to flow freely again. Today, the retrofitted dam is the centerpiece of a small park. From here, architecture aficionados may want to climb the steps to the top of the bridge above and take in some of the town's unique buildings.

On the western corner of River and Main Streets is Kent Free Library. The library was built in 1903, with Andrew Carnegie's money, on land donated by Marvin Kent. In 2006, the original building was incorporated into a substantially larger library, but you can still see the Carnegie library plaque on its exterior.

Looking east from the same corner, you can see the iconic two-story redbrick structure that was the city's original train station, built in 1875. The railroad's arrival here meant that the town would continue to grow, even as canal transportation declined. Marvin Kent was the person most responsible for bringing the new Atlantic and Great Western line to town; in 1864, the grateful citizens of Franklin Mills changed the town's name to honor him.

After descending from your observation point back to the park at the top of the dam, continue north on Riveredge Trail, crossing under the bridge, where the path is a wide brick walkway. Follow it about 0.3 mile, and you'll find a large rock, which purportedly marks the spot where Captain Samuel Brady leapt across the river—some 22 feet or more—to elude his would-be captors in 1780. (While it sounds like a tall tale, Captain Brady has this stretch of trail, and an Ohio Turnpike Plaza, named after him.)

Continue north on Riveredge Trail, either taking a set of stone steps to your left up to street level, or heading through the bridge underpass and then crossing Crain Avenue to see Kent's downtown. A variety of galleries, restaurants, and shops may draw your attention away from your walk for an hour or two. That's OK; you're here to explore.

When you're ready, you can return to Tannery Park by taking Franklin Avenue to Stow Street, where you'll turn right; or return to Riveredge Trail and go back along the river.

NEARBY ACTIVITIES

While children may not want to leave Fred Fuller Park's playground equipment, Kent is packed with more to see and do. The city and downtown merchants host numerous festivals and activities all year long. (For a schedule, see mainstreetkent.org.)

Many people enjoy kayaking or floating down the Cuyahoga River in the warmer months. Novices should be aware that some stretches of the river are challenging and can be dangerous. Get information from a reliable source, like cuyahogariverwater trail.org, before you plan to get on the water.

Kent State University is located 1 mile east of the John Brown Tannery Park parking lot. The Portage stretches from the eastern edge of downtown Kent directly onto the Kent State University campus. You can follow the wide redbrick trail to tour the very walkable campus and see a wide variety of stunning outdoor sculptures. Also take a moment to consider the somber, thought-provoking May 4 Site and Memorial. You may also want to visit the nationally known fashion museum (kent .edu/museum, 330-672-3450).

• •

TRAILHEAD GPS COORDINATES: N41.15055° W81.36325°

DIRECTIONS From Cleveland, take I-77 S to Exit 156, and merge onto I-480 E. Keep right to stay on I-480 E. In about 5 miles, keep right again to stay on I-480 E/OH 14. Continue on OH 14 for about 12 miles, into Streetsboro, where you'll turn right onto OH 43 to head south into Kent. In 6.3 miles, turn left (east) onto Main Street and then, in 0.3 mile, right (south) onto Water Street. Follow Water Street 0.3 mile south to Summit Street and turn right (west). John Brown Tannery Park is about 0.3 mile west on your left.

Riveredge Trail is just steps away from Kent's downtown business area.

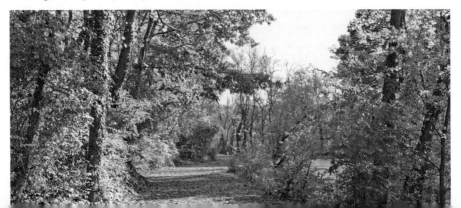

41 SENECA PONDS PARK

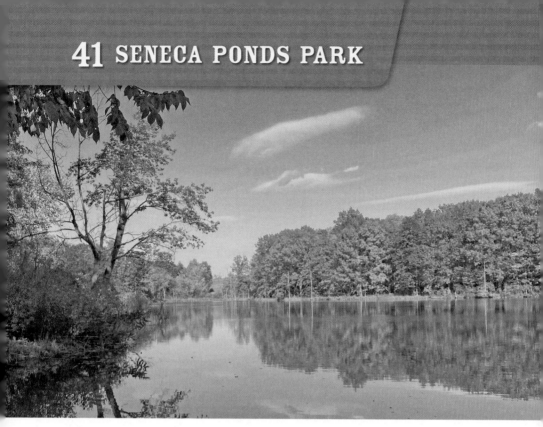

This park is popular with both anglers and hikers.

SURROUNDED BY CORPORATE offices and light industry, a small parcel of land protects woods, wetlands, and possibly our sanity.

DESCRIPTION

As has happened in countless outlying suburbs, Streetsboro's commercial district developed quickly. The urban sprawl steamroller of big-box retailers, manufacturers, and other employers threatened to engulf the entire city. Fortunately, Western Reserve Land Conservancy and Portage Park District were able to create a small preserve in the middle of an office and light industrial park. The trails loop around two of the three ponds on this rustic, 48-acre preserve.

While visitors can see neighboring businesses from at least two spots on the trail, and will never completely escape the droning sounds of traffic coming from the Ohio Turnpike, the unassuming little path through wetlands and forest has proven a welcome and popular addition to the neighborhood, drawing walkers from nearby businesses at lunchtime and evenings throughout the workweek. Seneca Ponds is also a popular fishing destination; bass and sunfish can be hooked here. (See tips for successful catch-and-release techniques at wildlife.ohiodnr.gov /fishing/fishing-basics.)

DISTANCE & CONFIGURATION: 1-mile loop

DIFFICULTY: Easy

SCENERY: Deciduous forest, wetlands, three ponds, beavers, wildflowers

EXPOSURE: Shaded in spring and summer, when trees are full

TRAFFIC: Moderately heavy on evenings and weekday lunchtimes

TRAIL SURFACE: Dirt, mulch, grass, and gravel

HIKING TIME: 35 minutes

DRIVING DISTANCE: 23 miles from I-77/I-480 exchange

ACCESS: Daily, sunrise–sunset

MAPS: USGS *Hudson* and *Twinsburg;* also at trailhead and park website

FACILITIES: None

WHEELCHAIR ACCESS: No

CONTACT: Portage Park District: 330-297-7728, portagecounty-oh.gov/portage-county-park -district/parks-maps/pages/seneca-pond

LOCATION: Mondial Pkwy., Streetsboro

I have had some spirited discussions with people who aren't entirely comfortable with saying that a short loop *in an industrial park, of all places,* qualifies as a hike. I hear that loud and clear. In each case, I've been grateful that my counterargument was fairly well received. In real estate, we've been told, the three most important things about a property are location, location, and location. In photography, even self-professed camera snobs will agree, the best camera is the one you have. And when I talk about hiking, I often say my favorite trail is the one I can hike today.

One of the reasons I love the *60 Hikes* series is because the books put so many trails in major metro areas on the radar of folks who would love to take a week off from work to hike—but they can't because life doesn't cooperate. If sticking a trail—even a short one—in the middle of an industrial park makes hiking around your work schedule a daily possibility, that's a win in my book, and reason enough to include Seneca Ponds here. Putting trails where people will use them is a fine idea, and I think Portage Park District deserves bonus points for forward-thinking and creative planning and development. Now without further ado, here's what you can expect.

Enter the Beaver Trail from the northern edge of the small parking lot, heading up a gentle slope to the first of many trail markers. Follow the trail as it curves to the left and you'll soon be on the edge of the largest of the three ponds. A bench is perched on the water's edge. Be quiet, look closely, and you may see beavers at work—and even if you don't, it's quite possible that you'll see (human) anglers at work. Proceed clockwise and note the different types of rocks you find along the trail. These erratics, typical of the area, were deposited by glacial activity 10,000 years ago, give or take a few decades. As you cross over a couple of footbridges to avoid some very squishy sections of the path, Beaver Trail meanders slightly west, and you can peer through the trees at a still-active railroad track. (Trains chug through infrequently, however.)

Since much of the trail and boardwalks were built by local Boy Scouts from the Seneca District, the park's name is a nod of appreciation to their hard work, which made this property more accessible without damaging its natural assets.

Seneca Ponds Park

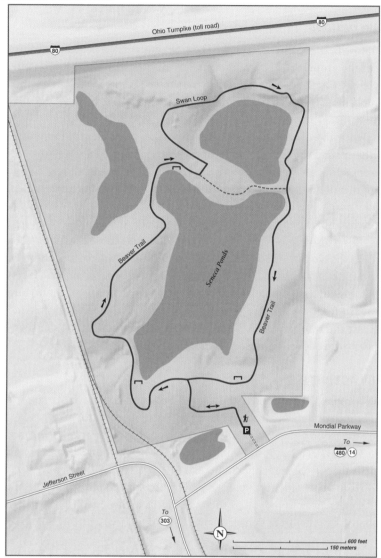

Soon you'll leave the woods to cross over a narrow strip of earth between two ponds, then return to the shaded path where another wooden park bench greets you. A sign alerts you to another trail, marked by a swan. Follow the Swan Loop north here.

YOU HAVE OPTIONS

If you follow Beaver Trail here to the right, you'll be taking a shortcut through the middle of the property. If you want to follow Beaver Trail—and it does offer a nice broad view of the pond—you can either shorten your total trek, or get creative and do a figure eight (which would lengthen your total distance to about 1.5 miles).

Following the description and map shown here, continue curving east around the northern edge of the large pond on the Swan Loop. You'll walk over a variety of different surfaces, including gravel, grass, and mulch, each doing a good job of keeping the trail dry in this wetland habitat. In the late summer and early fall, you'll step over a number of hickory nuts too. Numerous marsh-loving wildflowers can be found on this short stretch of exposed trail. Naturally, during most of the spring and summer, this is also a good spot to spy dragonflies and damselflies.

Back in the woods, and back on the Beaver Trail, now heading south, you'll find another park bench, this one ideally situated for enjoying a sunset. (Insect repellent will make the watching that much more enjoyable, as the mosquito population comes out in force on summer evenings.) The path rolls up a slight incline before veering east and returning you to your starting point, a stark reminder that you just might have to go back to work soon. (Better schedule another hike!)

NEARBY ACTIVITIES

I'm quick to admit I like to add a trail to my list of errands—and a park so close to big-box and other stores makes it easy to do. But if you don't have to follow a shopping list while in Streetsboro, you can spend more time on the trail! Herrick Fen State Nature Preserve (page 170) is just about 5 miles away; Towner's Woods' extensive trail system is about 8.5 miles from here; and Sunny Lake Park (page 197), with paved trails and a dog park, is about 7 miles northeast. And while Streetsboro may not be the most obvious place to get away from it all, in fact, you can: a highly rated KOA campground is just around the corner from Seneca Ponds, about 1 mile west on OH 303.

• •

TRAILHEAD GPS COORDINATES: N41.24988° W81.38211°

DIRECTIONS From Cleveland, take I-77 S to Exit 156, and merge onto I-480 E. In 6.6 miles, keep right to stay on I-480 E. In another 5.5 miles, keep right again to stay on I-480 E/OH 14. Go 10.6 miles and continue straight on OH 14 for another 0.5 mile. Turn right onto Mondial Parkway, following it about 1 mile to the park entrance on the north side of Mondial.

42 SUNNY LAKE PARK

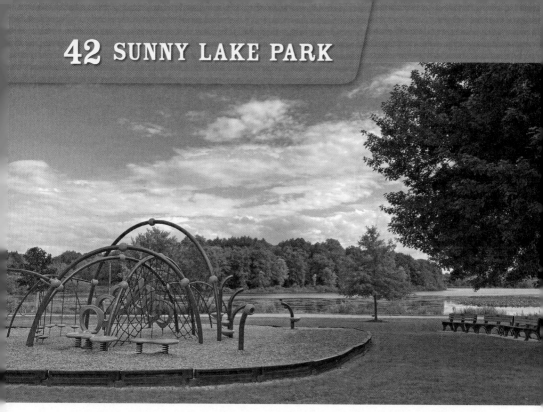

Active visitors of all ages can enjoy volleyball courts, seasonal boat rentals, and two playgrounds here.

SUNNY LAKE PARK serves many different interests. Want to soak up lazy lake views or watch great blue herons come in for long-legged landings? There are plenty of birds (and benches) to keep bird-watchers happy. Budding arborists will admire the Memorial Tree Garden on the park's south side. And a dog park on the west side of the park keeps tails wagging.

DESCRIPTION

From the main parking lot, head for the shelter and concession area, where visitors can rent kayaks, pedal boats, and rowboats during the summer season. Follow the paved path east across a short wooden bridge; then slow your pace to fully appreciate a tour of the Memorial Tree Garden. It features a wide variety of trees, including flowering crabs, "Ivory Silk" Japanese tree lilac, dawn redwoods, Kentucky coffeetrees, red buckeyes, and several varieties of oaks and ash. In 1999, the Aurora Garden Club planted a garden celebrating Aurora's 200th birthday. Daylilies, "Overdam" feather reed grass, "Autumn Joy" sedum, and flame grass grow there amid other decorative trees and bushes. As the garden evolves, and new trees are occasionally added, the unique park feature is an ever-changing tapestry.

The paved trail curves to the left, hugging the lake's eastern shore. In places, cattails grow so thick and tall that they obscure views of the lake. Sunny Lake is indeed sunny; most of the trail around it is exposed. That's not unusual for a lake trail.

DISTANCE & CONFIGURATION: 2-mile loop

DIFFICULTY: Easy

SCENERY: Arboretum, natural forest, birds, lake

EXPOSURE: Mostly exposed

TRAFFIC: Moderate–heavy, especially during warm weather

TRAIL SURFACE: Main loop, paved; optional footpaths, dirt and wood chips

HIKING TIME: 50 minutes

DRIVING DISTANCE: 19 miles from I-77/I-480 exchange

ACCESS: Daily, sunrise–sunset. If gate at main parking is closed, park at Memorial

Tree Garden, east of main entrance, off Mennonite Road.

MAPS: USGS *Aurora;* also available from City of Aurora Parks & Recreation Department

FACILITIES: Restrooms and water by main parking lot; picnic tables, shelters, grills, and playgrounds throughout park; dog park, volleyball court, and boathouse with boat rentals

WHEELCHAIR ACCESS: Yes; lake loop is paved, but nature trails are not.

CONTACT: 330-562-4333, auroraoh.com/departments/parks___recreation/parks/parks___trails/sunny_lake_park

LOCATION: 885 E. Mennonite Road, Aurora

But then, at about 0.5 mile, you can't see the lake for the trees. A couple of well-traveled but unmarked dirt trails on the left head through the woods toward the lake. (They're very short and loop back to the main trail quickly, so follow them if you want.) As the woods thin out, you'll be able to see most of the lake again from its midpoint. There's a lot to see.

Great blue heron sightings are almost guaranteed here. Birds often travel between here and Tinkers Creek State Nature Preserve, about 2.5 miles from here as the crow—or heron—flies. Gulls and goldfinches gather here as well. At 0.8 mile, you'll come to a small clearing and several birdhouses. A mown but unmarked utility path leads to your right (east). The paved path veers left, curling down to the lakeshore.

You may choose to leave the pavement here, as I did, and dive into the woods via a hard-packed dirt trail that winds through the oak and maple trees and over a couple of small hills, before leaving the woods, depositing you back on the paved path.

Back on the paved loop trail, the path begins to curve left as you continue counterclockwise. At the northern end of the lake, you'll find a small picnic shelter and a playset that will be almost irresistible to kids who love to climb. From this spot, you can just about see the whole lake. Lily pads cover the water in places; this is an ideal spot to listen as frogs, birds, and bugs sing to you. The woods are thick again as you round the lake's western edge; several park benches are placed to take advantage of the resulting shade and birding opportunities.

On the west side of the lake, you'll spot more birdhouses and also notice a large, fenced dog park area. Because it is most easily accessed from Page Road, most dog owners enter and leave from that parking area rather than from the main park entrance. As you reach the end of your counterclockwise loop, you'll pass by the boathouse (staffed seasonally) and volleyball courts.

Other than some basic grounds and trail maintenance, and the obvious care put into the Memorial Tree Garden, Sunny Lake's trees and vegetation have been left

Sunny Lake Park

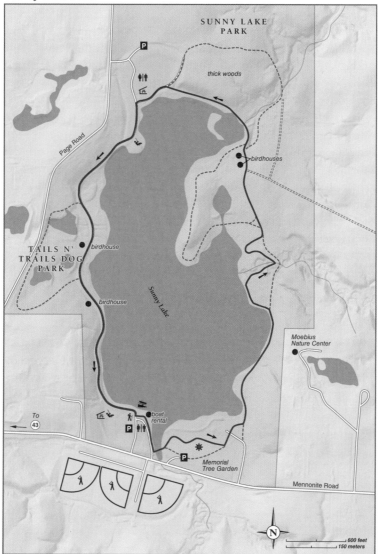

largely alone to shelter a large population of rabbits, black and gray squirrels, fat robins, noisy jays, singing spring peepers, and a few harmless snakes.

When you return to the main parking lot, you've logged at least 2 miles (plus another 0.5 mile or more if you explored any of the short nature trails). Over that distance, you've probably met up with a number of dog walkers, families with strollers, and maybe a bicyclist or two—even if you visit on a weekday. Sunny Lake's loop is also a popular spot at weekday lunchtimes, too, as workers escape the nearby industrial parks, if only for an hour.

NEARBY ACTIVITIES

Sunny Lake Park's 463 acres offer plenty of activities. On the western side of the main parking lot, there are swings, volleyball courts, and horseshoe pits, plus a sledding hill that's popular in the winter. Catch-and-release fishing is allowed with a permit from the city. Aurora residents can launch their own nonmotorized crafts here for free; nonresidents pay a nominal fee for the privilege. Details are available at the website, auroraoh.com/departments/parks___recreation/parks/parks___trails, or by calling 330-562-6131. Just east of the park and accessible by car off Mennonite Road, Moebius Nature Center hosts a variety of educational programs for folks of all ages, as well as tours by appointment. See the events schedule at the website, mymnc.org, or call 216-402-4361. For more hiking options, you can visit Tinkers Creek State Nature Preserve (page 201), about 2.5 miles southwest of Sunny Lake, or Paddock River Preserve (page 179), just about 3 miles to the north.

• •

TRAILHEAD GPS COORDINATES: N41.29121° W81.31826°

DIRECTIONS From the I-77/I-480 exchange, follow I-480 E 8.9 miles; keep right at the fork to continue on I-480 E for another 5.5 miles. Keep right at another fork to stay on I-480 E/OH 14 for another 9.7 miles, then take Exit 41 (Frost Road). Turn left (east) onto Frost Road and go 1.8 miles; turn left (north) onto OH 43/South Chillicothe Road. In 2.1 miles, turn right (east) onto Mennonite Road. Follow Mennonite about 1.5 miles east to the park's main entrance on the left at 885 East Mennonite Road. Additional parking is available on the north end of the park at 625 Page Road.

43 TINKERS CREEK STATE NATURE PRESERVE

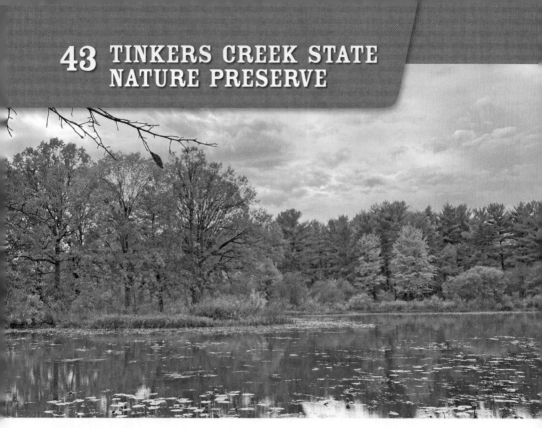

View from the Seven Ponds Trail

THIS 786-ACRE NATURE preserve offers great waterfowl and other wildlife viewing opportunities, as well as a peaceful, quiet marshland in which to be still and enjoy a bit of solitude.

DESCRIPTION

Though the parking area is on the north side of Old Mill Road, the main entrance to the preserve is across the street. But before you head south, make your way to the northeast end of the parking lot and follow the short Eagle Point Trail through the woods. The dirt path through young deciduous trees may not impress you at first, but once you reach the raised observation platform, you'll be glad you made the trip. The vista that greets you—a wide expanse of marshy wetlands—is outlined by tall trees that eagles like to call home, and many migrating species visit each year.

Retracing your steps back to and across Old Mill, you'll enter the preserve on a path that runs parallel to and just a few hundred feet from active railroad tracks. While that can mean a noisy distraction, they don't detract in the slightest from the views here.

The path narrows as it heads south. Not long after, about 0.3 mile south of the trailhead sign, the path forks—turn left (east). You'll soon step up on a wooden boardwalk. About half of this 0.5-mile loop is boardwalk, necessary because it travels over marsh. Ohio's early pioneers liked to hunt here, but they were also wary of the squishy

DISTANCE & CONFIGURATION: 2.5-mile balloon/figure eight

DIFFICULTY: Easy

SCENERY: Seven ponds, marshlands, herons, nesting Canada geese and wood ducks, beavers, raccoons, deer, snapping turtles

EXPOSURE: Mostly shaded

TRAFFIC: Light

TRAIL SURFACE: Dirt and gravel with some boardwalk

HIKING TIME: 1 hour for three trails and observation time at the overlook

DRIVING DISTANCE: 22 miles from I-77/I-480 exchange

ACCESS: Daily, 30 minutes before sunrise–30 minutes after sunset; pets not allowed

MAPS: USGS *Twinsburg;* also at trailhead and preserve website

FACILITIES: None

WHEELCHAIR ACCESS: No

CONTACT: Ohio Department of Natural Resources: 614-265-6453, ohiodnr.gov/go-and-do/plan-a-visit/find-a-property/tinkers-creek-state-park; Summit Metroparks: 330-867-5511, summitmetroparks.org

LOCATION: Old Mill Road, Aurora

ground. Some referred to it as a "perilous" place, full of sinkholes and quicksand. Though the thick peat is messy, deerflies and mosquitoes are really all that hikers in this area have to fear today—unless you suffer from ophidiophobia, the extreme fear of snakes. In that case, you should probably opt for a different trail. Almost every time I've been here, except in December and January, I've seen at least one snake.

You're also quite likely to come upon deer almost any time of year. If you're quiet, and lucky, you may hear the slap of a beaver's tail as you near the pond. The boardwalk ends just about the time the pond comes into sight.

The marsh, full of cattails, is on your right; the pond is on your left. The path can be quite muddy (this is a wetland, after all), and if your insect repellent fails here, you'll be sorry. Continue across the trail intersection and begin to circle the pond counterclockwise. Old-growth pines and young oak trees almost completely shade the trail. In spring and summer, an abundance of ferns and wild purple violets lines the path. Water in the pond itself is clean enough to watch crappie and turtles swimming around below the surface.

Several types of ferns dot the trail; in spring, expect to find a thick covering of mayapples here. Their umbrella-like leaves shade the pretty white flowers. On the north side of Lonesome Pond, grass and roots have overtaken much of the trail, making for less sloppy footing, even on wet days. After circling the pond, leave it lonesome once more and head south. A bench at the intersection of Lonesome Pond Loop and Seven Ponds Trail is a good place to contemplate what you've seen and consider your next steps.

Seven Ponds Trail heads south from here. Follow it as it weaves around the small ponds (which total seven, as advertised) and leads to a wooden observation deck. The deck faces east, and from here you can see almost all of the marsh. Herons like to fly between here and nearby Sunny Lake Park (page 197). It's a rare visit to either park that doesn't include a heron sighting.

Tinkers Creek State Nature Preserve

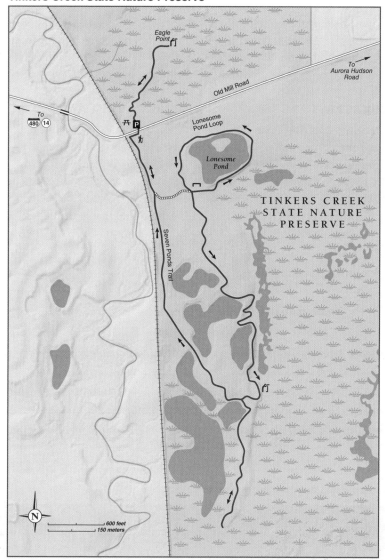

While this trail (and the whole preserve) sees little traffic, you may meet an avid birder or photographer here on the deck; it's popular with both.

When you can tear yourself away from the view, follow the path around a gentle bend to the right. Soon after, the path splits. Follow the left fork south to the tip of the "peninsula" surrounded by the open marsh. Shaded by beeches, oaks, and maples, this spur is especially pretty in the fall. When you return to the loop and head west, you'll make your way by and between the remaining ponds.

As you head north, the trail straightens out and, for the most part, it dries out as well. The railroad tracks are on your left, and the trail returns you to the intersection of Lonesome Pond Loop. With footsteps cushioned by the pine needles, you'll exit as quietly as you came in, slipping past the trailhead sign and crossing Old Mill Road.

NEARBY ACTIVITIES

If watching the waterfowl dive and splash makes you want to drop a line in the water, go around the corner to the Tinkers Creek Area of Liberty Park (formerly Tinkers Creek State Park). There, just off Aurora Hudson Road, you'll find plenty of fish-friendly spots and a completely different set of trails. Serious bird-watchers will want to visit Aurora Sanctuary State Nature Preserve, a 164-acre property owned by the Audubon Society of Greater Cleveland. Access is available through the Aurora Town Hall parking lot, 130 South Chillicothe Road. For more information, contact the local Audubon Society at 216-556-5441.

• •

TRAILHEAD GPS COORDINATES: N41.28481° W81.39163°

DIRECTIONS From Cleveland, follow I-480 E 8.9 miles; keep right at the fork to continue on I-480 E for another 5.5 miles. Keep right at another fork to stay on I-480 E/OH 14 for another 9.7 miles, then take Exit 36 (OH 82/Aurora Road). Turn left (east) onto OH 82/Aurora Road and go 0.8 mile. Make a slight right onto OH 82 and go 2.6 miles. Turn left (east) onto Old Mill Road and go 0.8 mile to the small parking lot on the left (north) side of the road.

This is a popular spot during bird-migration season.

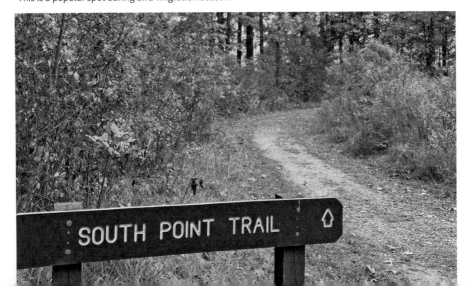

44 WEST BRANCH STATE PARK: Michael J. Kirwan Dam

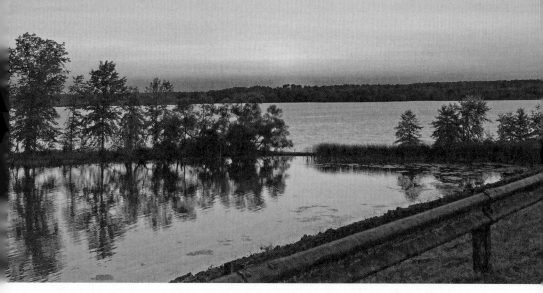

Michael J. Kirwan Dam is definitely one of the best sunrise (and sunset) spots in Portage County.

IF YOU CAN ignore all the fun that massive West Branch State Park has to offer and make it to the business end of the park—the dam—you'll find a place where time almost seems to stand still.

DESCRIPTION

With so much to explore in West Branch State Park, you might want to stay a few days. (No kidding—the campground is very popular, with choice campsites booked months in advance.) The park sprawls over more than 5,300 acres; the lake comprises another 2,650 acres. The dam is on the far east end of the park. In fact, it's not part of the park at all. Rather, the park is part of it.

Michael J. Kirwan Dam and Reservoir is a recreational area owned by the U.S. Army Corps of Engineers. The adjacent land and reservoir are leased to the Ohio Department of Natural Resources, which manages it as a park. Boring details aside, here's why you'll want to go: The dam provides one of the most sweeping vistas in northeast Ohio, and one that stretches out a sunset to the point that time seems to stand still.

From the parking lot, traipse up a short hill to the dam access road. It's closed to vehicular traffic but is as wide as a city street. Almost any time you go, you'll find a few other walkers, joggers, and cyclists here, but it never seems crowded at all.

DISTANCE & CONFIGURATION: 3-mile out-and-back

DIFFICULTY: Moderate

SCENERY: Heavily wooded beech-maple forest, a few stands of pine, lake views, overlook

EXPOSURE: Mostly shaded

TRAFFIC: Moderate on weekdays; heavy on weekends

TRAIL SURFACE: Partially paved

HIKING TIME: 1 hour

DRIVING DISTANCE: 35 miles from I-77/I-480 exchange

ACCESS: Daily, 6 a.m.–11 p.m.

MAPS: USGS *Ravenna* and *Windham;* also at trailhead and park office (5708 Esworthy Road)

FACILITIES: Restrooms, phone, picnic shelter, and grills by boat ramp

WHEELCHAIR ACCESS: No

CONTACT: Park office: 330-296-3239, ohiodnr.gov/go-and-do/plan-a-visit/find-a -property/west-branch-state-park; U.S. Army Corps of Engineers: 330-358-2247

LOCATION: Wayland Road, Ravenna

The dam access road really deserves a better name, but it is what it is. A rose by any other name, right? From the minute you're on the dam roadway, you have a bird's-eye view of the reservoir, or at least the eastern end of it. You'll be heading northwest as you cross the dam, and while it's always pretty, I highly recommend timing your visit to late afternoon or early evening, so you can stroll as the sun begins to set.

As hikes go, this one is as straight and flat as it gets—you're walking over a dam, remember? The sun playing over the vast stretch of water to your left as you head out can play tricks on your mind. Let it. That's part of the magic of this hike—you don't have to pay attention to where you're going; there's absolutely no way to get lost.

Thanks to the trail's unnatural straightness and unusual position, well above surrounding landmarks, it can also mess with your perception. Although it's just a little over 1.5 miles from one side of the dam to the other, at times as you walk across, it will seem as though you're nearly there; at other points, as if you'll never get there. And when you get there—the other side of the dam, that is—you'll turn around only to find that the return trip plays the same tricks on your mind. Again, let it. Hiking is at least as good for your mind as it is for your body.

Because timing is important with sunset hikes, here's some advice: Don't underestimate the time you'll need to cross the dam and return. It's tempting to stop, savor a view, watch a water-skier in the distance, gawk at a deer or a hawk . . . so allow some extra time in your plan. And take your camera. The sunset views here make almost every photographer look like a professional.

NEARBY ACTIVITIES

West Branch State Park—named for the west branch of the Mahoning River, which was dammed in 1965—offers a variety of wet and dry activities for folks of all ages and interests. In addition to some popular snowmobile/bike trails, an 8-mile segment of the Buckeye Trail loops through the park's western end. As of this writing, the Buckeye Trail Association was making great progress on moving most of the trail off road, and

West Branch State Park: Michael J. Kirwan Dam

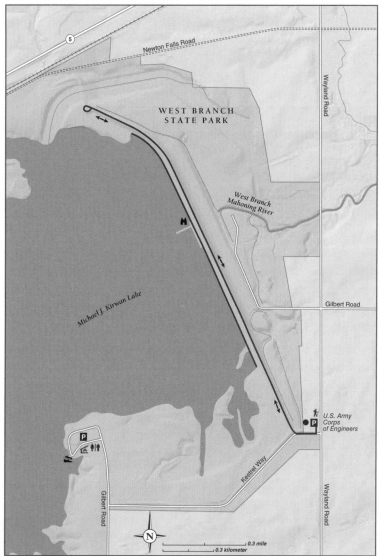

soon the trail at West Branch is expected to loop the entire reservoir. If you enjoy trails like that, consider joining and volunteering with the BTA. They'd love to have you!

Add to that mountain bike, nature, and bridle trails; numerous boat launches; a marina where you can rent jet skis; and a 700-foot swimming beach, and West Branch State Park might qualify as one of northeast Ohio's hidden gems.

The park's campground is extremely popular and hosts a variety of family-friendly events, including its beloved Christmas in July and the annual Halloween

Campout in October. For more information, see ohiodnr.gov/go-and-do/plan-a-visit /find-a-property/west-branch-state-park-campground.

To find out more about boat rentals, call the marina at 330-296-9209 or visit westbranchmarina.com.

• •

TRAILHEAD GPS COORDINATES: N41.14715° W81.07193°

DIRECTIONS From I-77, take Exit 156 and merge onto I-480, heading east. In 6.6 miles, keep right to stay on I-480 E, and in another 5.5 miles, keep right again to stay on I-480. Continue to follow I-480 E another 10.6 miles to OH 14 in Streetsboro. Follow OH 14 E 11.6 miles and exit onto OH 5. Merge onto OH 5 E, and in less than a mile, veer right to stay on OH 5. Follow OH 5 about 7 miles east of Ravenna and turn right (south) onto Wayland Road. Follow Wayland 1.3 miles, and turn right (west) onto Kestrel Way, where a small parking lot and the Corps office are located. (Because mapping apps tend to give directions to the boat ramp or swimming beach at West Branch State Park, use the address 8655 Kestrel Way to get accurate directions.)

The Dam—providing great views since 1965

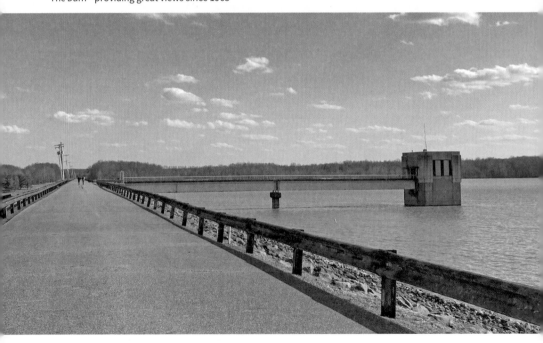

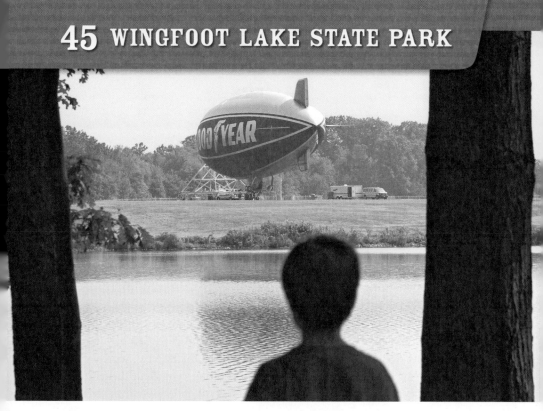

There's good reason this park is a designated site on the Ohio Air and Space Trail.

THIS PROPERTY WAS operated as a private recreation area for employees of the Goodyear Tire & Rubber Co. for several decades. When it opened (again) in 2010 as Ohio's 74th state park, interest in its history was revived, and the park has attracted a new generation of fans.

DESCRIPTION

It's a safe bet that most visitors to Wingfoot Lake State Park don't go just to hike the 800-plus-acre property. Land-based attractions here include a small nature center, a popular disc golf course, a fenced dog park, several large and well-appointed picnic shelters, plus numerous grills, picnic tables, and swings and benches set on the lake's edge. In addition, the 444-acre lake offers fishing and boating opportunities. And while hikers almost certainly won't find solitude here, they will find a wide and gently rolling paved path nearly circling the park, with some natural paths connecting its edges. In short, there are many vantage points from which visitors can gain a perspective on this interesting property and its place in history.

While Wingfoot certainly boasts a lot of amenities, a robust trail system isn't one of them. (At least, not yet—numerous developments are underway at this park, and new trails are on the drawing board.) For now, there are several ways to explore the

DISTANCE & CONFIGURATION: 1.6-mile loop, with optional 1 mile of paved/accessible walkways

DIFFICULTY: Easy

SCENERY: Lake and cultivated woodlands, unique view of the Goodyear Airdock

EXPOSURE: Mostly shaded

TRAFFIC: Moderate–heavy

TRAIL SURFACE: Paved

HIKING TIME: 35 minutes–1 hour

DRIVING DISTANCE: 41 miles from I-77/I-480 exchange

ACCESS: Daily, 6 a.m.–11 p.m.

MAPS: USGS *Suffield*; also at kiosk

FACILITIES: Nature center, boat rental, disc golf, miniature golf, playgrounds, sledding hill, volleyball courts, several restrooms and enclosed shelters, grills and picnic tables, and dog park

WHEELCHAIR ACCESS: Yes, mostly

CONTACT: 330-628-4720, ohiodnr.gov/go-and-do/plan-a-visit/find-a-property/wingfoot-lake-state-park

LOCATION: 993 Goodyear Park Blvd., Mogadore

park. Taking off from the parking lot nearest the entrance along the roadway, heading to the lake's edge, and making a counterclockwise loop around the property gives you a good look at the whole place—that's what's mapped and described here. Another option is to start from the main parking lot (marked by the historic Goodyear sign) and follow the paved paths that crisscross the park, darting from picnic shelter to putt-putt golf to Storybook Trail to lakeshore. This is a good option for wheelchairs and strollers. A third option, following the disc golf course from hole 1 to 18, is a great way to see the park and get a real appreciation for the rolling nature of the land. The caveat, of course: this is a very popular course, so you risk annoying a lot of disc golfers!

For this outing, we'll start from the northwest end of the first parking lot along the park road, directly across from the dog park.

From the parking lot, walk along the side of the park road south—toward the lake—until you see the imposing Goodyear sign. The historic stone slab sports the trademark Wingfoot logo, and although the dedication plaque doesn't definitively date it, it's certainly been around for the better part of a century.

After appreciating that unique piece of history, cross the roadway and find your way to the lake's edge. The grass is still mowed in much of the park, and it was land-scaped to welcome well-dressed visitors, so you'll find the drainage here is excellent.

As you meander toward the edge of Wingfoot Lake, under the shade of mature oaks, maples, and other deciduous trees, you'll soon come to the park's office and just beyond it, a kayak kiosk. Wingfoot was one of the first two Ohio State parks to test out the kiosk concept, whereby renters can download an app to rent a boat, paddle, and personal flotation device for an hour. (On the eastern edge of the park, a boat concession area, where visitors can rent pedal boats and small pontoon boats, is still staffed in the warmer months.)

Wherever you are on the edge of Wingfoot Lake, you're likely to encounter a few anglers hoping to hook bass, bluegills, crappie, brown bullheads, walleyes, or yellow perch. But while the landscaped grounds and lake views are sure to please

Wingfoot Lake State Park

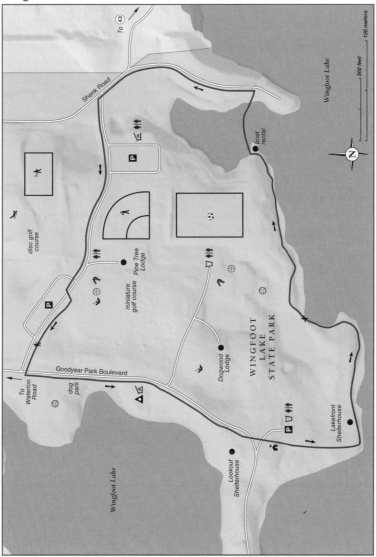

visitors, for most, those sights will take a backseat to the supersized structure on the southern edge of the lake: the Goodyear Airdock.

The massive blue-and-silver building where hundreds of airships have been erected is a rather obvious reminder that The Goodyear Tire & Rubber Co. makes more than tires. In fact, Wingfoot Lake Airship Base is the oldest airship base in the United States. In 1925, Goodyear built and operated the first US commercially licensed blimp flown using helium; it has sold several different airship models to the

U.S. Navy. On clear days from late spring through early fall, visitors will often see (and hear!) the company's blimps take off and land across the lake.

Regardless of the activity in the air, there's plenty to see and do on the ground on the north side of the lake. Continue to curve along the shore and then inland, following the (now paved) path eastward, over a pretty covered footbridge, then veering right to reach the new nature center building.

From here, you get to walk across a floating walkway to reach the peninsula of land where the nature center is located. Along the way you'll pass the (staffed) boat concession and, quite possibly, a few folks fishing off the platform.

When you get to the nature center, even if it's not open, there's plenty to see. Thanks to the lake's contours, with every curve of the path, your view changes.

As you turn left and follow the roadway north, you'll notice a couple of things right away. First, you can drive to the nature center if you choose (signs direct you from the main parking area), and a number of structures left over from the park's

There are plenty of places to drop a line along the shore at Wingfoot Lake.

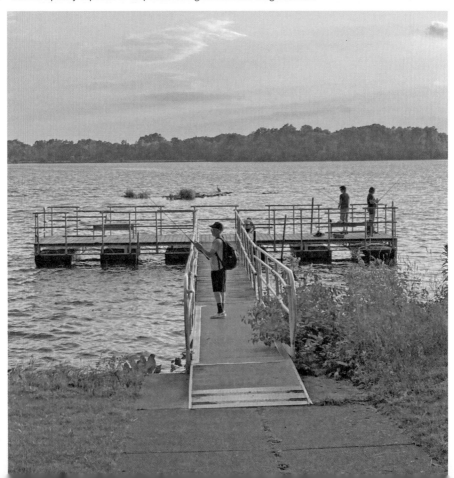

previous incarnation are still in use. Several structures that look like tiny houses were pump houses when Goodyear hosted its employees here; today, they are used by the park system for storage. In the middle of the park, the canteen, where Goodyear employees and their families once purchased candy and other items, is now used primarily for office space, and three large, enclosed picnic shelters are available for event rentals. But we're not quite there yet—rolling down a slight incline from the nature center, you'll come to a wide-open field that supports pollinators, purple martins, and disc golf enthusiasts. In other words, this is a good place to pay attention!

Cross the park road and find a narrow mown path heading north and up a slight incline. This trail was planned in cooperation with the Autism Society and Portage County Board of Developmental Disabilities to help make appreciating nature comfortable and accessible for people of different abilities. A Braille Trail is also in the works for this area, where braille descriptions will offer information about the unique scents and sounds along this stretch of the park.

From the mown path, you can loop around and return to the park roadway, making your way back to the parking lot along the road, but if the disc golf course isn't crowded, you can cross the park roadway and jump on at hole 14. Following the course is a good way to enjoy more of the park's rolling landscape on dirt and grass— but only if you're not interrupting a competitive group on the course! Following the course through to hole 18 will bring you back to your starting point. However, if you don't want to interrupt a game, you'll easily find your way back along the roadway, finishing your loop at just over 1.5 miles.

Unless you're out of daylight or energy, don't stop there! Almost a mile of meandering, paved paths crisscross the beautiful grounds, with constantly changing views of the lake.

NEARBY ACTIVITIES

If Wingfoot's rather buttoned-up nature leaves you longing for more rustic trails, consider Quail Hollow Park to the south (page 183) or Springfield Bog, a Summit Metropark property just about 3 miles east of here.

• •

TRAILHEAD GPS COORDINATES: N41.01808° W81.36178°

DIRECTIONS Follow I-77 S toward Akron, taking Exit 129 to I-76 W. In 1.7 miles, take Exit 18 to I-277/US 224 E toward Canton. In 3.9 miles, continue onto US 224 E and go another 6.7 miles. Turn right (south) onto Martin Road, and in 0.3 mile, turn left (east) onto Waterloo Road. Follow Waterloo about 1 mile east to the park entrance at Goodyear Park Boulevard.

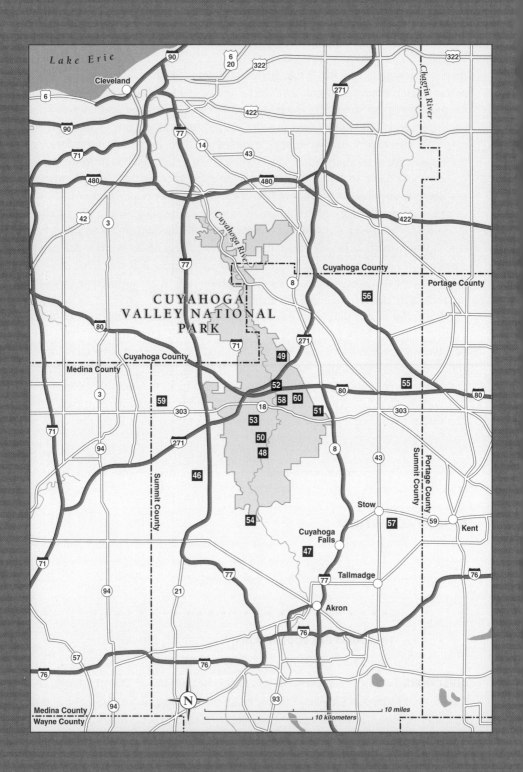

SUMMIT COUNTY

46 BATH NATURE PRESERVE

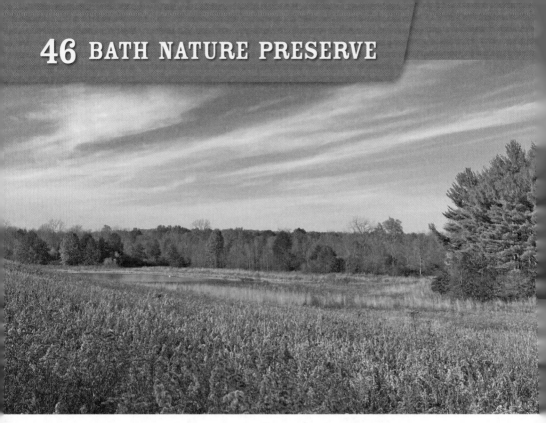

Visitors will appreciate the township's efforts to protect and restore the land in this large preserve.

THIS SUMMIT COUNTY nature preserve offers trails for hikers, a field station for biology students, and fun astronomy factoids for visitors of all ages.

DESCRIPTION

The 411-acre Bath Nature Preserve was once part of the Raymond Firestone Estate. Both Raymond and his father, Henry, who founded the Tire and Rubber company in 1900, were outstanding philanthropists in addition to being extremely successful businessmen. Although the family donated far and wide, their imprint on northeast Ohio is most impressive.

In 1997, Bath Township purchased this land, and since then the preserve has protected a variety of plant communities, including old-growth forest, wetlands, and grasslands. In 2001, the preserve opened for public use. In 2013, a long-term project to restore a tamarack bog began; visitors can now enjoy the thriving stand of deciduous conifers on the south end of the preserve.

In addition to preserving and restoring the land and some of its plant communities, Bath Township has created a space that allows locals to enjoy the passive recreational hobby of stargazing. When you enter the parking lot, you'll likely notice two large buildings that look a bit unusual: both have protruding supports for their roll-off

DISTANCE & CONFIGURATION: 3-mile figure eight with shorter (1.5 miles) and longer options (plus 3 miles of bridle trails)

DIFFICULTY: Moderate with several rolling hills

SCENERY: Deer and hawks in the oak-maple-hickory forest, frogs and other aquatic life in the ponds, bog-loving tamaracks, broad prairie hillsides

EXPOSURE: Mostly exposed

TRAFFIC: Moderate

TRAIL SURFACE: Some pavement, but mostly crushed limestone, dirt, and grass

HIKING TIME: Allow 2 hours

DRIVING DISTANCE: 17 miles from I-77/I-480 exchange

ACCESS: Daily, 7 a.m.–sunset

MAPS: USGS *West Richfield;* also at trailhead and at kiosk at Bath Community Activity Center off N. Cleveland-Massillon Road

FACILITIES: Restrooms and water fountain at trail kiosk and at picnic shelters at either end of trail

WHEELCHAIR ACCESS: No

CONTACT: Bath Township Parks: 330-666-4007, advkeen.co/bathtownshipparks

LOCATION: 4160 Ira Road, Bath Township

roofs. The buildings comprise the impressive Fairlawn Rotary Observatory, which is home to the Akron Astronomy Club. (For more information, see observatoriesof ohio.org/fairlawn-rotary-observatory.)

The University of Akron also operates a field station here, where students conduct hands-on studies in biology and ecology. (Occasionally, the university offers educational programming for the public; see fieldstation.uakron.edu/contact-us for information about upcoming events.)

But you're probably here to hike, so let's get started.

From the parking lot off Ira Road, step onto the North Fork Trail heading east. At first, you'll travel on pavement, and you can stop to appreciate a few informative signs that are part of the solar system trail. The 1.3-mile solar system trail follows the paved North Fork Trail, with signs sharing planetary knowledge and lore while marking the relative distance between the planets. If you follow this description, you'll miss a few of the signs but enjoy more of the preserve as you hike.

Remaining on North Fork for the time being, enjoy the view of wide open, prairie-like fields with native grasses and wildflowers in season. Birds, butterflies, and woodland insects offer their various trills, chirps, and songs along the way.

Soon, turn left at the fork in the path to reach the Creekside Trail split; then turn right onto the mown-grass path. Bird boxes are strewn along this trail and throughout the property, and some of the species that live here, like killdeer, make their nests near the ground, so you may feel more surrounded by your feathered friends than usual.

When you walk by an oil-and-gas well, it's a good time to check your expectations about preservation and restoration projects. The "preserved" label doesn't mean the land is pristine; and not all of the plants you'll see here are native. Nature preserves and protected areas are always works in progress; generally, however, the "preserve" label does prevent significant new development projects.

Bath Nature Preserve

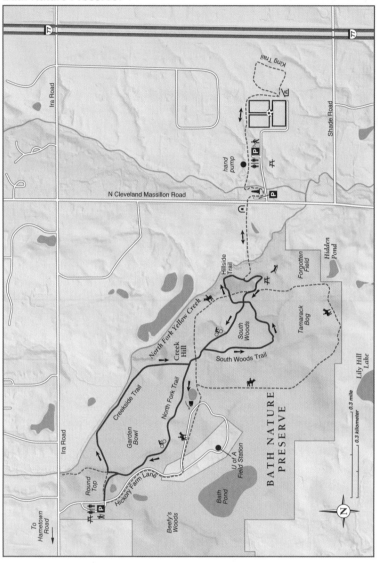

Continue past the oil well to stay on Creekside Trail, which, true to its name, follows a creekbed. It's not surprising that this trail can be slow to dry out after a good rain.

Cross over a small footbridge on Creekside, then follow the trail as it veers to the right. A utility road continues straight; make sure you follow Creekside Trail as it passes another oil well and climbs uphill at the aptly-named Creek Hill. Soon the grassy path intersects with the pavement of North Fork Trail. Turn left onto North Fork and follow it as the ground levels out, then turn right onto South Woods

Trail. You can confidently ignore unsigned trails (most likely used for field station research), as the sanctioned trails are well marked.

The wide, hard-packed dirt-and-gravel South Woods Trail wanders under oak, maple, and birch trees, offering more shade than most of the trails here, at least when the trees are fully leafed out. Follow South Woods Trail across North Fork Trail and continue northeast onto Hillside Trail, the southernmost of the nature trails here. True to its name, Hillside Trail twists and turns several times before rejoining the North Fork Trail. There, you'll turn right and begin the long, sloping trek back to your starting point.

As you continue north, you'll wander by the sledding hill, pass a footpath leading to a small fishing pond, and see a few more signs along the solar system walk. It's fitting because the Greek word *planetes,* from which we get "planet," means wanderer.

YOU HAVE OPTIONS

You probably caught sight of the bridle trails several times as you walked through the preserve. Hikers are permitted on the bridle trails here, and following them will add about 3 miles to your total distance. Alternatively, if you want to stick to the paved North Fork Trail, you can get the full effect of the solar system walk—about 1.4 miles, one way. To shorten the distance for new or beginning hikers, you could opt to park a second car at the Bath Activity Center lot off Cleveland-Massillon Road.

NEARBY ACTIVITIES

Depending on the season, you may want to bring along a fishing pole or your sled. For a completely different approach to the preserve, you can enter off North Cleveland-Massillon Road, where a larger-than-life-size statue of Chief Logan will welcome you to Bath Community Park. There you'll find tennis courts, soccer fields, and a paved trail that leads north, through a tunnel, then uphill about 0.25 mile to reach the sledding hill, where you can connect with Hillside Trail and the preserve's other hiking trails. From either entrance to the nature preserve, you're not far from Sand Run Metro Park, where more paved and nature trails await.

• •

TRAILHEAD GPS COORDINATES: N41.18729° W81.65549°

DIRECTIONS Follow I-77 S toward Akron and take Exit 143 for OH 176. Turn right onto OH 176, then left onto Brecksville Road. Continue onto North Cleveland Massillon Road for about 1 mile, then turn right onto Ira Road. The parking lot is located at 4160 Ira Road in Bath Township. To access trails from the south, find parking at Bath Community Activity Center (1615 N. Cleveland Massillon Road).

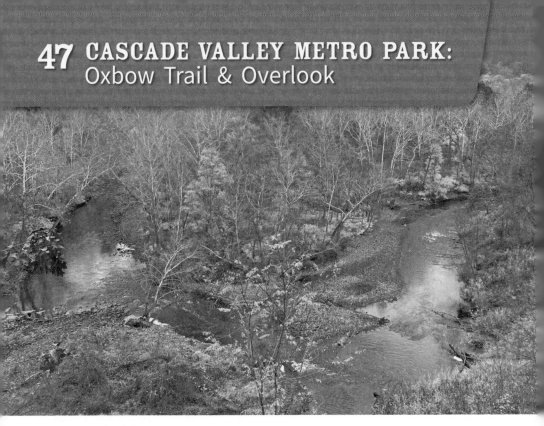

Oxbow overlook in fall

OXBOW TRAIL WINDS through the Cuyahoga River Valley, north of Akron. From the burbling rapids of the Cuyahoga River to a cardiac climb to a fabulous vista, this hike offers variety over a short haul. Looking past the sledding hill and ball fields nearby, hikers can enjoy the scenery of a wooded trail along the riverside, then gaze at the river and surrounding valley from above.

DESCRIPTION

If Oxbow Trail were a book—well, it would be a novella—you'd describe it to your friends by saying, "It started a bit slow, but before I was halfway through, I hoped it wouldn't end." In fact, Oxbow packs so much scenery in its little loop that you'll be glad you picked it up. It's also a great casual dining spot. Oxbow's many picnic tables are placed to provide comfortable space between diners. It's entirely possible to enjoy a picnic supper here, with the lilting of the Cuyahoga to entertain you, and never catch wind of the dinner conversation at another table.

Because the trail is damp along the river and shady throughout, it's a great place for insects to hang out, so it's advisable to apply some bug repellent when visiting. The insects attract birds, of course, and you're likely to hear, if not see, woodpeckers at work on some of the 60-foot-tall (and taller) trees along the way. Mostly deciduous varieties—tall oaks and black cherries—shade the trail.

DISTANCE & CONFIGURATION: 1.7-mile loop; 0.5-mile trip to overlook can be done as a stand-alone trail

DIFFICULTY: Moderate, with a steep hill to start (see "You Have Options" for a flat path to the overlook)

SCENERY: Marsh, river, woodlands, two different views of the rumbling Cuyahoga River

EXPOSURE: Mostly shaded

TRAFFIC: Moderate most days; bustling on evenings and weekends

TRAIL SURFACE: Dirt carpeted with leaves; first leg can be muddy; steps may be slippery when wet

HIKING TIME: 45 minutes

DRIVING DISTANCE: 35 miles from I-77/I-480 exchange

ACCESS: Daily, 6 a.m.–11 p.m.; leashed dogs allowed

MAPS: USGS *Peninsula* and *Akron West;* also at trailhead and park website

FACILITIES: Restrooms (may be closed in winter) and water; emergency phone at southernmost entrance; restrooms at Sackett Ave. trailhead

WHEELCHAIR ACCESS: No

CONTACT: Summit Metro Parks: 330-867-5511, summitmetroparks.org/cascade-valley-metro-park.aspx

LOCATION: Cuyahoga St., Akron

Head south-southwest (counterclockwise) from the trailhead to meander through several marshy turns (in dry weather) or large puddles (in wetter times). In the spring, you'll be met by white trilliums (Ohio's official state wildflower) and a variety of violets that like the wet ground along the river.

About 0.2 mile into the trail, the path turns sharply left, heading north, and meets up with the Cuyahoga River. Traveling along the river's edge, you'll soon hear several rapids providing a musical accompaniment to the sound of your feet on the dirt and leaves. Approach very quietly and you may see great blue or green-backed herons fishing for dinner. Crouch down to look into the clear water and you'll probably notice a handful of empty freshwater shells.

Soon you'll pass a small clearing with several picnic tables. (Here you can also see the parking lot to your left.) Continue past the tables along the main trail. It remains flat and almost entirely shaded until you come to a railroad-tie staircase. Take a deep breath—you're about to climb up 98 (or so) railroad-tie steps. At the top, pause, take another deep breath, and turn around. The view is good. And it's about to get better.

Once you've caught your breath, follow the trail as it makes a sharp bend to the right (east), and you'll find the overlook. A deck offering an impressive view of the river valley awaits. Once you're done enjoying that, you're faced with a decision: to do the Overlook Trail extension or not.

YOU HAVE OPTIONS

The Overlook Trail is actually a 0.5-mile stand-alone, paved, fully ADA-accessible trail with an entrance off Sackett Avenue. Because it winds under tall shade trees and offers the complete view from the accessible deck, it's a wonderful option for anyone not able to do stairs or longer hikes.

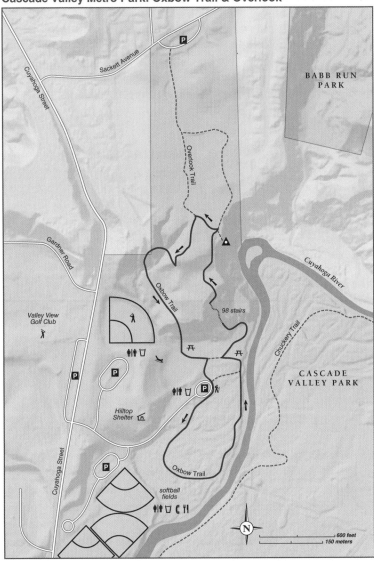

Cascade Valley Metro Park: Oxbow Trail & Overlook

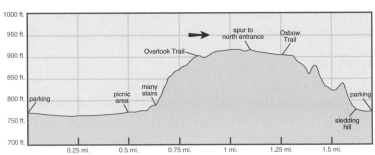

The short, paved loop may seem like a denouement to the rockier Oxbow Trail, but it also offers a chance to catch your breath and give your knees a break. If you take it—in either direction—you'll soon rejoin Oxbow.

If you choose to skip the paved Overlook Trail, admire the view again before you return to Oxbow.

From the overlook deck, follow Oxbow Trail as its dirt path veers left and then works its way down, with a few stairs here and there as you twist your way back to the trailhead.

As you descend on Oxbow Trail, the sledding hill comes into view. During the winter and early spring, thanks to the lay of the land, you'll be able to keep an eye on the sledding hill—and your car in the parking lot—during most of the final third of the loop. In the summer, you'll have less of a view but will continue to enjoy the trees' air-conditioning effect.

When there's no snow and no ball game, you'll still have company on the trail. This is a popular spot for families, especially during the Metro Parks' annual hiking sprees. Hilltop Shelter, above the sledding hill, is available for free on a first-come, first-serve basis. The shelter, which holds about 40 people, can also be reserved for a fee by calling 330-867-5511.

NEARBY ACTIVITIES

Oxbow's sledding hill is popular after a good snowfall. The park service maintains a 24-hour seasonal information line at 330-865-8060. Across the street from the Chuckery entrance, you'll see Himelright Lodge, where the park system is developing the new Valley View area on a former golf course property. At the time of this writing, trails there were under development.

While you're here in Cascade Valley Park, you may want to take an extra hike to see the Signal Tree. Local lore says that Indigenous peoples purposefully formed the lowest branches of the burr oak tree, which has grown here for at least three centuries, so the branches would grow at right angles to signal the way to an important trail. Whatever its past (the tree isn't talking), this much is clear: It's a beautiful tree, so if you have an opportunity, go see it for yourself. At the time of this writing, both trails leading to the tree were closed due to work connected with the Gorge Dam removal project. Although both of those spots may be closed through the end of 2025, there are other opportunities to hike nearby.

Babb Run Bird and Wildlife Sanctuary, a Cuyahoga Falls city park, is about 2 miles to the north. (When you look down and to the left from the overlook, you're seeing the western edge of Babb Run.) Downtown Cuyahoga Falls is very pedestrian-friendly, and the Highbridge Glens Park, with a boardwalk and lovely view of the river, is smack in the middle of town, at 1817 Front Street. Numerous locally owned restaurants with outdoor seating dot the street, as well. You'll also find several more miles of hiking through the woods at nearby Munroe Falls Metro Park (page 264).

• •

TRAILHEAD GPS COORDINATES: N41.12201° W81.52048°

DIRECTIONS Cascade Valley Park: Chuckery/Oxbow Area entrance is located at 1061 Cuyahoga Street, between Uhler and Sackett Avenues, in North Akron. From Cleveland, follow I-480 E to I-271 S. From I-271, in 3.4 miles, take Exit 18A (OH 8). Merge onto OH 8 S and go 11.3 miles. Exit at Broad Boulevard. Turn right (west) to follow Broad for 1.7 miles, and then turn left (south) onto 26th Street. In 0.2 mile, turn right (southwest) onto Sackett Avenue. In 0.6 mile, turn left (southeast) onto Cuyahoga Street. Follow Cuyahoga Street for about 0.5 mile; the park sign will be on your left. (*Note:* There are two entrances to the Chuckery/Oxbow Area on Cuyahoga Street; take the northernmost entrance. The Overlook entrance can be found at 354 Sackett Avenue.

This way to the Cuyahoga River!

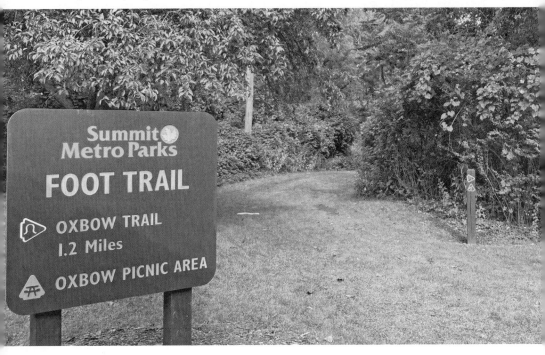

48 CUYAHOGA VALLEY NATIONAL PARK: Beaver Marsh Boardwalk & Indigo Lake

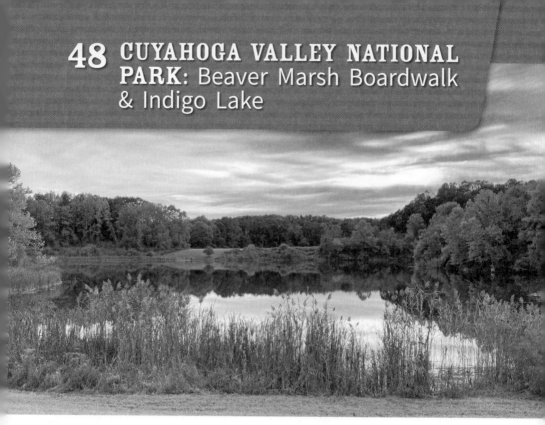

Indigo Lake

ONCE A (REAL) DUMP, this area was transformed by some enterprising beavers who turned it into a viable habitat, and not only for themselves. Today more than 50 bird species nest here each year, and countless national park visitors enjoy the boardwalk's serenity. It's also a natural connection to other attractions in the park and beyond.

DESCRIPTION

Can you say "extreme makeover"? In the early 1980s, what is now the Beaver Marsh Boardwalk—a wildly popular attraction in the national park—was a soggy dumping ground, full of junk from a nearby car repair shop and assorted other trash. Even before volunteers from the Portage Trail Group, Sierra Club, and National Park Service (NPS) could reclaim the land, a couple of beavers took matters into their own, um, paws. Park volunteers and employees helped the beavers by clearing out the debris, and the NPS opened a stretch of boardwalk across the marsh. From a single dam to a community of beavers, muskrats, mink, and many other animals and birds, the marsh and its adjacent land constitute one of the most diverse spots in the 33,000-acre Cuyahoga Valley National Park (CVNP), a reclaimed habitat for more than 500 types of plants and more than 50 bird species.

DISTANCE & CONFIGURATION: 3.5-mile out-and-back with options up to 6 miles

DIFFICULTY: Easy, flat

SCENERY: Beaver marsh and pond, more than 500 types of plants and animals

EXPOSURE: Boardwalk, almost entirely exposed; southernmost section of hike, shaded; Indigo Lake, exposed

TRAFFIC: Moderate–heavy (expect some bikes)

TRAIL SURFACE: Towpath Trail, wooden boardwalk and paved; trail connector and Indigo Lake, dirt and grass

HIKING TIME: 2.25 hours for walking and watching; add 30 minutes for Hale Farm connector.

DRIVING DISTANCE: 17 miles from I-77/I-480 exchange

ACCESS: Daily, 7 a.m.–11 p.m.

MAPS: USGS *Peninsula*; also at nps.gov /places/000/hunt-house-trailhead.htm

FACILITIES: Restrooms at Hunt House Visitor Center, Indigo Lake, and Ira Road trailhead

WHEELCHAIR ACCESS: Boardwalk, yes; Indigo Lake connector and Hale Farm, no

CONTACT: Cuyahoga Valley National Park: 330-657-2752, nps.gov/cuva

LOCATION: Bolanz Road, Peninsula

The marsh's diversity and its accessibility (wheelchairs and strollers can easily navigate the wide, 530-foot-long boardwalk via the hard-packed, crushed-limestone surface of the Towpath Trail) have earned it a spot on the Ohio Division of Wildlife's list of Watchable Wildlife sites. It's also popular with photographers, so don't be surprised if you have to dodge a tripod here and there as you walk along.

For this trek, start from the Hunt House Trailhead, just south of another popular attraction. Szalay's Farm Market, at the corner of Bolanz and Riverview Road, began as a vegetable farm in 1931. The market, which is still worked by the Szalay family, features a corn maze and live music throughout the summer, drawing throngs from greater Akron and Cleveland.

Depending on when you walk by the fields, you may be surprised by the loud shots of corn cannons sounding periodically. They're just trying to scare away the crows and other animals who eat the corn without paying for it. Stop into the market to see why they're willing to put up with the noise—the corn really is some of the best in northeast Ohio.

As you make your way toward the boardwalk, you'll see signs pointing to Hunt House Trail. Note that it leads to Indigo Lake, and it's worth the extra mile it will add to your hike—farther if you continue to Hale Farm. But for now, you're on your way to this hike's namesake attraction.

When you reach Beaver Marsh, you're sure to notice the cattails. They are an important food source for many animals, and when this area was first settled, they were also a staple in the diets of the Indigenous peoples and early settlers, who made meal from their long stems. (Speaking of diets, this might make you grateful for your next salad.)

Now that you've reached Beaver Marsh, you want to see beavers, right? Here are some basic tips: First, beavers are nocturnal. That means they do most of their home building and repair work in the evening. Visit near dusk and look for them as they

Cuyahoga Valley National Park: Beaver Marsh Boardwalk & Indigo Lake

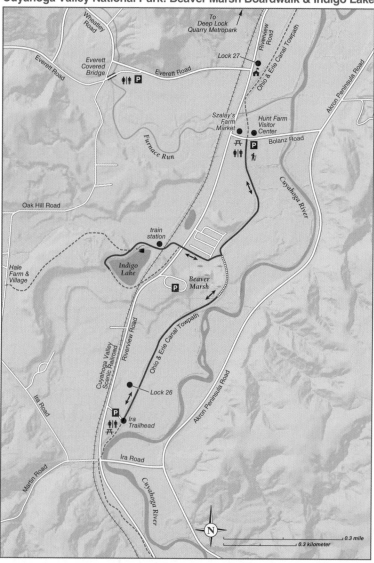

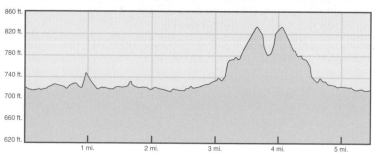

swim. Watch for a wake, the V-shaped disturbance in the water created by a beaver's tail as it swims. Keep an eye on the water lilies, and you may see a hungry beaver grab a leaf to eat. It will roll the leaf and hold it in its paw like a green cigar as it nibbles. Also look for mink and muskrats that live in and around the water. Muskrats build their homes along the banks of ponds and streams and occasionally on top of beaver lodges.

Even if you don't see any beavers, you're almost certain to see herons, a variety of ducks, and numerous smaller birds—active almost anytime, in any season, on this stretch of the Towpath. Many benches dot the boardwalk, offering places to sit and watch.

The boardwalk offers such beautiful scenery, and so much to see, that you may not want to leave at all. And as you head south from the boardwalk, Ira Road trailhead (just past Lock 26) makes a natural turnaround point, giving you a chance to revisit the boardwalk. (Of course, if you don't turn around, you can follow the Towpath Trail into Akron, south into Zoar, and beyond.) But turn around you must to visit Indigo Lake, and to return to your car.

YOU HAVE OPTIONS

To shorten this hike, park a shuttle vehicle at Lock 26. The large lot, often crowded with Towpath cyclists, has several interpretive displays offering a glimpse into life in the late 19th and early 20th centuries. Following the trail west to Indigo Lake is worth the extra steps (about a mile), and following the trail farther, you'll reach Hale Farm.

As you cross back over the boardwalk, even on a second (or third or fourth) look, it's still hard to imagine that this spot was once a dump. Clearly, this was a successful makeover. The beautiful result: a safe haven for hundreds of animals and plants and a great escape for the humans who make their homes on either side of the valley.

Just north of the boardwalk, you can take a pleasant excursion to Indigo Lake by following the signs to Hale Farm and Indigo Lake Station. The Cuyahoga Valley Scenic Railroad train stop is less than 0.5 mile due west. You might be tempted to catch the train; even if you give in and take a ride, make sure to admire the lake first.

Indigo Lake is small but lovely; its name was inspired by its deep-blue hue. I am often surprised when I talk with frequent visitors to CVNP who are not familiar with Indigo Lake. In my opinion, it's one of the prettiest, most tranquil spots in the park. So let's just keep that between you and me, OK?

Walking around the lake will add about a mile to your Towpath trek. Follow the limestone path and signs pointing to Hale Farm & Village until the path is paved as it heads uphill. Before you reach the top, the path splits. (The paved portion rolls on to Hale Farm.) Follow the grassy trail as it bends to the left, rising above the lake.

The trail continues curving to the east and begins rolling downhill, depositing you in a broad, open field with a wide-open view of the southern end of Indigo Lake. As picturesque as it is now, it's hard to believe that this lake started life as a gravel pit and quarry. Today, it's another successful makeover story—a spot that provides satisfying views for park visitors, as well as a home for many birds, butterflies, and insects.

Once you've soaked up the loveliness of Indigo Lake, retrace your steps up the hill and back to the train station and Towpath. (The grass-and-dirt trail heads into the woods and then crosses the railroad track and Riverview Road, providing an alternate route if you'd prefer to complete the lake loop, but it will require you to walk north on the berm of Riverview Road a few hundred feet to return to the Towpath Trail.) Once back on the Towpath, head north to return to the lot.

NEARBY ACTIVITIES

Of course, when Szalay's Farm Market is open, it's a great place to visit. In addition to fresh produce—from spring strawberries and summer sweet corn to apples and fall pumpkins—the market features live music and a corn maze (in season).

If you choose to visit Hale Farm & Village, you'll find yourself way, way back in time. The working museum is owned and operated by the Western Reserve Historical Society. It offers an accurate representation of life in the Western Reserve, circa 1826. Candle-making, glassblowing, and pottery demonstrations are regular fare; special seasonal events, such as Civil War reenactments and Holiday Lantern Tours, draw large crowds. For hours, admission, and events information, call 216-721-5722 or visit wrhs.org.

Hunt House, on the north side of Bolanz Road, highlights the role of the small family farm as a force in the valley's development. Even when the historic home/visitor center isn't open, you can pick up a map and activities brochures at the information kiosk, or check the online calendar at nps.gov/cuva.

• •

TRAILHEAD GPS COORDINATES: N41.20030° W81.57210°

DIRECTIONS Follow I-77 S toward Akron and take Exit 143 for OH 176 (toward I-271). Turn left (east) onto Wheatley Road/OH 176. Go about 2.9 miles toward Riverview Road. Veer left onto Everett Road, and then in 0.6 mile, turn right onto Riverview Road, heading south. In 0.3 mile, turn left onto Bolanz Road. Find trailhead parking on the south side of Bolanz Road.

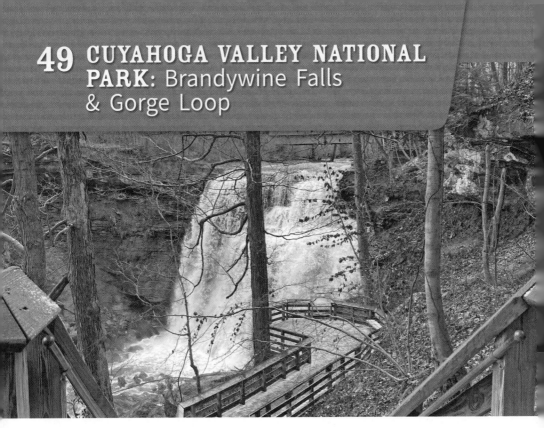

49 CUYAHOGA VALLEY NATIONAL PARK: Brandywine Falls & Gorge Loop

Gorge Loop gives you a chance to see the falls from several vantage points.

THIS SHORT TRAIL packs a wallop in terms of scenery—and a respectable cardiovascular workout, thanks to an elevation change of more than 150 feet.

DESCRIPTION

Brandywine Falls tumbles 65 feet to crash into the otherwise mild-mannered creek that runs through the ravine below. After a heavy rain, the noise can complicate conversation on the boardwalk. No worries; you'll have plenty of quiet time on your hike. While the falls are one of the park's most-visited sights, the crowds don't all head for the trail. (Their loss.)

But before you hit the trail, you'll need to find a parking place—and sometimes, the lot is full. Locals come in droves on fall weekends, and during the summer you'll often see out-of-state plates in the lot. It's nice to know our local national park attracts so many visitors, but it means you may have to get creative to enjoy this spot. Getting to the lot early (before 11 a.m.) on weekends, or going almost anytime during the week, is usually all it takes to find a parking spot. If that fails, you can park at the Boston Mills Visitor Center and hike to the falls, taking the Towpath north to Stanford Trail, which joins the Gorge Trail to the falls, for a round-trip of about 4 miles.

But let's assume you got a parking spot at the top of the falls, and you're ready to hike. From the trailhead on the north end of the parking lot, take the sloping

DISTANCE & CONFIGURATION: 1.7-mile loop, with options to extend to 7 or more miles

DIFFICULTY: Moderate

SCENERY: 65-foot-high waterfall, ravine, great birding opportunities

EXPOSURE: Mostly shaded

TRAFFIC: Busy

TRAIL SURFACE: Wooden boardwalk and dirt trails

HIKING TIME: Minimum of 1 hour

DRIVING DISTANCE: 13 miles from I-77/I-480 exchange

ACCESS: Daily, sunrise–sunset

MAPS: USGS *Northfield;* also at trailhead, park visitor centers, and park website

FACILITIES: Restrooms and water at trailhead

WHEELCHAIR ACCESS: No

CONTACT: Cuyahoga Valley National Park: 330-657-2752, nps.gov/cuva

LOCATION: Brandywine Road, Northfield

wooden boardwalk to the right to visit the falls right away. No sense in waiting to see the main attraction!

Follow the boardwalk trail alongside the sandstone walls that are almost always perspiring and dripping with spider webs. From the top viewing platform, you'll take wooden stairs down another 300 feet or so to get close enough to the falls that they can properly impress you. They are popular for a reason—they really are beautiful—so once you've had a chance to appreciate the view (and probably taken a few pictures), move on with confidence that the trail is also delightful.

On the last stretch of boardwalk as you work your way (counterclockwise) around the falls, you'll find some interpretive signs that explain how the falls were put to work in the early 1800s. The first sawmill was built here in 1814, and the village of Brandywine Falls quickly grew up around the new industry provided by the falls. When I-271 was built, the village all but disappeared. Area leaders, particularly Akron's John Seiberling, tried to balance the transportation needs of a growing region with preservation of spots like Brandywine Falls. Eventually, while Seiberling was serving as a U.S. Congressman, this area was deemed a national recreation area before it was redesignated as a national park.

The boardwalk deposits you on a bridge that crosses over the top of the falls. This stretch of trail is paved, as it is part of the Summit County Bike & Hike Trail, so expect to share the trail with some bicycle traffic. Once you've reached the north side of the falls, you'll get a good look at the iconic Inn at Brandywine Falls. The popular bed-and-breakfast is private property, but the trail on park property allows you a good look at the small farm the innkeepers operate.

Shortly after passing the farm, you'll veer left on the Brandywine Gorge Loop, while cyclists continue to the right. The trail surface is dirt and rock from here, and at this point, you're heading downhill and into the ravine.

Tall hemlocks and oak trees are thick on the north side of the trail but sparse enough on the other side that you can enjoy a view of the creek below almost the entire length of the trail, until it bottoms out and crosses the creek on a narrow footbridge.

Cuyahoga Valley National Park: Brandywine Falls & Gorge Loop

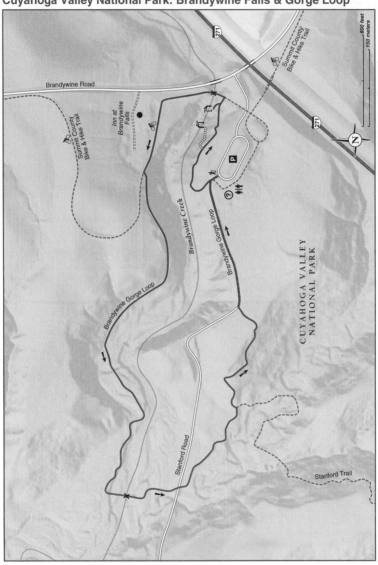

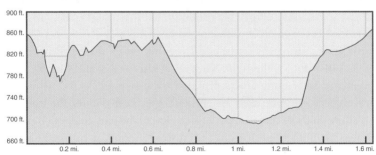

If you're returning to the trail for the first time in many years, you might think, "What footbridge?" Don't worry, your memory is right—a couple of decades ago, there was no bridge here, and we all enjoyed crossing on several large, strategically placed rocks. But today, the footbridge takes us safely across instead. (And our thank-you note to the trail builders is long overdue.)

From the bridge, the trail heads south and off into the woods far enough that you'll lose sight of the creek. Soon, you'll arrive at the junction with Stanford Trail, where you have options to lengthen your hike (see below). But for this hike, stay on Brandywine Gorge Loop to climb back to the Brandywine Trailhead on the south side of the ravine. The climb is very pretty, through thick woods, and while you won't be able to see the creek or falls on this side of the gorge, you will find the way sprinkled with a variety of seasonal wildflowers.

Returning to the parking lot, enjoy your feeling of accomplishment, but not for too long; other visitors are probably wanting your parking space.

YOU HAVE OPTIONS

At the junction with Stanford Trail, you can take that path to visit Stanford House, a little more than a mile away. As noted in the parking information earlier, Stanford Trail connects with the Towpath about 1.5 miles west of here, so if you're wanting a much longer hike, here's your chance. Going from Brandywine Falls to Blue Hen Falls is a real treat. If you depart the Gorge Loop and follow Stanford Trail to the Towpath, heading south, you'll reach Boston Store on Brandywine Road. From there, just on the west side of Riverview Road, you can pick up the Buckeye Trail to Blue Hen Falls. From there, it's just about 1.5 miles to Blue Hen, but round-trip, it packs a nearly 600-foot elevation change—a steep set of stairs accounts for a fair portion of that climb. That particular stretch of the Buckeye Trail got a major overhaul in 2021, and again, the trail builders did a great job. The total distance from Brandywine to Blue Hen and back on this route is about 9 miles, and combining those routes is an excellent way to see two special spots in the park.

NEARBY ACTIVITIES

Want to bike? Several parking areas specifically for the Summit County Bike & Hike Trail are nearby—and of course, hikers can use those lots too! One particularly "cool" spot on the Bike & Hike Trail runs parallel to OH 8, just north of OH 303. The trail cuts through some tall rock ledges, and it feels like someone left the air-conditioning on there, all year long. The parking area, at 64 W. Streetsboro Street in Hudson, is about 2.5 miles south of the Brandywine Falls parking lot.

The Boston Mills Visitor Center, Boston Store, and The Gallery on Brandywine Road are also good places to stop and extend your visit in the national park.

• •

TRAILHEAD GPS COORDINATES: N41.27661° W81.53998°

DIRECTIONS Follow I-480 E to I-271 S, then take OH 8 south to Highland Road. Turn right onto Highland Road, then right onto Olde Eight Road, following it to West Highland Road, where you'll turn left, heading west. Turn left again on Brandywine Road, following it south for about 1 mile. Brandywine Falls Trailhead parking lot will be on your right, immediately south of the Inn at Brandywine Falls.

You can start the loop here and go either way, but why wait to visit the falls?

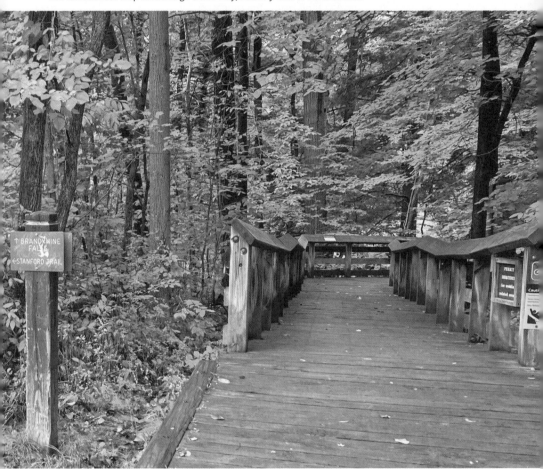

Everett Covered Bridge has been built, repaired, and rebuilt several times since 1877.

EVERETT COVERED BRIDGE enjoys a bittersweet distinction: It is the only covered bridge that remains in Summit County, and one of few tangible reminders of the once-bustling community of Everett. The bridge spans Furnace Run and serves as the trailhead for several of the park's hilliest trails.

DESCRIPTION

From the parking lot off Everett Road, find your way to the bridge, where a series of interpretive signs explains why and how it was built. As you walk across the bridge, you may try to imagine the village of Everett, which was a vibrant place long before the bridge was built . . . the first time.

In the 1820s, Everett was a tiny hamlet, with fewer than 10 residents. The Ohio & Erie Canal, built between 1825 and 1832, changed all of that. By 1888, Everett had about 200 residents, and the Akron and Summit County Directory described it as "a small village and station on the Valley Railway/Ohio Canal and Cuyahoga River . . . surrounded by a very hilly country and in the bottoms the land is very fertile."

In the late 19th and early 20th century, visitors to Everett would find a self-sufficient village with a blacksmith, cemetery, dance hall, general store, saloon, and one-room schoolhouse.

DISTANCE & CONFIGURATION: 2.3-mile balloon or 1.9-mile loop

DIFFICULTY: Moderate; hilly

SCENERY: Streambed, old- and new-growth forest

EXPOSURE: Almost entirely shaded

TRAFFIC: Fairly busy

TRAIL SURFACE: Dirt and stone

HIKING TIME: 1 hour

DRIVING DISTANCE: 16 miles from I-77/I-480 exchange

ACCESS: 24/7

MAPS: USGS *Peninsula*

FACILITIES: Restrooms at trailhead

WHEELCHAIR ACCESS: No

CONTACT: Cuyahoga Valley National Park: 330-657-2752, nps.gov/cuva

LOCATION: 2247 Everett Road, Peninsula

The railroad that spurred the village's growth and connected it to other towns was good for the region, but ultimately, not for Everett. By the mid-1900s, the school in the village closed and students were sent to school in nearby Peninsula. Everett began to lose its population and identity.

In the 1980s, the National Park Service conducted an architectural survey of many of Everett's remaining homes and businesses. Some of the properties were purchased by the park system for preservation, and others for conservation, as the Cuyahoga Valley National Recreation Area was redesignated as a national park in 2000.

Today, there are a few vestiges of Everett left, the bridge over Furnace Run being the best known. Depending on when you visit, you might wonder why such a stout bridge was needed to cross the usually mild-mannered Furnace Run. While it rarely looks formidable, Furnace Run flows swiftly enough after a good rain (or spring thaw) to make fording the stream dangerous. It's thought that the bridge was built in response to the drowning death of local farmer John Gilson in the winter of 1877.

The bridge's crisscrossing beams and large open triangle at its center are typical of the Smith Truss Design. The covered roof was intended to protect the beams from weather damage and extend the bridge's life, but it had a run of bad luck. It was repaired after a flood in 1913, then again after it was hit by a truck in 1970. A 1975 flood swept the bridge into Furnace Run.

The bridge that you see now was built after members of the community and the foundation that would become the Conservancy for Cuyahoga Valley National Park raised funds for a historically accurate reconstruction.

And, history lesson now concluded, it's time to hike the trail that takes its name from the creek. If you follow Furnace Run Trail as described here, you'll complete it as a balloon, just a bit more than 2 miles in length. If you follow the trail across Oak Hill Road, you'll enjoy much of the same scenery and cover just a tad less than 2 miles. Either way, you're in for a short, hilly excursion.

From the north side of the bridge, follow Furnace Run (the trail) as it skirts Furnace Run (the creek). This short, flat stretch of trail is especially beautiful in the spring, when it's awash with bluebells.

Cuyahoga Valley National Park: Everett Covered Bridge & Furnace Run

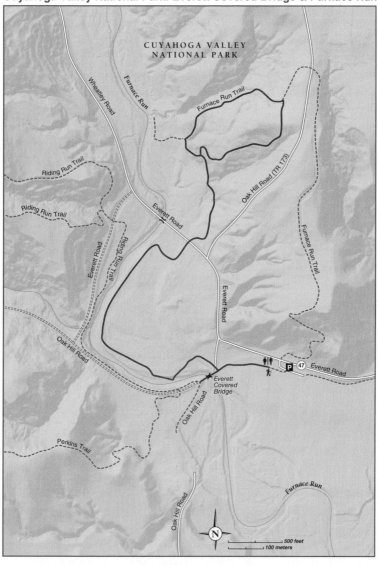

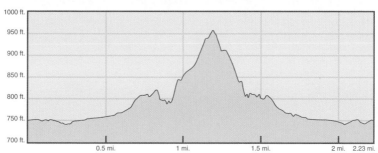

As soon as you cross Everett Road, the trail begins to take you uphill, slightly at first. After you cross a footbridge, you'll begin a fairly steep ascent, made a little easier with a couple of switchback sections. If you have to stop to catch your breath, use the excuse that you want to appreciate the ravine views (they're really lovely). Regardless of the season, you'll find the trail blanketed by pine needles and complicated by the tree roots.

Once you've topped out, you can choose to follow the trail left, completing the loop, or turn right, finishing the balloon configuration. If you turn left, you'll cross Oak Hill Road and head down through the woods before crossing Everett Road to return to the parking lot.

If you turn right, you'll soon find yourself heading down to Furnace Run (the creek) and retracing your steps back to the base of the bridge, where, if you like, you can pick up the bridle trails to hike a few more miles.

NEARBY ACTIVITIES

Looking for a longer hike? Riding Run and Perkins Bridle Trails begin on the west side of the bridge; their combined distance is about 7 miles. Also, just a short drive from here, you'll find the shady (but slightly less hilly) Plateau Trail (page 248). And if you'd prefer a much flatter trek, try the Towpath. The popular Beaver Marsh Boardwalk, just around the corner, is a good option (page 225). Also just around the corner: Szalay's Farm Market. The iconic, family-owned farm on Riverview and Bolanz Roads is open seven days a week during the growing and harvesting seasons.

• •

TRAILHEAD GPS COORDINATES: N41.20430° W81.58103°

DIRECTIONS Take I-77 S approximately 12 miles to Wheatley Road (Exit 143). Turn Left onto Wheatley Road, heading east about 2 miles, before continuing onto Everett Road. The parking lot will be on your right. (Use 2247 Everett Road in Peninsula as a street address to reach the trailhead parking lot.)

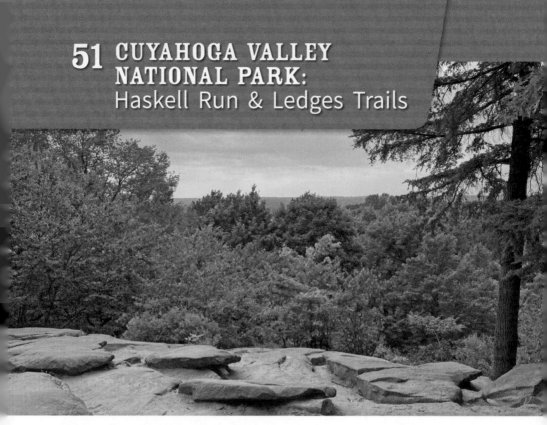

51 CUYAHOGA VALLEY NATIONAL PARK: Haskell Run & Ledges Trails

Looking west from Ledges Overlook

TAKE A TUNNEL to visit a pioneer cemetery and then on to some awe-inspiring caves and ledges. These hilly trails visit some of the most-photographed spots in Cuyahoga Valley National Park's ledges, including what is arguably the best spot in the valley to watch a sunset.

DESCRIPTION

The main parking lot for Happy Days Lodge is on the north side of OH 303. To reach the trailhead, you'll walk down a flight of stairs and cross under OH 303 via a 200-foot-long lighted tunnel. When you emerge, you'll find yourself on the edge of the Mater Dolorosa Cemetery, which dates to 1869. Its inhabitants include Civil War soldier Thomas Coady and his parents, who lived to be 93 and 83 years old. (We'll never know the secret to their longevity, but we can guess that they walked a lot.)

Wandering through the cemetery, you'll notice that the majority of its other souls rest in mystery, their names having long since faded from the sandstone markers.

On the southern end of the cemetery, you'll step onto the short but steep Haskell Run Trail. Follow the path as it veers left and then right, dropping about 30 feet before crossing a short wooden footbridge. That's Haskell Run, the meandering creek for which the trail is named. From here, the trail bends sharply left, working its

DISTANCE & CONFIGURATION: 3-mile figure eight with option to add 2 more miles

DIFFICULTY: Moderate, with difficult sections

SCENERY: Large sandstone ledges, forest ravines, valley overlook

EXPOSURE: Almost entirely shaded

TRAFFIC: Moderate; the overlook can be crowded

TRAIL SURFACE: Mixed—from large stones to dirt and gravel

HIKING TIME: 1.5 hours

DRIVING DISTANCE: 23 miles from I-77/I-480 exchange

ACCESS: Daily, sunrise–sunset

MAPS: USGS *Peninsula;* also at park visitor centers and park website

FACILITIES: Permanent restrooms located in Happy Days Lodge parking lot; restrooms and water available at Ledges and Octagon Shelters

WHEELCHAIR ACCESS: No

CONTACT: Cuyahoga Valley National Park: 330-657-2752, nps.gov/cuva

LOCATION: OH 303, Hudson

way up toward the base of the Ledges Trail. Arriving at the top of 20 or so steps, turn left onto Ledges Trail.

NEED A SHORTER OPTION?

Haskell Run Trail is a favorite with families and a great choice if you are very short on time for a hike. This trail packs a couple of respectable hills, some history, and a handful of interpretive signs in just about a half mile. If you complete the loop on Haskell Run and return to the parking lot, you can drive to the Ledges Overlook to enjoy that famous view.

Footing on the Ledges Trail can be challenging because you'll climb over too many rocks (and steps) to count. Some were left by glaciers; others were placed by human hands.

In the 1930s, the Civilian Conservation Corps (CCC) created countless stairways out of the indigenous stones here; the vast majority are still in use, providing hikers with a safer path. You will appreciate their work for both its form and its function. A 1918 report of the U.S. Department of the Interior declared that "particular attention must be devoted always to harmonizing of these improvements with the landscape." Along this trail and throughout the park, you'll see evidence of the CCC's adherence to this goal.

As you continue south, the giant walls of sandstone and Sharon Conglomerate line Ledges Trail. The 300-million-year-old rock, formed of cemented sand and small quartz pebbles, has created a playground of sorts for modern-day visitors like us. It also has a cooling effect, and in the summer many seek relief from the heat here thanks to the stone and thick forest.

Continuing south, several footbridges (also of the CCC era) help you across mild-mannered streams feeding Haskell Run. Farther south, the trail veers right and leads you across the park's driveway, Ledges Road, to reach the overlook area.

Cuyahoga Valley National Park: Haskell Run & Ledges Trails

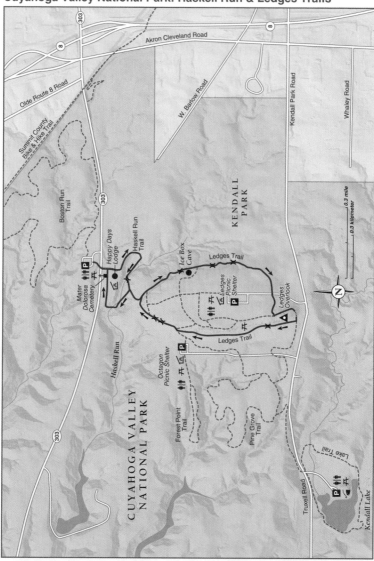

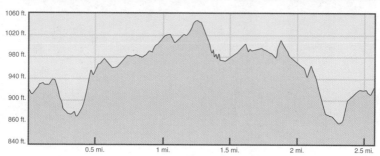

241

If you brought a dog and a Frisbee, you're in luck: as the trail rises a bit, you'll arrive at a large, open field just perfect for playing with your pup, flying a kite, picnicking, or reading on a blanket. (Conveniently, restroom facilities are also found here.)

As you follow the path up another 30 yards or so you'll spot a sign directing you left (south) to the Ledges Trail or straight ahead to visit the Ledges Overlook. The overlook is a sunset-watcher's paradise, and almost anytime is a good time to sit on the flat expanse of rock, facing west, to gaze across the valley. On most days, you can see well past the communities of Bath and Brecksville.

If you ever find yourself alone here, appreciate the rarity of that moment. On many nights, a crowd gathers here to catch the short sunset performance, and sometimes viewers actually applaud as the sun slips out of sight. It is an almost-magical spot in this beautiful valley. Move on for now (you won't want to finish the hike without the benefit of daylight), and plan to come back another time to enjoy the nightly show.

From the overlook point, the Ledges Trail continues a bit south, then heads west, dropping down several dozen steps into the forest. A sign at the bottom of the steps steers you to the right (north) to complete the Ledges Trail loop, but you can add a couple of miles to your overall trip here, if you want.

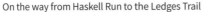

On the way from Haskell Run to the Ledges Trail

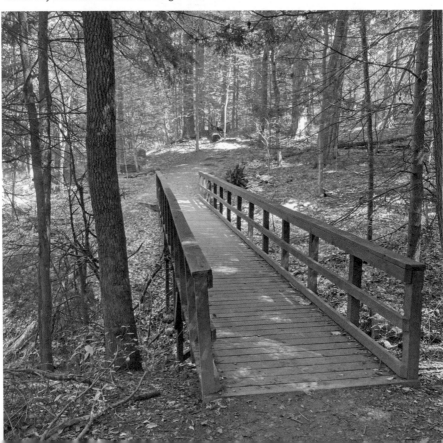

YOU HAVE OPTIONS

If you continue straight through the cool forest, and follow the signs for Pine Grove Trail, you'll cross the park road that leads to the Octagon Shelter from Truxell Road. The approximately 2-mile loop trail is flatter than Ledges Trail but just as lovely. After winding through the aspen, beech, maple, and pine tree forest, you'll see a sign noting the connector to Lake Trail, offering you an even longer extension if you choose to take it.

If you're staying on the Ledges Trail, continue in your clockwise loop heading north, climbing gradually and then descending again to find a sign directing you back to Haskell Run Trail and Happy Days Lodge. When you get back to Haskell Run, veer left to complete your clockwise, figure-eight jaunt around this cool and rocky place.

On the final 0.25 mile of Haskell Run, you'll enjoy one more good climb up a gravel trail and then a dozen stone steps to arrive on the western edge of the field adjacent to the lodge. Several grills and picnic tables here may seem rather inviting at this point, as you have likely worked up an appetite on the trail. Go back through the tunnel to return to your car, where you can take a breather before you pick your next destination.

NEARBY ACTIVITIES

Formerly a visitor center, Happy Days Lodge is a reservable events site that also hosts concerts and forums and speakers on topics related to the Cuyahoga Valley and other national parks. To find out what's going on at Happy Days Lodge and elsewhere in the park, call 330-657-2752 or visit nps.gov/cuva/planyourvisit.

On the north side of the Happy Days Lodge parking lot, you'll find the trailhead for Boston Run, a rolling 2-plus-mile trail popular with hikers, runners, and cross-country skiers. Of course, you can hike or bike for miles on the Towpath. The closest Towpath Trailhead parking lot is off OH 303, about 2 miles to the west (in Peninsula). Parking for the paved Summit County Bike & Hike Trail is located just east of here, at the intersection of OH 303 and Olde Route 8 Road. And if you're hungry or want to shop, head to Peninsula, where several well-loved, independently owned restaurants and stores are waiting for you. Also nearby: the park visitor center (6947 Riverview Road in Peninsula) is open daily, 9:30 a.m.–5 p.m., year-round.

• •

TRAILHEAD GPS COORDINATES: N41.23156° W81.50785°

DIRECTIONS From the I-77/I-480 exchange, take I-480 E to I-271 S. Take Exit 18 to follow OH 8 south to OH 303. On OH 303, head west to find Happy Days Lodge parking lot, on the north side of OH 303, approximately 1 mile west of OH 8.

52 CUYAHOGA VALLEY NATIONAL PARK: On the Buckeye Trail from Pine Lane to Boston

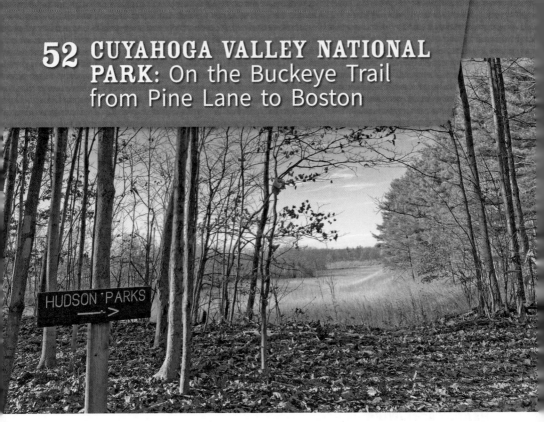

This section of the Buckeye Trail passes through Wildlife Woods, a Hudson city park.

ONE OF THE least-crowded stretches of trail in the national park, the Buckeye Trail from Pine Lane to Boston Store packs a lot of hills and a variety of scenery into just over 3 miles.

DESCRIPTION

This hike starts on a shady, quiet stretch of the Buckeye Trail (BT), but don't expect an easy outing. It's a hilly trek with some steep sections, two creek crossings, and a variety of terrain. You can hike it as a 7-mile loop by following the Towpath back to Lock 29 in Peninsula, then taking the BT (which follows Dell Road) back to the trailhead. Alternatively, you can park a shuttle vehicle at the Boston Store/Boston Mills Visitor Center lot and cut your distance in half. That's what I describe here.

Starting from Pine Lane Trailhead and heading north, you'll follow the ridgeline a short distance, ducking into a row of pines, then begin a descent that will take you deeper into the valley before a number of steep climbs brings you back up.

Fred Kelly, who owned much of this land in the 1940s, planted many of the pines you'll see here. The newspaper columnist and Wright Brothers' biographer was also a humorist who apparently had a big personality. Supposedly, he regularly carried an axe around the area so he could chop up tacky billboards. We can thank Kelly for a good anecdote and for the pine trees, which inspired the trailhead's name.

DISTANCE & CONFIGURATION: 3.6-mile one-way (requires shuttle vehicle) or 7-mile loop

DIFFICULTY: Moderate

SCENERY: Dense forest, creek crossings, excellent spring wildflower displays, sweeping valley views

EXPOSURE: Almost entirely shaded

TRAFFIC: Very light

TRAIL SURFACE: Mostly dirt, some gravel

HIKING TIME: 1.5–3 hours

DRIVING DISTANCE: 16 miles from I-77/I-480 exchange

ACCESS: 24/7; parking lots that close at sunset are clearly posted.

MAPS: USGS *Peninsula;* nps.gov/cuva /planyourvisit/upload/Cuyahoga_Valley _Trails_2022_South_508.pdf; buckeyetrail.org

FACILITIES: Restroom at Pine Lane Trailhead; water and restrooms at Boston Store

WHEELCHAIR ACCESS: No

CONTACT: Boston Mills Visitor Center: 440-717-3890; nps.gov/cuva

LOCATION: Pine Lane, Peninsula

As you roll up and down the hills, you'll notice many hemlocks, oaks, and—during spring—a number of woodland wildflowers. In most places this section of trail is fairly narrow, often just wide enough for a single person, which is typical of many stretches of the BT.

Just past the first creek crossing, over a little tributary to Boston Run, is a potentially confusing spot on the trail where I've missed the sign—not once, but twice. Save yourself the same confusion: stay right to remain on the BT. Soon you'll hear the bells from the church in Peninsula, and the next thing you know you'll take a little footbridge across a second small creek crossing.

Less than 2 miles from the trailhead, you will arrive at another notable stand of pines and find yourself in Wildlife Woods, on the edge of the Ohio Turnpike, where three trails converge. The BT and Valley Bridle Trail both meander through this park owned by the city of Hudson (page 277). The city's trail forms a little loop here at the top of the hill on the south side of Boston Mills Road (and the turnpike), and just east of here, it leads down to a small parking lot off Boston Mills Road.

To your left is an open expanse of native grasses, in what is called the Borrow Pit. When the Ohio Turnpike Commission was building the east–west roadway, it authorized the digging of dirt alongside the turnpike's planned route, and after it was built, prairie grasses were planted in the pits left behind.

On the edge of the prairie, the turnpike, and the pines, several route options are available. You could take the city's loop around Wildlife Woods and return to Pine Lane for a total of just over 3 miles. Or, if you stayed on the Buckeye Trail, you would continue onto Boston Mills Road, turning left, and then ducking into the woods again in a few hundred feet. Or, to follow this hike description, take the Valley Bridle Trail to your left, heading west through the prairie that grew out of a Borrow Pit.

This portion of trail, with its asphalt and concrete surface, offers a significant change in scenery from the first section of this hike. As you walk down the gentle slope, tall grasses and sun-loving wildflowers wave to your left and the turnpike rises

Cuyahoga Valley National Park: On the Buckeye Trail from Pine Lane to Boston

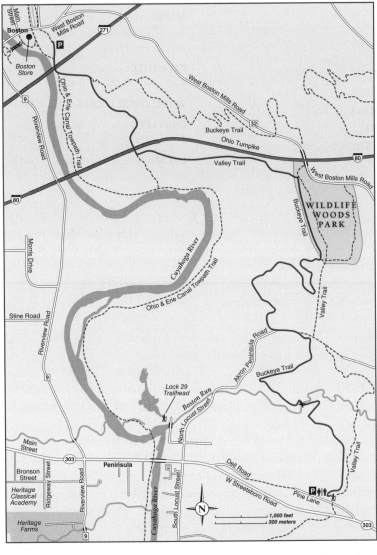

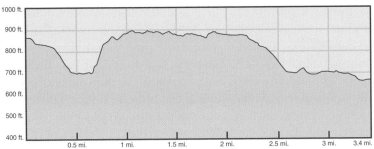

above you to the right. As you continue walking downhill toward the west, a broad view of the valley appears to your left. Continue following signs for the Valley Bridle Trail. This section of the hike is completely exposed, and if you decide to return on the Towpath, most of the rest of the trip will also be fully exposed from this point.

The bridle trail, now a wide dirt path, converges again with the BT and Towpath before delivering you to the Boston Store parking lot. If you left a shuttle vehicle here, you're done! If you want to add a few more miles, you can continue to follow the Valley Bridle Trail to Brecksville stables and beyond—the trail extends for more than 24 miles in the national park. Or see below for other ways to add to or shorten this particular hike.

YOU HAVE OPTIONS

Want to add some miles? From Boston Store, you can go see either or both of the valley's best-known waterfalls. From the Boston Mill Visitor Center across the river, head west to pick up the Buckeye Trail to Blue Hen Falls for a 3-mile (round-trip) trek and over 500 feet of elevation change. The trail got a serious upgrade in 2021, so if you appreciate trail building, you may find the trail almost as impressive as the waterfall! If you follow the Towpath north from Boston Store, you can pick up Stanford Trail and follow it to Brandywine Falls (page 230). You can also shorten this hike (to just about 3 miles) by parking a shuttle vehicle at Wildlife Woods (page 277).

NEARBY ACTIVITIES

Whether the Boston Store marks the midway point of your hike or the end, if The Gallery across the street (1565 Boston Mills Road) is open when you get there, go in—you'll be glad you did. Formerly known as Trail Mix, The Gallery is operated by The Conservancy for Cuyahoga Valley National Park and features new and local artworks. See conservancyforcvnp.org/experience/gallery for hours and exhibit info.

Hungry? Peninsula, just west of here, and Hudson, to the east, offer a variety of restaurants, ice-cream shops, and markets to replace the calories you've burned. If you've timed your hike to finish just before sunset, consider heading to the Ledges Overlook (page 239) to enjoy the view from there.

• •

TRAILHEAD GPS COORDINATES: N41.23953° W81.53838°

DIRECTIONS From I-480 E, take I-77 S about 7 miles to Exit 146, following signs for OH 21 to Richfield. Turn right onto OH 21, then in about 1 mile, turn left onto Boston Mills Road. Turn right onto Black Road, following it about 1 mile to OH 303 (Streetsboro Road). Turn left onto OH 303 and then turn left onto Pine Lane to find the trailhead.

A change of scenery greets you at almost every turn on this loop trail.

WHILE CUYAHOGA VALLEY National Park is full of great scenery, the Oak Hill area offers a special treat for the eyes. Here you'll encounter a series of S-curves that wiggle through the woods, following a ravine.

DESCRIPTION

Enter the trailhead at the eastern end of the Oak Hill parking lot. A trail map is posted there on a park bulletin board. Both the shorter Oak Hill Trail and the outer loop of Plateau Trail begin to the left, or north, of the sign. A few grassy steps and a short wooden bridge later, the trails diverge. Oak Hill Trail turns to the right and loops around the highest point of the plateau in just 1.5 miles. But the shorter loop skips most of the hills, and much of the fun, of the longer trail.

So stay on Plateau Trail, heading north, as the path bends left and climbs gradually beneath the cover of hemlock trees. For a few paces, the old trees give way to meadow bushes and growth. This is one of the few stretches of trail where you'll be able to see the sky, as much of the way is completely shaded by hemlocks and deciduous trees. Half a mile into the trail, you'll come to Chestnut Pond.

Small and easy to dismiss, the pond is a haven for amphibians who apparently take quite a bite out of the local insect population. (Translation: mosquitoes probably won't bother you here.) As you turn and leave the pond, the trail turns sharply to the

DISTANCE & CONFIGURATION: 5-mile loop

DIFFICULTY: Moderate

SCENERY: Pine and deciduous forests, three ponds, lush hemlock ravine

EXPOSURE: Mostly shaded

TRAFFIC: Light

TRAIL SURFACE: Dirt, with short stretches of grass and gravel

HIKING TIME: 2 hours

DRIVING DISTANCE: 16 miles from I-77/I-480 exchange

ACCESS: 24/7. Two restricted trails, one on either side of Meadowedge Pond, are clearly signed. They lead to the Cuyahoga Valley Environmental Education Center (CVEEC) and are authorized for CVEEC use only.

MAPS: USGS *Peninsula;* also at trailhead kiosk, most park visitor centers, and park website

FACILITIES: Restrooms at trailhead

WHEELCHAIR ACCESS: No

CONTACT: Cuyahoga Valley National Park: 330-657-2752, nps.gov/cuva; Cuyahoga Valley Environmental Education Center: conservancyforcvnp.org/education

LOCATION: Oak Hill Road, Peninsula

right. You're about to have one of those aha moments, or perhaps more accurately, an ooh-and-aah moment. Only a few steps from Chestnut Pond you'll find a long, long corridor of tall pines as visually stunning as they are fragrant. As you stroll through the hallway of pines, gaze up at their tops, 60 feet or so above you.

At the western end of the pine corridor, the path veers right again. Gravel and grass work together to keep this stretch of trail nice and dry. Heading north, you'll begin to see evidence of the hard work put into this trail, which was completed in 1997. More than a dozen small culverts have been created alongside and underneath the trail. They are both unobtrusive and necessary. As you round the loop and head east, the ravine is only a few feet from the trail. It's worth a few careful side steps to peer over the edge along here. The ravine is only about 10 feet deep here, but keep an eye on it; it grows wider and deeper as you continue on the trail.

At 1.5 miles, you'll pass a sign indicating a connector trail to Sylvan Pond. If you follow it, you'll also find the short (1.5-mile) inner loop, Oak Hill Trail. But for now, stay on the Plateau Trail; you have a lot to look forward to.

Less than 2 miles into the trail, tree buffs will find a section of the path loaded with multitrunked trees. Is there a proper name for this? If there is, it's elusive, but children—who tend to name things more expediently than botanists—call them two-headed and three-headed trees. Call 'em what you will, but noticing them along this section may take your mind off the fact that you're heading uphill for most of the next 0.8 mile. As the trail bends to the right, you'll pass over a feeder stream to Sylvan Pond (unnoticeable during dry periods) and head south, easing downhill. Soon you'll cross another footbridge, this one high enough to warrant leaning over the railing for another look at the ravine.

Just past the 3-mile mark, you'll climb a bit more and veer left to Hemlock Ravine, where a sign directs you to a short side trip. The 0.2-mile, out-and-back trail to Hemlock Point is to your left. Take the opportunity to enjoy the overlook. Back

Cuyahoga Valley National Park: Plateau Trail

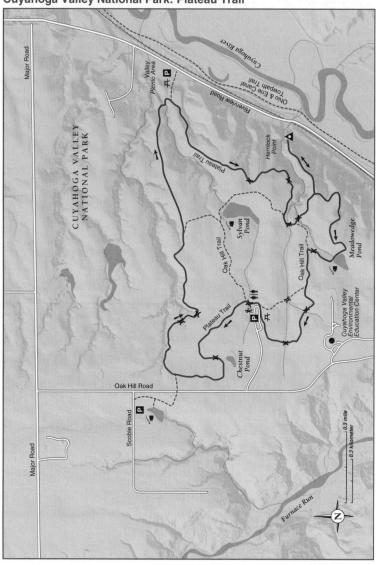

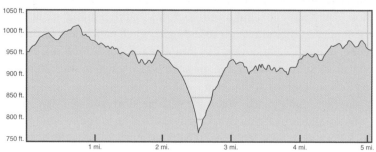

on the main trail, you'll follow a series of S-shaped curves. In fact, the trail turns you this way and that, barely righting itself (and you) before it crooks left again, then right, where you'll see the twists served a purpose: Directly in front of you is the beautiful Meadowedge Pond—and you didn't even see it coming.

Meadowedge Pond is especially impressive in the late spring and summer. The pond vista is an oasis of color and song and a treat for your senses: orioles, goldfinches, and yellow warblers fly around the pond, while frogs splash and cattails wave. Don't hurry by; soak it up.

The colors and sounds offer a nice contrast to the quiet, forested trail behind you. When you're ready for yet another change of scenery, follow the wide, grassy trail to the right, heading north into the shade of pines and hemlocks. The trail unfurls again in a series of S-curves to reach a sign indicating the Oak Hill Trail straight ahead. You can follow it from here back to the parking lot or continue on Plateau Trail by turning left. For the sake of finishing what you've started, stay on Plateau Trail.

The ravine is on your right at this point, and the trail is at its flattest. Still, it's not straight, snaking along the last 0.75 mile in the now familiar S pattern. Near the end of the trip, you'll ease down a gentle slope, in the company of young hemlock trees, to emerge in an open grassy area surrounded by picnic tables and—in the spring and summer, at least—a lovely show of wildflowers, including oxeye daisies, coltsfoots, and clovers. It's somehow fitting that Plateau Trail manages to get in this final change of scenery as the curtain goes down on your hike. The show is over, and the parking lot is on your right. You can leave, but you probably can't forget what you've seen here.

NEARBY ACTIVITIES

Nearby Ledges Trail (page 239) offers different dazzling views. The village of Peninsula (page 268) offers historic architecture and more, including several locally owned restaurants that can satisfy a variety of dining preferences.

• •

TRAILHEAD GPS COORDINATES: N41.21961° W81.57605°

DIRECTIONS Follow I-77 S toward Akron and take Exit 143 for OH 176 (toward I-271). Turn left (east) onto Wheatley Road/OH 176. Go 2.8 miles and turn left onto Oak Hill Road. Go north about 1 mile, and the entrance to Oak Hill Picnic Area is on your right. (East Siders may prefer to take OH 8 south to OH 303, heading west 3.5 miles to Riverview Road, and then following it 0.6 mile south to Major Road. Turn right, following Major Road west for 1.5 miles; then turn left onto Oak Hill Road, and go about 1 mile.) The entrance to Oak Hill Picnic Area (and the trails) is on the eastern side of Oak Hill Road. Follow the driveway 0.2 mile east to the parking lot.

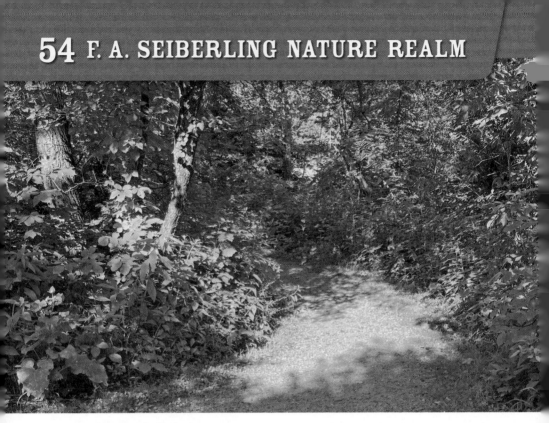

This way to the suspension bridge!

INSIDE THE VISITOR center, you can learn about pond life and enjoy watching birds from a large viewing window. When you're done, step outside to explore the Nature Realm's wealth of trails and habitats.

DESCRIPTION

F. A. Seiberling cofounded The Goodyear Tire & Rubber Co., and if that was all he had done, you'd probably expect to find a park in Akron named after him. But Seiberling did much more. He served as an early member of the Board of Park Commissioners, and over the years he donated more than 400 acres to help establish the county park system. In 1964, the park district purchased the 100-acre plot on which the nature realm now sits; interestingly, Seiberling himself owned the land from 1920 to 1948. Seiberling, who served as a U.S. representative from Ohio, was also instrumental in establishing the Cuyahoga Valley National Recreation Area (later, National Park) in 1974. But enough history for now.

Today, the grounds of the Nature Realm offer a variety of pretty ornamental trees and many more native plantings. From the crabapples that bloom in early spring to May and June's rhododendron blossoms to the rich explosion of fall perennials, you can always find color here. Most of the well-groomed trails have a country-garden style to them, and the park serves as a popular spot for novice and professional

DISTANCE & CONFIGURATION: 1.9-mile loop

DIFFICULTY: Easy

SCENERY: LEED-certified nature center, woods, small ponds, herb and flower garden, bouncy suspension bridge

EXPOSURE: Mostly shaded

TRAFFIC: Moderate, sometimes crowded on weekends

TRAIL SURFACE: Pavement, stone, dirt, and mulched paths

HIKING TIME: Allow an hour

DRIVING DISTANCE: 21 miles from I-77/I-480 exchange

ACCESS: Grounds open daily, 6 a.m.–11 p.m. Visitor center open Tuesday–Sunday; closed holidays but open most Monday holidays, 10 a.m.–5 p.m. Pets, bikes, and other recreational equipment not permitted.

MAPS: USGS *Peninsula;* also at visitor center

FACILITIES: Restrooms and water at the visitor center

WHEELCHAIR ACCESS: Yes, the visitor center and several trails

CONTACT: 330-865-8065, summitmetroparks .org/fa-seiberling-nature-realm.aspx

LOCATION: Smith Road, Akron

photographers. Once you get onto the trails, the crowds thin out noticeably, and on the south end of the park, you have a chance to connect to the rugged Mingo Trail and hike all the way to Sand Run Metro Park. Ready to go?

When you enter the park from the southwest corner of the parking lot and head for the visitor center, you'll notice you're looking down on it. You're not looking down because the hill is steep—it's more of a gentle slope—but because the building is partially underground. As you approach, you'll also notice some large solar panels near the building's entrance.

While the center was originally designed to be environmentally friendly, major renovations in 2009–2010 made the building a shining example of green building principles. Go inside to learn more about those principles, and you'll also have an opportunity to meet several live reptiles, amphibians, and other Ohio natives. Additional educational opportunities await inside—for children and adults. Stay as long as you like, but remember, you're here to hike, and there's much to see outside.

Leave the building by the same door you entered, and head south, veering left to cross Seneca Pond on a short footbridge. As you continue south, you'll pass an inviting campfire ring. Watch the park's events calendar, as naturalists host programs here throughout the year. As you continue south onto Cherry Lane Trail, the pavement soon changes to a hard-packed dirt surface, and you'll notice you're going down a slight grade. (All of the trails here are fairly level, however, making the Nature Realm an easy introduction to hiking for young children or even adults who haven't done much exploring outdoors.)

As you pass Echo Pond, Cherry Lane and Fernwood Trails share the same path. Immediately after passing the pond, the trail makes a sharp left, and soon you'll have an option to turn right to continue on Fernwood to connect with Mingo Trail. Mingo, which leads to Sand Run Metro Park, is a much hillier, more rugged trail than those here at the Nature Realm. If you head off on Mingo, know that it's 3 miles

F. A. Seiberling Nature Realm

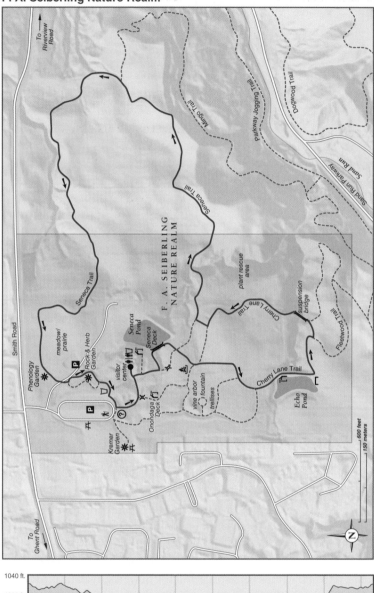

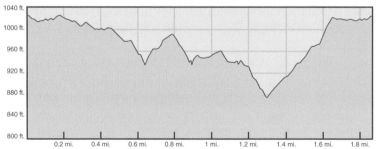

long and one of the park system's most challenging trails. (*Tip:* Download a map of Sand Run before you go.)

To follow the hike described here, stay on Cherry Trail—you're almost to the suspension bridge! The long wooden bridge supported by cables spans a 45-foot-deep ravine. You may find that you're torn between running across it to feel it bounce or stopping to take in the beauty of the ravine. (*Tip:* Do both!)

Once across the bridge, you'll head north on Cherry Lane Trail (signs marked with a carving of two cherries), which soon joins up with Seneca Trail.

Turn right on Seneca Trail to briefly venture beyond the Nature Realm's border, up a few rolling hills, to an overlook that gives you a good view of the Sand Run Valley. A bench there is an ideal place to enjoy the view—and maybe catch your breath. (If anyone in your hiking party complains, you can assure them that the remaining 0.25 mile or so is mostly flat and easy compared to the previous 0.1 mile or so.) As Seneca Trail bends left, heading west, back to the Nature Realm grounds, you'll be walking through prairie and meadow plantings—not in the woods—for the first time on your trek so far.

When the trail bends left again, you'll realize that you've almost reached the end of the trip. If you want to linger awhile, you're in a good place to do just that: your hike concludes in the Rock and Herb Garden, where almost all the herbs and other plants are labeled for easy identification.

NEARBY ACTIVITIES

For more hiking, visit Sand Run Metro Park. You can drive to the main entrance, just about 2 miles south of the Nature Realm. You're also not far from the Towpath and from Oxbow and Overlook Trails in Cascade Valley Metro Park (page 220).

If you'd like to learn more about the Seiberlings, you may want to visit beautiful Stan Hywet Hall. The 65-room mansion with equally impressive grounds was the Seiberlings' home for many years. There is an admission fee to tour the house and grounds; call 330-836-5533 or visit stanhywet.org for details.

TRAILHEAD GPS COORDINATES: N41.13933° W81.57576°

DIRECTIONS Follow I-77 S to Exit 138 (Ghent Road). Turn right (southeast) onto Ghent Road and go 1.5 miles. Turn left onto Smith Road. Travel approximately 2 miles to find the park entrance (1828 Smith Road) on your right.

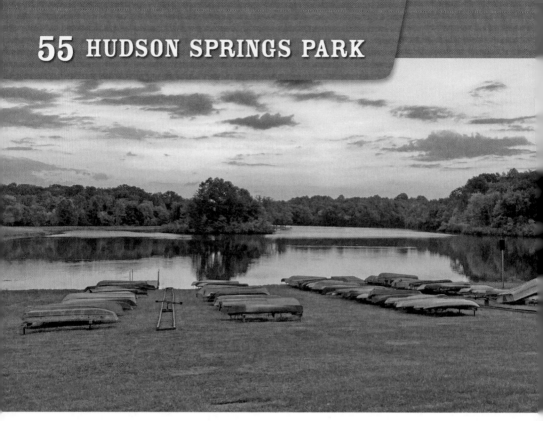

Contact the city of Hudson for details on boating here.

BRING THE FAMILY: After circling the lake on the shady crushed-limestone trail, young hikers will be rewarded with a great view of a playground on the northwest edge of this park. Those who've outgrown playgrounds can enjoy a round on the disc golf course or take in a sunset from one of many benches or decks on the lake's north side. And if your kids have paws, bring 'em along. A fenced dog run is on the northeast side of this city park.

DESCRIPTION

Hudson Springs Park spans 260 acres, including a 50-acre lake. Fishing and small (nonmotorized) boats are allowed here. Hudson residents can rent space on the lakeshore to keep their canoes and rowboats handy; nonresidents may bring their own nonmotorized boats to enjoy the water.

Though the lake is the park's largest feature, most visitors come to enjoy the trail, so you will certainly have company as you travel around the lake.

To follow the trail counterclockwise, head south from the parking lot, entering the trail just to the right of the shelter and boat launch area. Before the dirt-and-gravel path curves to the east, you'll have an option to veer left and cross Stow Road to meander through the 33 acres of Bicentennial Woods. The almost entirely flat, 0.5-mile trail stretches out under one of the city's few remaining stands of hardwood trees.

DISTANCE & CONFIGURATION: 2-mile loop

DIFFICULTY: Easy

SCENERY: Lake views, lush woods, a small island

EXPOSURE: Three-quarters of the trail is shaded

TRAFFIC: Moderate

TRAIL SURFACE: Crushed limestone

HIKING TIME: 50 minutes

DRIVING DISTANCE: 30 miles from I-77/I-480 exchange

ACCESS: Daily, sunrise–sunset

MAPS: USGS *Hudson* and *Twinsburg*

FACILITIES: Restrooms in the parking lot; three picnic shelters within the park

WHEELCHAIR ACCESS: No

CONTACT: City of Hudson Parks & Recreation Department: 330-653-5201, hudson.oh.us /Facilities/Facility/Details/4

LOCATION: 7095 Stow Road, Hudson

From that trail junction, keep going, following the wider, relatively flat Hudson Springs trail as it approaches a well-disguised culvert. From there, you'll start up a slight rise. As the path curves east, you'll have a good view of the entire lake and its little island.

Soon after, you'll notice an unmarked path on your right, leading east to Deer Hollow, a residential neighborhood adjacent to the park. It's one of several such footpaths here, most of which are unmarked. Just past this one, however, to the left of the trail, a sign points visitors to an overlook. Follow the 0.3-mile detour off the main trail to enjoy a good look at the lake. After the fairly steep descent, you'll find a wooden deck with built-in benches overlooking the lake's calm waters.

Returning to the main trail, turn left to roll up and over several small hills before the path turns left. The trail continues to roll up and down over a few hills, 10 feet or so at a time, offering a little workout if you're accustomed to walking on flat ground. As you round the eastern edge of the lake, you'll come to another observation deck, this one raised and facing west, making it perfect for sunset viewing. For a less-direct (but equally beautiful) view of the sunset, follow the loop a little farther northeast to another slightly larger deck.

As you continue (now west) on the trail, you'll come to a dog run area (which is posted as such) and then to a pole-hole on the disc golf course. Both are popular with park visitors.

Just a bit farther west, on the south side of the trail, two pieces of land jut into the lake. A small memorial arboretum is here, along with a few park benches and picnic tables, situated so that you can enjoy a peaceful lake view with your back to the action at the disc golf course and playground. Ah, but peaceful contemplation is only fun for so long. Heading west on the path again, you might find it hard to resist the playground's charm.

The northwestern corner of the park boasts play equipment for kids of all sizes and abilities, with a small obstacle course, swings, and slides—and they're all fun. But perhaps most inspired is the little hedge maze, perfect for pint-size explorers.

Hudson Springs Park

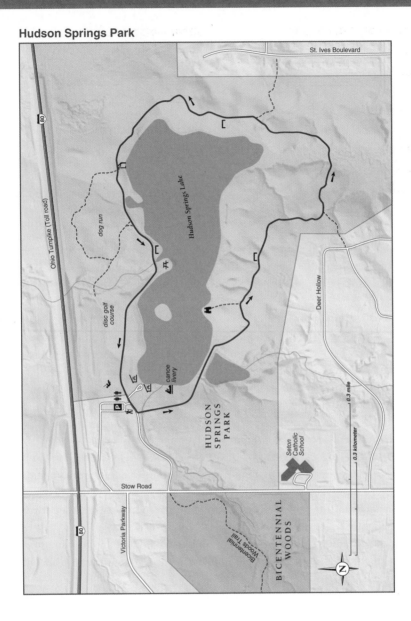

The maze was dedicated in 1988 "To all children . . . from the Hudson preschool parents." The playground is adjacent to the parking lot, so when you're finished playing, you're free to leave. Bet you'll be back, though.

NEARBY ACTIVITIES

If the hedge maze, trails, bocce courts, disc golf course, and playgrounds don't tucker you out, cross Stow Road to pick up the 0.5-mile hiking trail through Bicentennial

Woods. Or, if you prefer a bit of history with your hike, drive into the heart of Hudson and admire its many well-preserved, century-old homes and other reminders of the city's Western Reserve heritage. Western Reserve College was established in Hudson in 1826. In 1882, the college moved to Cleveland, and Hudson took the loss hard. By 1906, Hudson had no water service, and the business district went bust. Then Hudson native James Ellsworth stepped in. He told local officials that he'd help out, provided they rescind all liquor licenses in town. The officials complied, and by 1912, Hudson was once again a thriving town. And, today, Western Reserve Academy, a private high school, is situated on the former college grounds.

• •

TRAILHEAD GPS COORDINATES: N41.25148° W81.40775°

DIRECTIONS From Cleveland, take I-480 East to Exit 41 (Frost Road). Turn right (northwest) onto Hudson Aurora Road; in 1.8 miles, turn left (south) onto Stow Road. The park entrance is on the eastern side of Stow Road, just south of the Ohio Turnpike, in less than 1 mile.

Be sure to visit this overlook for a beautiful view of the lake.

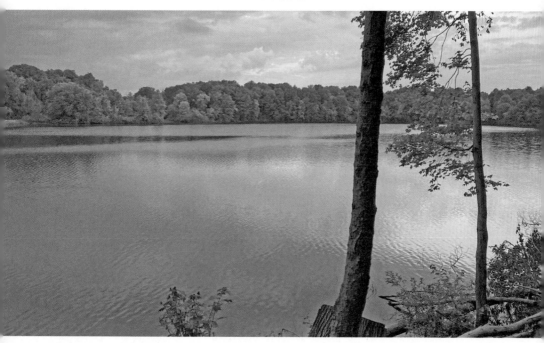

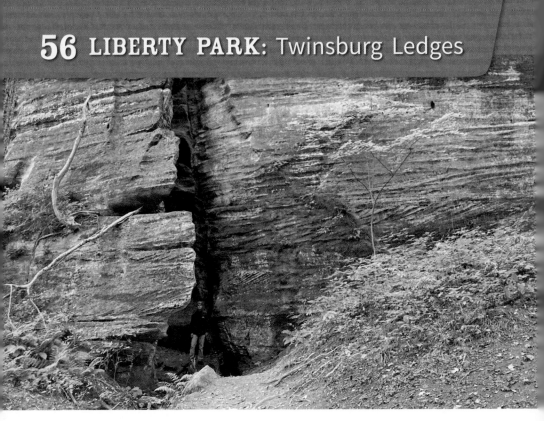

Glacier Cave

TWINSBURG LEDGES HAS been a popular spot since it opened in 2011. And no wonder—a short but exciting trail makes the thrilling ledges more accessible than others in the area, such as those in the national park and Nelson-Kennedy Ledges State Park. There are also some displays designed with accessibility in mind for visitors to the nature center.

DESCRIPTION

From the parking lot, make your way north to the nature center, which is usually open Wednesday through Sunday. If you can go inside, you'll find that the park system took "accessible" to heart in its design of the nature center, which opened here in 2015. In addition to the exhibits that pay homage to the site's former uses as a gathering spot for Indigenous peoples and a maple sugaring operation, there are several displays designed with help from the Cleveland Sight Center. Those displays are specially created to be accessible to people with low vision. Other exhibits incorporate sensory elements that may improve the experience for visitors who are on the autism spectrum.

After exploring the inside of the nature center, make sure to consider the displays just outside the entrance that highlight black bears. Here you can see how you measure up to the impressive mammal. While sightings are not exactly commonplace,

DISTANCE & CONFIGURATION: 1.6-mile figure eight

DIFFICULTY: Moderate, with one steep hill and stretches of uneven footing

SCENERY: Ledges, prairie, indoor nature center

EXPOSURE: Almost completely shaded

TRAFFIC: Fairly busy

TRAIL SURFACE: Limestone, dirt, wooden boardwalk

HIKING TIME: Allow at least an hour

DRIVING DISTANCE: 14 miles from I-77/I-480 exchange

ACCESS: Park open daily, 6 a.m.–11 p.m.; see website for nature center hours

MAPS: USGS Twinsburg; also posted at trailhead

FACILITIES: Restrooms and water at trailhead and inside nature center

WHEELCHAIR ACCESS: 0.25-mile Maple Loop Trail, yes; Ledges Trail, no

CONTACT: Liberty Park: 330-487-0493, summitmetroparks.org/liberty-park.aspx

LOCATION: 9999 Liberty Road, Twinsburg

each spring, black bears are reported throughout northeast Ohio, and Twinsburg has had its share of sightings, particularly around the Ledges.

Now, who's ready to go for a hike?

Just outside the nature center, the flat, 0.25-mile Maple Loop Trail gives visitors a look around from this relatively high vantage point in northern Summit County. As you loop around, you'll see a few nature play stations just off the trail. The interactive stops have special appeal to kids, but visitors of all ages can stop and play.

As you step on to Ledges Trail and begin a shady and somewhat steep descent, you'll see the stunning sandstone ledges for which this trail was named. It's worth noting that this stretch is the most difficult of the Ledges Trail; the path soon levels out. As you near the bottom of the hill, you'll see a sign inviting you to explore the small Glacier Cave. Go! Don't worry if you're afraid of the dark; cracks overhead allow sunlight to peek through.

Once you've marveled at the cave's surprisingly roomy inside—and natural air-conditioning—return to the main trail, which soon bears left (north) to reach a small observation deck overlooking a wetland. As you continue in a counterclockwise direction, you'll travel across the wetland via a long boardwalk. The boardwalk not only contributes to the trail's relatively easy (moderate) rating, it also helps ensure visitors stay on the trail and avoid damaging the ferns, mosses, lichens, and other natural resources that are preserved here.

Once you've reached the end of the boardwalk, you'll return to the bottom of the hill and begin to climb back up to the trailhead.

Is this the best example of northeast Ohio's marvelous ledges? Although Nelson-Kennedy Ledges (page 175) and the Ledges Trail in Cuyahoga Valley National Park feature more extensive ledges, Twinsburg's ledges absolutely are as lovely as the others. And, while I personally like my hikes a little longer and more challenging than this one, there's a lot to be said for trails that are easier to navigate. Liberty Park's trails are a great place to test a young hiker's abilities; to work back to longer, more

Liberty Park: Twinsburg Ledges

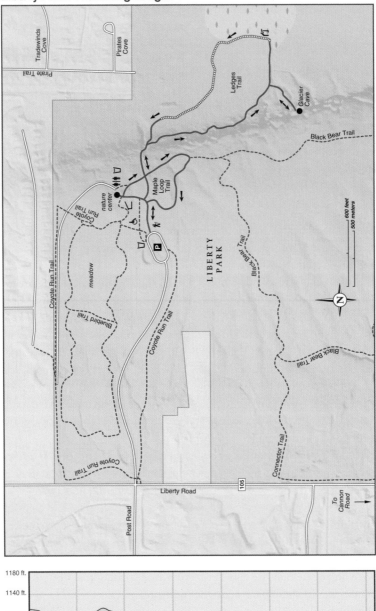

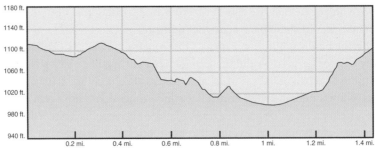

difficult hikes after an injury; or just to increase your endurance—and that's a very good thing.

YOU HAVE OPTIONS

The interpretive signage in and around the nature center, combined with the accessible Maple Loop Trail and nature play areas, make this a fun and easy outing for very young children or anyone with mobility issues. Those who want to add some distance to their outing can follow two other trails here, Coyote Run and Black Bear Trails, for a combined total of about 3.3 miles, or take the connector trail into the conservation area to create a longer out-and-back hike.

NEARBY ACTIVITIES

There's another side of Liberty Park just a few blocks away, at 9385 Liberty Road. There, visitors can enjoy several ball fields; a dog park; and the flat, 0.6-mile Sugarbush Trail, traveling through a beech-maple forest. Just south of here, at 3973 E. Aurora Road, you'll find a different experience at Pond Brook Conservation Area, where an easy, 1.6-mile trail follows Pond Brook through a wetland environment.

Also nearby, you'll find Twinsburg's historical city square. It has served as the center of town festivals since the early 1800s. A bandstand, historic church, and war memorial grace the square, located at the junction of OH 91, Ravenna Road, and Church Street. A local point of pride is that the internationally famous Twins Days celebration has been held in Twinsburg since 1976. For information about the town's most famous festival, see twinsdays.org.

• •

TRAILHEAD GPS COORDINATES: N41.33241° W81.41155°

DIRECTIONS Take I-480 E to Exit 36 (OH 82/Aurora) and turn left (east) onto OH 82, toward Twinsburg. In 0.7 mile, turn left toward Cannon Road, then turn left again onto Liberty Road. The park entrance will be on your right in 1.5 miles.

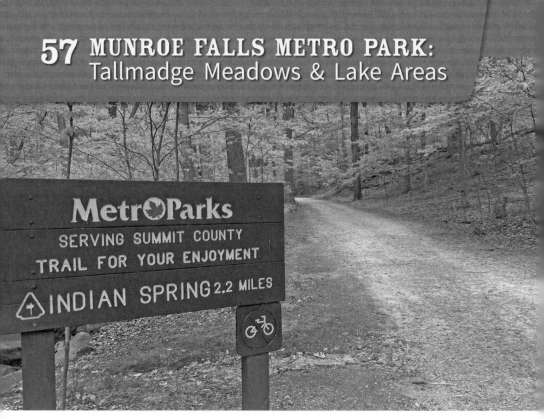

You'll find Indian Spring Trail in the Lake Area of Munroe Falls Metro Park.

CONNECTING TWO AREAS with different ecosystems within Munroe Falls Metro Park, this trail combination gives hikers a chance to enjoy a variety of scenery—and more miles. Both areas also offer paved, accessible trails for visitors.

DESCRIPTION

Munroe Falls Metro Park has two distinct personalities, and two distinct entrances: Tallmadge Meadows, located off OH 91, and the Lake Area, off South River Road in Munroe Falls. Both have ample parking. I like to start and finish at Tallmadge Meadows, especially if I've timed my outing to catch a sunset at the end of the trail.

From the Tallmadge Meadows Trailhead, follow the paved path as it curves toward the prairie meadow for which it is named. You'll soon come to a trail intersection: if you go to the right, you can continue on pavement and loop around the paved, accessible, 0.35-mile Meadow Loop Trail. This is a great option for folks working up to longer treks, and almost every point on the entire loop is a good place to watch a sunset.

If you're up for a longer hike, turn left instead.

On your left, at the bottom of a slight hill, you'll notice a few grave markers. The area, purchased by the parks in 2007, is the site of the former County Home, an institution for those considered mentally ill, who did not have family or who were

DISTANCE & CONFIGURATION: 5-mile figure eight

DIFFICULTY: Easy–moderate

SCENERY: Woods, wildflowers, prairie, and a great sunset view

EXPOSURE: Mostly shaded

TRAFFIC: Moderate

TRAIL SURFACE: Dirt, roots, and some boardwalk

HIKING TIME: 1.5–2 hours

DRIVING DISTANCE: 31 miles from I-77/I-480 exchange

ACCESS: Sunrise–sunset

MAPS: USGS *Hudson;* also on park website

FACILITIES: Restrooms, water, and covered picnic area at Tallmadge Meadows Trailhead; restrooms, grills, picnic tables, and kayak launch by the lake; sledding hill west of Indian Spring Trailhead; additional parking and map by Indian Spring Trailhead

WHEELCHAIR ACCESS: Main trails in description, no; shorter paved loop at Tallmadge Meadows and Firefly Loop at Lake Area, yes

CONTACT: Summit Metro Parks: 330-867-5511, summitmetroparks.org /munroe-falls-metro-park.aspx

LOCATION: 1088 North Ave., Tallmadge

otherwise unable to care for themselves. Sadly, only a few of the gravestones have names or other identifying information.

Once you've considered this spot, head back to the trail and continue to your left, with the meadow on your right. The pavement soon ends, and you have another choice: go straight to complete the shortcut for the 2-mile Meadow Trail or turn left to head into the woods. Go left.

The hard-packed dirt trail bends around to the left again, heading east, then goes down a slight hill and over a footbridge. At the top of a short rise, you'll see a sign directing you to follow the Meadow Trail to your right—but you can go left here, and you should, if you want to pick up the trail that connects to the park's Lake Area.

The trees are taller here, and the ground is a little softer. At the bottom of a little hill, you'll come to a wide dirt-and-gravel path that connects to the 2.2-mile Indian Spring Trail. Turn right and you'll soon walk by the Beaver Pond. (It may, in fact, be inhabited with beavers, but I'd wager the turtle population vastly outnumbers the mammals that call this pond home.) The trail bends a bit to the right to rise slightly above the edge of the pond.

YOU HAVE OPTIONS

Immediately east of the pond, you can continue straight on an old service road. If you choose to follow that wider, more exposed path, you'll cut about 1.3 miles off your total distance but otherwise not change your route.

To complete the hike as described here, continue on the dirt path to the right, rising above the water's edge. As Indian Spring Trail winds through hardwood forest, you'll encounter a few gentle hills along the way. The trail can be a little slow to dry out after a good rain (or during the spring thaw), but it's never impassable.

Munroe Falls Metro Park: Tallmadge Meadows & Lake Areas

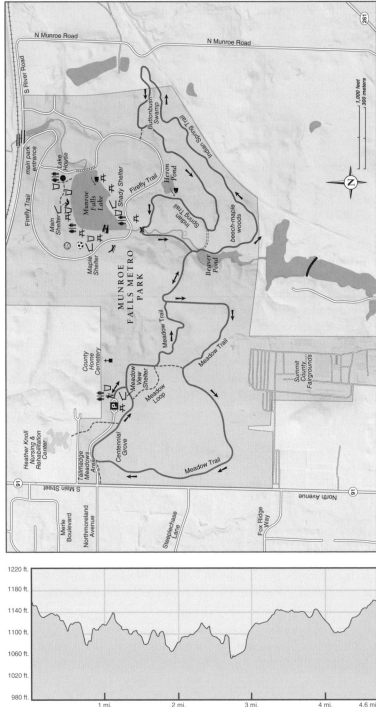

The upside is that the rich soil supports a decent population of spring wildflowers, including mayapples, some trilliums, and the occasional jack-in-the-pulpit.

When you reach Heron Pond, you'll be able to see the park road, but the pond is serene. Continuing on Indian Spring Trail from the pond, you'll veer slightly left and wander through the mature beech-maple forest until you reach a stone staircase taking you down to the Lake Area's trailhead parking lot. Here, you may notice people heading to the park road, which has been modified to serve as part of the easy Firefly Trail. The 1.3-mile loop is partially paved and offers an easy, short hike with lake views. Whether you choose to follow it or not, you'll need to return to the south end of the trailhead parking lot to make your way back to the Tallmadge Meadows area.

At the Indian Spring Trailhead kiosk, continue a few hundred yards south. You'll pass a small natural spring, then see your connector trail on the right, heading up a slight hill. Follow it back to the Meadow Trail, where you'll turn left.

The Meadow Trail wiggles through the woods on hard-packed dirt. A couple of footbridges carry you across the streams that feed the wetlands on the western side of the park. As you leave the woods and circle to the right, you'll find yourself back on the edge of the meadow, and, if you've timed it right, watching a sunset as you finish your hike.

Even if you don't catch the sunset, you'll have plenty of birds and insects to entertain you, as this stretch of native plantings is a great attraction for redwing blackbirds, goldfinches, various dragonflies and damselflies, and other fun-to-watch species as you begin to head uphill, now back on pavement. At the top of the hill, follow the path (and the signs) to the left to return to the trailhead.

NEARBY ACTIVITIES

Hungry? Across the street from the park, Cornerstone Market specializes in local produce, meats, and cheeses—it's a great place to get snacks or a full meal for a picnic. If it's more hiking you want, you can go north to the Summit Metro Park Brust Park Trailhead to walk along the Cuyahoga River on the paved Bike & Hike Trail. Prefer unpaved trails? Adell Durbin Park, about 2 miles north on OH 91, offers about 3 miles of hilly, woodland trails, plus a playground for smaller children.

• •

TRAILHEAD GPS COORDINATES: N41.13077° W81.43555°

DIRECTIONS: Follow I-480 E, staying right to take I-271 S for about 3.5 miles. Stay left to continue south on OH 8 for about 10 miles to Exit 7/Graham Road. Turn left onto Graham and go almost 2 miles to OH 91/S. Main Street in Stow. Turn right onto OH 91 and continue about 2 miles. The entrance to Tallmadge Meadows will be on your left.

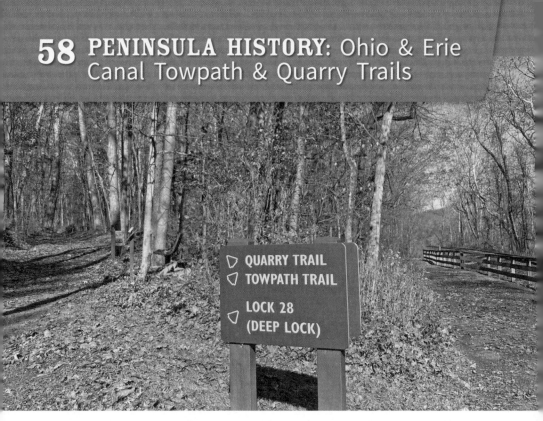

Does Peninsula have a lock on history? Actually, it has two—and you'll see both on this hike.

PENINSULA DISPLAYS THE well-preserved vestiges of a canal-era and railroad town, while serving as a portal into Cuyahoga Valley National Park.

DESCRIPTION

Change steamed through Peninsula in the form of a canal in the 1820s, and it then rolled through again in the 1880s when the railroad came to town. The changes kept coming, with the dedication of the Cuyahoga Valley National Recreation Area (now National Park) in 1974. And when the federal government comes to town to claim more than 30,000 acres, *change* is putting it mildly.

While other towns might buckle under the strain of being a gateway to a national park, Peninsula has worked to maintain its own identity. Many of the town's historical buildings have been restored and are still in use—you'll see some of them on this hike. At the same time, in some ways, Peninsula also serves as an extension of the park. Lock 29 along the Ohio & Erie Towpath Trail literally deposits thru-hikers and bikers into the heart of Peninsula. The local bike shop is a welcome beacon to cyclists in need of minor repairs. Peninsula's restaurants are so popular with train riders that the Cuyahoga Valley Scenic Railroad frequently features a layover lunch stop here.

Start your tour at the trailhead sign and map at Lock 29. Take the steps up to the bridge that literally and figuratively connects the relatively new Towpath Trail and

DISTANCE & CONFIGURATION: 3.7-mile balloon with "T"

DIFFICULTY: Moderate (Quarry, somewhat challenging; Towpath and village portions, easy)

SCENERY: Two canal locks, sandstone quarry, historical architecture, wildlife along the river

EXPOSURE: Trail, shady; sidewalks, exposed

TRAFFIC: Typically heavy in town, moderate on Towpath Trail, and light on Quarry Trail

TRAIL SURFACE: Asphalt, sand, dirt, crushed limestone, sidewalks in village

HIKING TIME: 1.5 hours

DRIVING DISTANCE: 16 miles from I-77/I-480 exchange

ACCESS: Towpath Trail, 24/7; Quarry Trail, 6 a.m.–11 p.m.

MAPS: USGS *Peninsula;* architectural tour guide at Peninsula Library & Historical Society, 6105 Riverview Road

FACILITIES: Restrooms, water, and drink machine at Lock 29 parking

WHEELCHAIR ACCESS: Peninsula sidewalks, yes (most businesses, no); Quarry Trail, no

CONTACT: Summit Metro Parks: 330-867-5511, summitmetroparks.org/deep-lock-quarry-metro -park.aspx; Cuyahoga Valley National Park: 330-657-2752, nps.gov/cuva

LOCATION: Mill St. W, Peninsula

national park to the historical town of Peninsula. An interpretive sign on the bridge highlights the building of the Ohio & Erie Canal. When construction began in 1825, workers had to devise it so that boats could negotiate the 395-foot elevation difference between Akron and Cleveland. Locks 29 and 28 were key to leveling the ride, and the canal was key to Ohio's economy.

Go below the bridge and walk into the now earth-filled lock. The mason's marks on some of the blocks are still visible, indicating the quarry and the work group from which the stone came.

Once over the bridge, continue south on the Towpath Trail and under OH 303/ Main Street, where the paved path gives way to crushed limestone. The river runs on your left; beyond it, railroad tracks carry passengers on the Cuyahoga Valley Scenic Line. About 0.5 mile into the trail, a sign points to Deep Lock Quarry. Take the cue and venture off the Towpath heading west. Cross a narrow, wooden footbridge and then head up a steep hill. Follow the dirt path under tall pines and right over the rocky but now level ground. You'll reach the quarry shortly.

Sandstone dug here helped build many local homes and businesses, as well as several locks along the canal. Today, leaf litter covers the quarry's floor, but the sheer stone walls leave no doubt where you are.

The adventurous may want to climb into the quarry, and it's allowed, but all should take care near the edges, as gravel and sand can make for slippery footing. The rim trail skirts the western edge of the quarry. As you round back to the eastern side of the quarry, you'll see Summit County Metro Parks trail markers (in yellow) leading to the Deep Lock Quarry Metro Park parking lot, off Riverview Road. Unless you want to explore the park further, however, stay on the trail heading south and retrace your steps to the Towpath.

Peninsula History: Ohio & Erie Canal Towpath & Quarry Trails

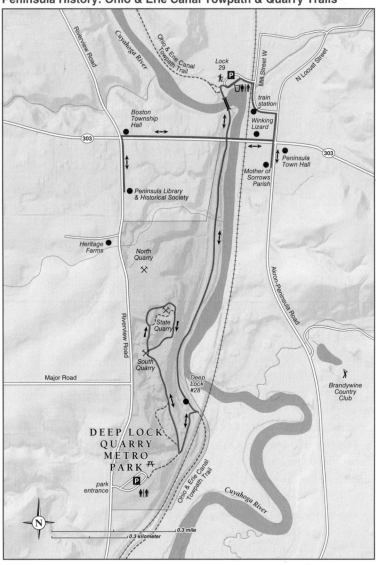

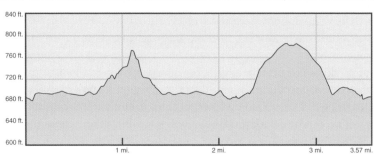

Turn left (northeast) on the Towpath Trail and take a good look at Lock 28, also known as Deep Lock. While a typical lock would move a boat up or down 8 or 9 feet, Deep Lock could raise and lower boats 17 feet. A historic civil engineers' landmark plaque, displayed inside the lock, recognizes it for being the deepest lock on the canal.

Continue north on the Towpath toward Peninsula. The calls of geese and other birds blend with the bubbling of the river, now on your right. As you head back to the center of this historical village, ignore a few unmarked but well-used paths leading off the Towpath. Most lead to private properties along Riverview Road, so stay on the Towpath to return to OH 303/Main Street. There, you can cross the street north and return to your parking spot if you want to end your hike, or continue on the village sidewalks, where you'll get a different view of the village and its history.

From OH 303/Main Street, turn left (west) and head into the Peninsula Village Historic District, listed on the National Register of Historic Places. There's no sign to alert you to the history of some of the homes here, but several are worth a good look. Perhaps the biggest bargain on the block, a Vallonia model Sears Roebuck kit home, sold for $2,076 in 1926. Its steep roof and signature columns have been maintained so that it's easily recognized as a Sears Roebuck model.

Around 100,000 kit homes were built in the United States between 1908 and 1940. Most models came entirely as precut and numbered pieces of lumber. The homes were affordable and efficient to build. The Sears catalog boasted that a kit home could be built in about 60% of the time required to build a traditional home.

As you continue west and up a gentle hill, consider the girth of the maples that line the yards here. Most of them were planted around the time the village was established. If they could talk!

Just before the intersection of Riverview Road and OH 303/Main, you'll see the Boston Township Hall and its distinctive bell tower at 1775 Main Street. Built as a school in 1887, today it houses Boston Township offices, community meeting rooms, and the Cuyahoga Valley Historical Museum. Turn left (south) on Riverview to visit the Peninsula Library & Historical Society, where you can learn more about the area.

Retrace your steps to OH 303/Main and turn right. As you cross the bridge and the railroad tracks, you'll pass a variety of shops, cafés, and galleries. The sign for the old PENINSULA NITE CLUB hanging at 1615 Main Street has been around for many years; the building was a nightclub and a dance hall in the 1930s and '40s. Today, the restaurant is the Winking Lizard, proudly displaying the cool antique sign (next to its own).

About a block east of the Lizard, turn right and walk one block south on Akron-Peninsula Road to Mother of Sorrows Parish. Originally built in 1882, the church was enlarged in 1935 in a rather clever way. The building was literally cut in half, the west end was moved back, and the middle was filled in to enlarge the sanctuary.

Now turn around and go north on Akron-Peninsula Road (also known as Locust Street). You'll pass Peninsula Town Hall, constructed with sandstone from the local quarry in 1851. Cost to the taxpayers? About $600. It's still used to house village services—talk about a long-term investment.

From there, you can conclude your village tour by heading north on Locust Street to Mill Street to return to the Lock 29 parking lot. Or continue to explore Peninsula. Its history is still unfolding.

NEARBY ACTIVITIES

Peninsula hosts family-friendly events year-round; you can find the current schedule at villageofpeninsula-oh.gov.

Cuyahoga Valley Scenic Railroad offers numerous excursions. Get schedules and ticket information at 330-439-5708 or cvsr.com.

Want to learn more about farming in the valley? Heritage Farms on Riverview Road has been operated by the same family since 1848. It hosts a variety of events, including a farmers market. The farm even has a few private campsites; call 330-657-2330 or visit heritagefarms.com to find out more.

• •

TRAILHEAD GPS COORDINATES: N41.24316° W81.55038°

DIRECTIONS From Cleveland, take I-77 S to Exit 146 (toward I-80) and keep right to OH 21/Richfield/Brecksville. Turn right (south) onto OH 21/Brecksville Road. Go 2.2 miles and turn left (east) onto OH 303/West Streetsboro Road. Go about 5 miles. Turn left (north) onto Akron-Peninsula Road/North Locust Street after crossing the river, and then immediately turn left again on Mill Street and into the lot. (A sign directs you to Lock 29 Trailhead Parking.)

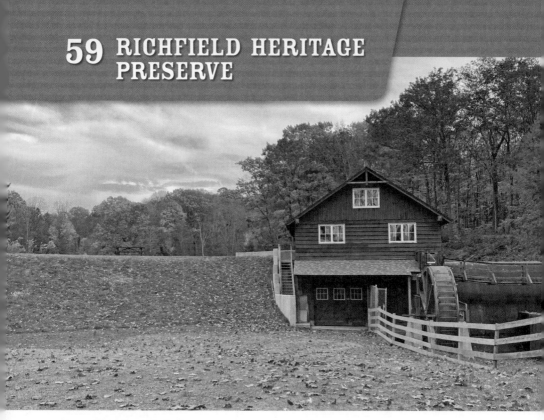

Kirby's Mill was built in 1922.

ONCE THE HOME of a prolific inventor, then a Girl Scout Camp for 74 years, this 336-acre property is now open for all to enjoy. With more than 7 miles of hiking and bridle trails, the rolling landscape also features a kayak launch and several historic buildings.

DESCRIPTION

The Richfield Joint Recreation District is a cooperative effort between the Village of Richfield and Richfield Township that was formed when Crowell Hilaka Girl Scout Camp closed in 2011. After that, voters passed levies to purchase and operate the land, which prevented it from being developed. Between the work of park board members and a team of volunteers, today the property has over 7 miles of hiking and bridle trails, plus a section of the Buckeye Trail (BT). Some of the buildings and amenities that speak to the land's previous uses are in the process of being restored. While some of the trails were still under development at the time of this writing, it's clear that there's much to enjoy and learn here.

And here's a piece of trivia to take away: The entrance to the park is at the highest point of elevation in Summit County.

From the parking lot, head toward the lodge, where you'll find a large, inviting fire pit, then go past a sign for the kayak and canoe launch. Continue on the

DISTANCE & CONFIGURATION: 3.5-mile balloon

DIFFICULTY: Moderate, with optional walking on creekbed and rocks

SCENERY: Woodlands, two small lakes, historic mill, camp buildings

EXPOSURE: Mostly shaded

TRAFFIC: Fairly busy

TRAIL SURFACE: Dirt, limestone

HIKING TIME: Allow at least an hour

DRIVING DISTANCE: 13 miles from I-77/I-480 exchange

ACCESS: Sunrise–sunset

MAPS: USGS *West Richfield*; also posted at trailhead and on website

FACILITIES: Restrooms at trailhead; several reservable shelters

WHEELCHAIR ACCESS: No

CONTACT: Richfield Joint Recreation District: 330-888-0511, richfieldheritagepreserve.com

LOCATION: 4374 Broadview Road, Richfield

hard-packed dirt-and-gravel trail, past a restroom facility, to pick up the Buckeye Trail heading south to the Lower Lake.

YOU HAVE OPTIONS

If you want to explore all of the park land, you can follow the Blue Trail to the right to get a look at the Upper Lake and then connect with the Red Loop or bridle trail to return to the southern half of the property. For this outing, I was eager to head south to see some of the remnants of the camp buildings and the home of the former owner.

The BT is narrow as it follows the creek. Shortly after crossing a footbridge, you'll go up a gentle hill and then veer right to pick up a connector trail to the Green Trail. Look for a sign pointing to HIGH LEA/SUMMER BARN, and then turn left, heading south. Continue over another narrow footbridge, then into a thick pine planting.

Where the path splits, continue straight, and you'll soon pass a sign directing you to Lower Lake. The small buildings you pass along here are left over from the property's days as a Girl Scout Camp. Volunteers are working to remove some of the buildings and to restore others. Before you leave the collection of buildings behind, the trail begins down a gentle slope. Turn left on the White Trail, which takes you farther downhill, and soon you'll see Lower Lake. As you continue south, you'll get a look at the Kirby home.

Born in Cleveland in 1884, James B. Kirby is probably best known around northeast Ohio as the inventor of the vacuum cleaners that bear his name. But Kirby was a serial inventor—holding more than 160 patents—and he left his mark on this land. The home he built in 1921, in the Swiss-chalet style, made use of fieldstone found on this property to build the massive fireplace. Kirby built the lakes, too, and, true to his inventor's nature, he designed them to have a unique, built-in filtration system to avoid the need to dredge them. In fact, he patented the system and the lake's name: Lake Jinelle was a combination of his wife's first name, Nellie, and the first initial of his own name.

Richfield Heritage Preserve

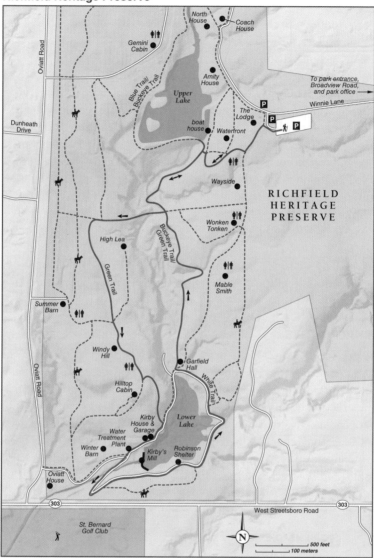

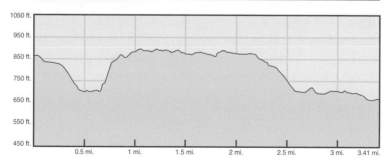

As you continue to the south end of the lake, still on the White Trail, you'll walk parallel to OH 303 and get a good look at Kirby's Mill. Although it was patterned after ancient gristmills, when he built it in 1922, Kirby implemented new, more-efficient hydroelectric power generation.

As you head uphill, stay on the path closest to the lake, crossing over a footbridge and returning to the BT. When the trail takes you to the top of the lake, you'll find Garfield Dance Hall, also known as the "Bounce House." Another of Kirby's innovative experiments, the structure was built on streetcar springs so it would bounce as guests danced. (As of this writing, it is also slated for restoration.)

As you continue north on the BT, the path is narrow and a little uneven as it takes you past several more buildings that remain from the former Girl Scout Camp. Camp Hilaka was open for 74 years, from 1937 to 2011, so countless area residents have special memories of this place.

Once the Buckeye Trail crosses the utility clear-cut, you can turn right to retrace your steps to follow it back to the lodge, and then to the parking lot, or take a left and continue past the kayak launch and around Upper Lake if you want to put another mile or two on your boots today.

NEARBY ACTIVITIES

Looking for more trails? From here you're just a short drive from Cleveland Metroparks' Hinckley Reservation, where you can find a flat lake loop trail, as well as some interesting ledges and carvings (page 148). If you've worked up an appetite, you're in luck, as a wide variety of local restaurants, wineries, and ice-cream shops in both Richfield and nearby Peninsula will satisfy a wide range of tastes. Wondering about the lodge and other buildings here? The lodge is a reservable event center that can accommodate up to 200 guests. Some of the other buildings can be reserved too; contact the preserve for more information.

• •

TRAILHEAD GPS COORDINATES: N41.24986° W81.67464°

DIRECTIONS: From I-480 E, take I-77 S to Exit 146. Stay right and turn onto OH 21/ Brecksville Road. Follow OH 21 south about 1.4 miles to Brush Road. Turn right onto Brush Road, staying on Brush until reaching Broadview/Richfield Road, where you'll turn left. The parking lot for the preserve will be on your right.

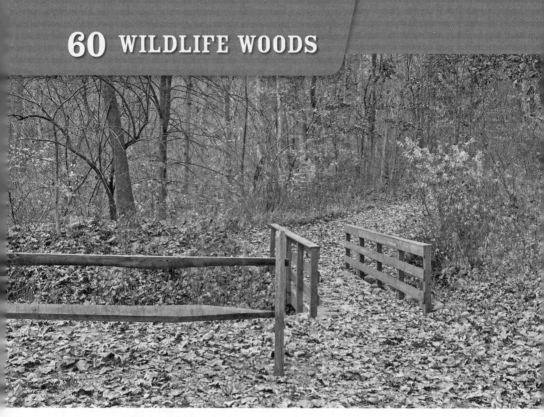

The trailhead at Wildlife Woods

TUCKED BETWEEN CUYAHOGA Valley National Park and the Ohio Turnpike, this 58-acre razorback hill was preserved by the city of Hudson. The fully forested wildlife preserve features a heart-pounding hill and a short trail that, in spite of the sounds from the freeway, really feels like a getaway from the daily grind.

DESCRIPTION

It's a good bet that countless people have zipped by Wildlife Woods without a thought about stopping, or to question its past. That's a shame because the small parcel of land has quite a lot to offer, both in terms of hiking fun and historical relevance.

Although it is just slightly outside of the city limits of Hudson, it was not only the city's first park, but it was also the impetus that led to the development of the city's parks department.

Like many park properties, we have a generous donor to thank for its preservation: William B. Shilts, who moved to Hudson in 1919, purchased the property. He and his family used the parcel of land as a retreat until 1959, when they offered to donate the land to the city of Hudson. The offer spurred the first meeting of the city's provisional park board, and by June of 1961, Wildlife Woods was Hudson's first city park.

A decade and a half later, the Federal Government purchased the land surrounding Wildlife Woods, which would become Cuyahoga Valley National Park.

DISTANCE & CONFIGURATION: 1.5-mile balloon

DIFFICULTY: Moderate

SCENERY: Woods, wildflowers, prairie, and turnpike

EXPOSURE: Almost entirely shaded

TRAFFIC: Very light

TRAIL SURFACE: Heavy leaf litter on dirt trail (can be slippery)

HIKING TIME: About an hour

DRIVING DISTANCE: 16 miles from I-77/I-480 exchange

DIFFICULTY: Moderate

ACCESS: Sunrise–sunset

MAPS: USGS *Northfield;* also on park website

FACILITIES: None

WHEELCHAIR ACCESS: No

CONTACT: 330-653-5201, hudson.oh.us /Facilities/Facility/Details/19

LOCATION: 313 Boston Mills Road, Peninsula

Today, the little pocket of land perched just east of one of the national park's busiest visitor centers, and on the edge of the Ohio Turnpike, is a surprisingly quiet spot—at least as a starting point for a hike. Even if the small parking lot is empty when you arrive, you're likely to encounter other hikers while you're in the park, as Wildlife Woods' short trail intersects with other trails that crisscross the valley.

From the parking lot, head east over a short footbridge. Once you're across, you'll immediately start climbing south up the steep, narrow hill (or "razorback"). If you were expecting an easy little hike, think again: you'll gain about 130 feet in the first 0.25 mile of this outing. You'll want to wear shoes or boots with good traction, since heavy leaf litter and the uneven trail surface can make the footing a little slippery.

At the top of the hill, there's little question about how to follow the trail, as the narrow path veers to the right, heading west through a dense growth of mostly oak and birch trees. Continue west until you reach a Hudson Parks sign that tells you to turn right (north). By the time you see the wooden sign with a yellow arrow, you'll have passed a few other trail markers for a section of the Buckeye Trail. Here the city's trail and the Buckeye Trail share the same path. Follow them as you continue to walk through a corridor of pine trees.

Soon your scenery changes to a rather eclectic mix: to the west, you'll see the edge of a wide prairie planting; directly in front of you, traffic whizzes by on the turnpike. And while you'll probably be enjoying the distinct smell of pine, you might be stumbling over the roots of those trees, well disguised by a thick carpet of pine needles.

When you reach the edge of the Hudson Park property, you'll find several signs telling you where you can go: the signage is a mix of national park markers, the Buckeye Trail's blue blazes, and the city park's signage. Before you follow the yellow arrows to the right and back to the parking lot, you might want to take a moment to consider this crossroads.

Wildlife Woods was preserved and established as a park before the Ohio Turnpike butted up against it. The prairie grasses waving to your left were planted during the construction of the turnpike, in a borrow pit where dirt was excavated during

Wildlife Woods

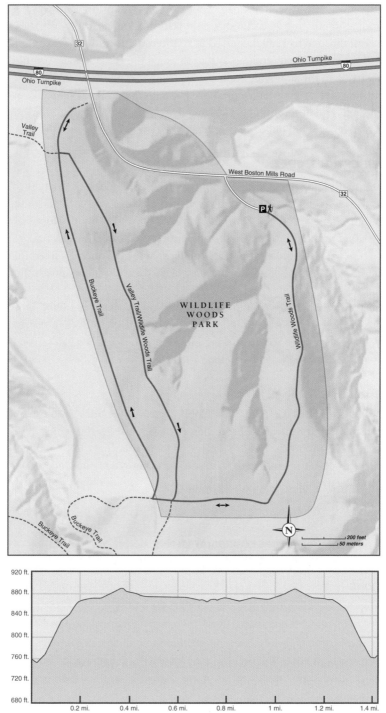

the building process. It wasn't until 1974 that the surrounding land was designated as a National Recreation Area (and later, a National Park). And while the Buckeye Trail was established in 1959, it started in southern Ohio and worked its way north. In 1983, the local Buckeye Trail organization asked the Hudson Park Commission to allow a portion of the statewide trail to pass through Wildlife Woods.

So, while this little park may not be very well-known, it has seniority over all of the other trails and developments you can see from this spot. If Wildlife Woods were to need a slogan, "Small but Mighty" seems like a good fit.

YOU HAVE OPTIONS, BUT . . .

It's worth mentioning that, from this point, you could hop on the Valley Bridle Trail, heading west to reach the Towpath Trail, or follow the Buckeye Trail south to Pine Lane, or north and west to the Boston Store (and beyond). But, because larger parking lots exist at numerous other trailheads, leaving your car in the city park's small lot doesn't seem like the best idea. In fact, you'll probably encounter a few other hikers who wander through Wildlife Woods as they make their way along those other routes.

Once you've gawked at the turnpike traffic as long as you care to, return to the city trail, turning right to finish the balloon on top of the hill, then veering left to begin your descent back to the parking lot. Remember that it's just as steep on the way down as it is on the way up, so don't rush your return trip.

NEARBY ACTIVITIES

While Wildlife Woods is definitely a "big bang for your buck" trail, many longer hikes can be had in the valley. From here, you're close to the iconic Brandywine Falls (page 230) and to the historic village of Peninsula (page 268). This short trail also makes a nice companion activity if you come here to try out the national park's mountain bike trails.

• •

TRAILHEAD GPS COORDINATES: N41.25514° W81.53673°

DIRECTIONS: Follow I-77 S, and take Exit 146, staying right to get on OH 21/Richfield. Turn right onto OH 21, traveling about 0.5 mile, then turn left onto Boston Mills Road. In about 1 mile, turn left onto Black Road, then turn right and continue on Boston Mills Road. Follow Boston Mills Road, veering right at the intersection of Hines Hill Road to stay on Boston Mills Road. The small parking lot will be on your right, about 1 mile east of the park visitor center. Note that the street address for Wildlife Woods is 313 Boston Mills Road, Peninsula (not Hudson).

APPALACHIAN OUTFITTERS
60 Kendall Park Road
Peninsula, OH 44264
330-655-5444
appalachianoutfitters.com

THE BACKPACKERS SHOP
5128 Colorado Ave./OH 611
Sheffield Village, OH 44054
440-934-5345
backpackersshop.com

CABELA'S
35685 Chester Road
Avon, OH 44011
440-723-5600
cabelas.com

EVERYTHING OUTDOOR CAMPING & TACTICAL
3823 Pearl Road
Medina, Ohio 44256
234-200-3135
everythingoutdoorcamping.com

GEIGERS
50 Shopping Plaza Dr.
Chagrin Shopping Plaza
Chagrin Falls, OH 44022
440-247-4900

14710 Detroit Ave.
Lakewood, OH 44107
216-521-1771
shopgeigers.com

REI
411 Park Ave., Suite 143
Beachwood, OH 44122
216-591-9770
rei.com

This scene awaits at the top of the hill at Wildlife Woods.

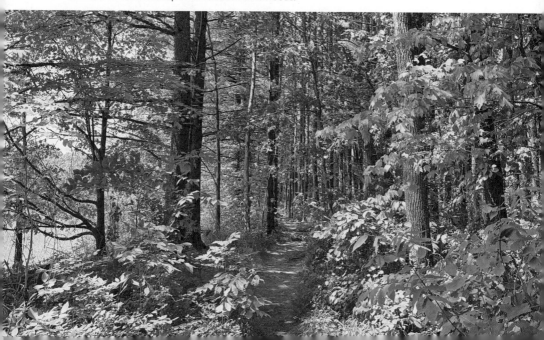

APPENDIX B: Places to Buy Maps

Also see the shops listed in Appendix A.

BUCKEYE TRAIL ASSOCIATION
shop.buckeyetrail.org/bt_trailshop/shop/home

CLEVELAND METROPARKS NATURE SHOPS
clevelandmetroparks.com

North Chagrin Nature Center
3037 SOM Center Road
Willoughby Hills, OH 44094
440-449-0511

Rocky River Nature Center
24000 Valley Pkwy.
North Olmsted, OH 44070
440-734-7576

Hinckley Lake Boathouse & Store
1 West Dr.
Hinckley, OH 44233
330-278-2160
This location is seasonal.

CUYAHOGA VALLEY NATIONAL PARK
nps.gov/cuva

Boston Store
1550 Boston Mills Road
Peninsula, OH 44264
330-657-2752

Canal Exploration Center
7104 Canal Road
Valley View, OH 44125
216-524-1497
Canal Exploration Center is closed for the winter November 1–May 5

F. A. SEIBERLING NATURE REALM
1828 Smith Rd.
Akron, OH 44313
330-865-8065
summitmetroparks.org/gift-shop.aspx

APPENDIX C: Hiking Clubs & Events

AKRON BICYCLE CLUB
(hikes off-season)
akronbike.org

APPALACHIAN OUTFITTERS
60 Kendall Park Rd.
Peninsula, OH 44264
330-655-5444
appalachianoutfitters.com

CLEVELAND HIKING CLUB
clevelandhikingclub.org

PORTAGE TRAIL WALKERS
330-673-6896

APPENDIX D: Other Resources

ASHTABULA COUNTY METROPARKS
440-576-0717
ashtabulametroparks.com

BUCKEYE TRAIL ASSOCIATION
740-832-1282
buckeyetrail.org

CLEVELAND METROPARKS
216-635-3200
clevelandmetroparks.com

CUYAHOGA VALLEY NATIONAL PARK
330-657-2752
nps.gov/cuva

GEAUGA PARK DISTRICT
440-286-9516
geaugaparkdistrict.org

LAKE METROPARKS
440-639-7275
lakemetroparks.com

LORAIN COUNTY METRO PARKS
800-526-7275
metroparks.cc

MEDINA COUNTY HISTORICAL SOCIETY
330-722-1341
medinacountyhistoricalsociety.com

MEDINA COUNTY PARK DISTRICT
330-722-9364
medinacountyparks.com

THE NATURE CONSERVANCY
614-717-2770
nature.org

OHIO & ERIE CANALWAY COALITION
330-374-5657
ohioeriecanal.org

OHIO DEPARTMENT OF NATURAL RESOURCES, OHIO STATE PARKS
614-265-6561
ohiodnr.gov

OHIO OUTDOOR SCULPTURE INVENTORY
oosi.sculpturecenter.org

PORTAGE COUNTY HISTORICAL SOCIETY
330-296-3523
pchsohio.org

PORTAGE PARK DISTRICT
330-297-7728
portageparkdistrict.org

STARK COUNTY PARK DISTRICT
330-477-3552
starkparks.com

SUMMIT COUNTY HISTORICAL SOCIETY
330-535-1120
summithistory.org

SUMMIT METRO PARKS
330-867-5511
summitmetroparks.org

BIBLIOGRAPHY

Abercrombie, Jay. *Walks and Rambles in Ohio's Western Reserve*. Woodstock, VT: Backcountry Publications, 1996.

Bartsch, William W. "Lake View Cemetery Trail Guide." Eagle Scout project, Troop 656, Cleveland Heights, OH, 1988.

Bobel, Pat. *The Nature of the Towpath*. Akron, OH: Cuyahoga Valley Trails Council, Inc., 1998.

Canalway Partners. "Towpath Trailheads in Cuyahoga County." Accessed May 12, 2024. canalwaypartners.com/discover/towpath-trailheads-in-cuyahoga-county.

Chojnacki, Linda. "Do you know the history of Squire's Castle?" Cleveland.com, January 13, 2012. Accessed May 12, 2024. cleveland.com/our-town/2012/01/do_you_know_the_legend_of_squires_castle.html.

Cleveland Hiking Club. "Cleveland Outreach and Engagement." Copyright © 2024. Accessed May 12, 2024. clevelandhikingclub.org/about/community-outreach-and-engagement.

Cleveland Metroparks. "Hinckley Spillway Dam." Accessed May 7, 2024. clevelandmetroparks.com/parks/visit/parks/hinckley-reservation/hinckley-spillway.

"Cuyahoga County Courthouse." Accessed May 12, 2024. case.edu/ech/articles/c/cuyahoga-county-courthouse.

Cuyahoga Valley National Recreation Area Trail Guide Handbook. Akron, OH: Cuyahoga Valley Trails Council, 1996.

Directory of Ohio's State Nature Preserves. Columbus, OH: Ohio Department of Natural Resources, 1998–2000.

Drost, Erik. "Iconic Cleveland: The History Behind Cleveland's Guardians of Traffic." *Cleveland Magazine*, July 23, 2021. Accessed May 12, 2024. clevelandmagazine.com/in-the-cle/articles/the-guardians-of-traffic.

Durr, Zachariah. "Worden's Ledges Hide Secrets—Odd Ohio." Cleveland.com, May 19, 2016. Accessed May 12, 2024. cleveland.com/entertainment/2016/05/wordens_ledges_hide_secrets_-.html.

Fakhari, Mohammad. "Geology of Nelson-Kennedy Ledges State Park." Ohio Department of Natural Resources. Accessed May 7, 2024. dam.assets.ohio.gov/image/upload/ohiodnr.gov/documents/geology/EducationGuide_NelsonKennedyLedges_2021.pdf.

"Fairlawn Rotary Observatory." Observatories of Ohio. Accessed May 12, 2024. observatoriesofohio.org/fairlawn-rotary-observatory.

Geiss, Julie. "Ohio's Quail Hollow Park has a rich history." May 19, 2022. Accessed May 12, 2024. farmanddairy.com/columns/ohios-quail-hollow-park-has-a-rich-history/718616.html.

Gross, W. H. (Chip). *Ohio Wildlife Viewing Guide*. Helena, MT: Falcon Publishing, 1996.

Hallowell, Anna C. and Barbara G. *Fern Finder*. Rochester, NY: Nature Study Guild, 1981.

Hannibal, Joseph T. and Schmidt, Mark T. "Rocks of Ages." *Earth Science* 41, no. 1 (Spring 1998): 19–20.

Henry, Tom. "Perry Nuclear Plant seeks 20-year operating extension." *The Blade*, January 31, 2024. Accessed May 7, 2024. toledoblade.com/business/energy/2024/01/31/efforts-are-underway-to-block-perry-nuclear-plant-s-license-extension/stories/20240130127#:~:text=Perry%20went%20online%20Nov.,7%2C%202026.

Hernández, Jo Farb. "Worden Ledges, Hinckley Reservation Noble Stuart (1882–1976)." *Spaces*. 2017. Accessed May 12, 2024. spacesarchives.org/explore/search-the-online-collection/noble-stuart-worden-ledges.

"James A. Garfield Memorial, The." Accessed May 12, 2024. lakeviewcemetery.com/visit/garfield-memorial.

Jeffers, Richard. *Ohio Magazine*, May 2023. "Ohio Finds: Moon-Shaped Face Stone Carving." Accessed May 12, 2024. ohiomagazine.com/ohio-life/article/ohio-finds-moon-shaped-face-stone-carving.

Kent Historical Society & Museum. "Stow Street Pioneer Cemetery." Copyright 2021. Accessed May 12, 2024. kentohiohistory.org/collections/historic-landmark.

Lanese, Jim. "Cleveland Lakefront Nature Preserve," Cleveland Historical, accessed May 12, 2024. clevelandhistorical.org/items/show/433.

Litt, Steven. "Lakewood Solstice Steps give city a quietly spectacular lakefront amenity." Cleveland.com, Oct. 26, 2015. Accessed May 12, 2024. cleveland.com/architecture/2015/10/lakewood_solstice_steps_give_c.html.

Latimer, Jonathan P., and Nolting, Karen Stray. *Backyard Birds* (Peterson Field Guides for Young Naturalists). Boston: Houghton Mifflin Company, 1999.

Leedy, Walter C. Jr. "Cleveland's Terminal Tower—The Van Sweringens' Afterthought." *The Gamut,* no. 8 (Winter 1983). Accessed May 10, 2024, clevelandmemory.org/cut2/gamut.pdf.

Manner, Barbara M. and Corbett, Robert G. *Environmental Atlas of the Cuyahoga Valley National Recreation Area.* Monroeville, PA: Surprise Valley Publications, 1990.

"Monument to Samuel Brady." *Ohio History Journal.* Accessed May 12, 2024. resources.ohiohistory.org/ohj/search/display.php?page=11&ipp=20&searchterm=crawford&vol=18&pages=578-582.

National Park Service. "Basic Information: Welcome to the Cuyahoga Valley!" Accessed May 12, 2024. nps.gov/cuva/planyourvisit/basicinfo.htm.

National Park Service "Everett." Last updated: December 5, 2021. Accessed May 7, 2024. nps.gov/cuva/learn/historyculture/everett.htm.

National Park Service. "Everett Road Covered Bridge." Last updated: November 22, 2021. Accessed May 7, 2023. nps.gov/cuva/learn/historyculture/everett-covered-bridge.htm.

"Pathfinder—A Guide to Cleveland Metroparks." Cleveland, OH: Cleveland Metroparks, 1996.

"Peninsula Village Architectural Tour." Peninsula, OH: Peninsula Area Chamber of Commerce (n.d.).

Roy, Christopher. "Camp Cleveland." *Encyclopedia of Cleveland History.* Last updated: August 12, 2019. Accessed May 12, 2024. case.edu/ech/articles/c/camp-cleveland.

Roy, Christopher. "Parma." *Encyclopedia of Cleveland History.* Last updated: October 22, 2019. Accessed May 12, 2024. case.edu/ech/articles/p/parma.

Sidaway, M.K. "Bath Nature Preserve to celebrate 20 years with new Solar System Walk." *Bath Country Journal,* February 26, 2021. Accessed May 12, 2024. scriptype.com/2021/02/26/bath-nature-preserve-to-celebrate-20-years-with-new-solar-system-walk.

Socha, Linda Hoy. "Area Cemeteries Rich in Historic Milestones of City," *Sun Newspapers,* 4 June 1998.

Towpath Companion. Akron, OH: Ohio & Erie Canal Corridor Coalition, 2001.

Watts, May Theilgaard. *Tree Finder.* Rochester, NY: Nature Study Guild, 1998.

West Side Market. "Market History." Accessed May 12, 2024. westsidemarket.org/about/market-history.

Yost, Lania. "Elyria Council weighs future of closed Two Falls Bridge." *The Chronicle,* Sep. 14, 2021. Accessed May 12, 2024. chroniclet.com/news/274629/elyria-council-weighs-future-of-closed-two-falls-bridge.

Zulandt, Carolyn. "Everett Road Covered Bridge." Cleveland Historical. Accessed May 13, 2024. clevelandhistorical.org/items/show/342.

Zulandt, Carolyn and Roy, Christopher. "Frazee House A Pioneering Home-made Home." Published December 8, 2011. Last updated September 27, 2023. Accessed May 12, 2024. clevelandhistorical.org/items/show/360.

INDEX

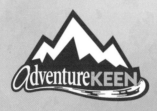

The Story of AdventureKEEN

We are an independent nature and outdoor activity publisher. Our founding dates back more than 40 years, guided then and now by our love of being in the woods and on the water, by our passion for reading and books, and by the sense of wonder and discovery made possible by spending time recreating outdoors in beautiful places.

It is our mission to share that wonder and fun with our readers, especially with those who haven't yet experienced all the physical and mental health benefits that nature and outdoor activity can bring.

In addition, we strive to teach about responsible recreation so that the natural resources and habitats we cherish and rely upon will be available for future generations.

We are a small team deeply rooted in the places where we live and work. We have been shaped by our communities of origin—primarily Birmingham, Alabama; Cincinnati, Ohio; and the northern suburbs of Minneapolis, Minnesota. Drawing on the decades of experience of our staff and our awareness of the industry, the marketplace, and the world at large, we have shaped a unique vision and mission for a company that serves our readers and authors.

We hope to meet you out on the trail someday.

#bewellbeoutdoors

ABOUT THE AUTHOR

Diane Stresing grew up in Columbus, moved to the Cleveland area in 1989, and currently lives in Kent. A genuine Buckeye, Stresing received a BA in journalism from The Ohio State University. When she's not hiking or biking in northeaast Ohio, Diane writes marketing content and features for a variety of clients.

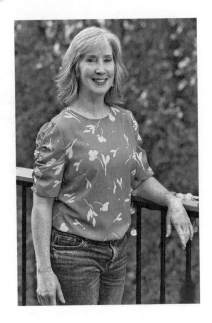